PRAISE FOR NOURISH YOUR TRIBE

"This is a terrific book from a nutrition expert who knows how to cut through confusion to provide clear evidence of what is helpful and what is toxic. I love the many charts, tips, principles, and real life stories. It will be a blessing to so many people."

—Kathi Kemper, MD, Executive Director, Center for Integrative Health and Wellness, Ohio State University Medical Center

"There was a time when providing healthy food to our families was a simple matter. Now we face a maze of information and misinformation where the long-term implications of our own food choices for our children may be much more important than we ever realized. *Nourish Your Tribe* guides parents along a holistic and integrative path toward nutrition that ensures that children grow biologically, physically, and emotionally to their full potential. Nicole Magryta has done a masterful job of showing us the way with a book that is easily understood, very readable and based on the latest ground-breaking peer-reviewed scientific research."

—John E. Wear, Jr., PhD, Executive Director, Center for the Environment at Catawba College

"Nicole Magryta weaves a gentle, rational message for parents about healthy food in *Nourish Your Tribe*. She emphasizes science over hype yet keeps the discussion understandable. She favors helpful resources and easily actionable tips over lengthy recipes. And she guides us not from a place of fear about what to eat but from a love for all children, and their parents. Food should be a source of nourishment and joy. This book makes that goal a whole lot easier."

—Russ Greenfield, MD, Director, Integrative Medicine at Novant Health

"Busy parents—is there any other other kind—face daunting odds to get their kids to follow a healthy, nutritious diet, starting with a culture that endlessly hawks bad food and ending with that 5 year-old boss at the kitchen table whose sole food group is mac 'n cheese. Help is on the way. In *Nourish Your Tribe*, Nicole Magryta gives us an invaluable, practical guide to building smart, healthy, pleasurable family eating habits that even the busiest parents can master."

—Ken Cook, President, Environmental Working Group

"*Nourish Your Tribe* is a comprehensive, educational tool that empowers parents to maximize nutrition and health for themselves and their families. A book that parents can regularly refer back to for continuing knowledge about health. A must read for all parents."

—Jennifer Hudson, MD, pediatrician and founder of Witty Bit World

"This is the best book that I have read on nutrition. It's an excellent reference book for every physicians library."

—Wayne Koontz, MD, 50 year veteran of pediatrics

"This is an excellent book for parents and professionals alike. It covers in a scientific but easily readable manner the most current thinking concerning all aspects of nutrition. I would recommend this book for parents, pediatricians, nutritionists and anyone involved in the care and feeding of children."

— Sanford C. Newmark MD, Director of Clinical Programs, Osher Center for Integrative Medicine, University of California San Francisco

NOURISH *Your* TRIBE

Empowering Parents to Grow Strong, Smart, Successful Kids

Nicole Magryta, MBA, RDN

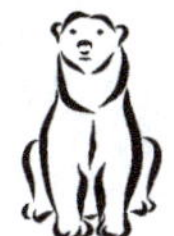

PURPLE BEAR PUBLISHING

North Carolina

FIRST EDITION

Editor: Paula Sarson
Proofreader: Kimberley Mulder
Cover Photograph: Maya Kellman Photography
Cover Design: Aaniyah Ahmed
Interior Design: Christina Gaugler

Illustrations: Seminole Indian comparison provided page 37 by © Price-Pottenger Nutrition Foundation, Inc. www.ppnf.org; Agouti mouse comparison page 47 provided by Randy L. Jirtle, Ph.D. Reprinted by permission. All rights reserved.

10 9 8 7 6 5 4 3 2 1

ISBN: 978-1-7328296-0-2 (Paperback Edition)
ISBN: 978-1-7328296-1-9 (Hardcover Edition)
ISBN: 978-1-7328296-2-6 (ebook)

This book may be purchased for educational, business, or sales promotional use. For information about special discounts for bulk purchases, please visit www.nourishyourtribe.com.

Library of Congress Cataloging-in-Publication Data is available upon request.

Printed and bound in the United States of America

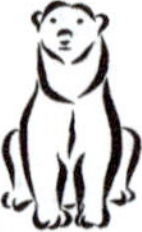

PURPLE BEAR PUBLISHING

Inspiring wellness and stewardship in humankind

DEDICATION

To my children, Thomas and Bella.
Keep learning how to love and honor your minds and your bodies.

To the children of my family and friends, those I work with,
and those I have yet to meet.
You all deserve a fair chance to be healthy and whole.

And to parents.
This is for your bravery and your thirst for knowledge.

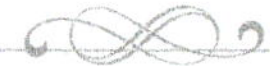

*Nutritious food is to the body
what pixie dust is to Neverland.*

—N. Magryta

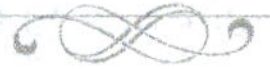

CONTENTS

INTRODUCTION

We get only one chance to support the growth of a child's body.

We are all witnesses to the obesity epidemic and the chronic health issues that plague our children, such as type 2 diabetes, autoimmune conditions, developmental disabilities, behavior and learning challenges, depression, and dental diseases. Our cultural environment has changed so dramatically over time that our now *socially accepted* norm is a diet of processed and convenience foods, both in and away from home. The result: Americans are experiencing a nourishment crisis.

So how did we get here? Have we been fooled by food companies' manipulative marketing to believe that what we are eating is good for us? Just how complicit is our government in the harmful practices of industrialized agriculture? Are we so distracted with the demands of daily life that we've lost track of what is truly nourishing for our families? There are a lot of players in our nourishment crisis: the food industry, industrialized agriculture, changing scientific recommendations, and ineffective—or nonexistent—government regulations are just a few examples of the forces that undermine our quest for healthy food choices. No wonder we parents are overwhelmed and confused! We have learned by now that we can't rely on our government to improve our food supply for us, and we can't count on corporations to choose our health over their profits.

One thing is clear: as parents, we need to take responsibility for our families' health. It's up to us to educate ourselves and our children as we navigate our rapidly changing environment. And it all begins with food. Our eating habits are influenced by our environment and our awareness. When we prioritize conscious healthy living in our own homes, we create powerful tribes that can lead by example, empowering us to share knowledge with our communities, where it is most needed. This book provides optimal nutrition advice that will help you give your children the best chance to reach their true potential.

As a clinical nutritionist and parent, good, *healthy* food makes me happy. From years of studying nutrition science and disease, I see the answers to our obesity epidemic. I understand the daily effort it takes to make a positive difference in our children's lives. I see the great potential we have to become a healthy society, but I am saddened by the collective choices we make in our communities, in our schools, and in our homes. Our food climate changed for the worse a long time ago. But the tide is slowly turning. Americans are starting to educate themselves about our current food supply, our environment, and the epidemic of disease. This education has fostered an awareness that we have a major problem in the world of nourishment. Now we need to act with greater fortitude to improve our choices. Choice is a muscle, and we need to exercise it!

MY STORY

I knew early on that I wanted to study nutrition science because of my curious and intuitive nature about food and how it affects our health. In college and graduate school, I was awestruck by the magnificent orchestra of events that happens in our ten trillion cells. I realized that everything is dynamic. Our cells are always morphing, responding quietly—without us noticing—to our ever-changing, external food environment. Over the past twenty years, I have had the privilege to learn from some of the greatest contributors to the field.

When my beloved husband and I first met, we were both interns at the University of Virginia Health Sciences Center in Charlottesville. I was studying clinical nutrition; he was studying pediatrics. I realized even then how little physicians were taught about nutrition science and the healing power of foods. I recall a heated discussion, early in our relationship, about cholesterol and heart disease. At the time, my dangerously bright doctor boyfriend argued that food had only a minor influence on cardiovascular health and reducing cholesterol. I, on the other hand, firmly believed otherwise. At the time, I quoted Dr. Dean Ornish and his dietary reversal of heart disease and Dr. Andrew Weil's approach to optimal wellness. I added my own experience of working with patients in cardiac rehabilitation. Nonetheless, my arguments were not taken seriously. My doctor boyfriend continued to think eating well meant one healthy entree a day; a salad at lunch afforded him Taco Bell for dinner.

Even in the kitchen, he used to surprise me. After making me his famous spaghetti sauce with Italian sausage, he left it in the refrigerator to cool. The next morning, when I went to skim the solidified fat off the top of the chilled sauce, he got all worked up and yelled, "No, stop! That's where all the flavor is!" At the time I thought, "Is this guy serious? Surely, he's not telling me all the flavor is locked up in this saturated yellow fat!"

I don't mean to pick on my now husband. In fact, he is one of the brightest, most dedicated physicians I know. I share this story to illustrate how our Western medical model fails to educate our physicians on the most powerful tool we have to fight disease: food. He will gladly tell you himself that his fifteen-credit-hour mandatory nutrition class at Emory Medical School was regarded among the students as a "blow-off" class that was given very little attention. In fact, a 2010 study from the Academy of Medicine found that on average, medical students received only 19.6 hours of nutrition education in their entire four years of basic medical school.[1] Today, most allopathic physicians who are well-versed in nutrition have either learned the science independently or now follow integrative or functional medicine approaches, which are in part what this book is going to help teach you about.

Four years into our marriage, my husband was forced to reevaluate his diet. He developed signs of hereditary cardiovascular disease: high LDL cholesterol (the bad kind), low HDL cholesterol (the good kind), and high triglycerides. For nine months, he tried a standard course of Lipitor and niacin, two medicines used to reduce his triglyceride levels and LDL cholesterol. This approach worked, but he was frustrated with the notion of relying upon medication for the rest of his life coupled with the "niacin flush," a common side effect, which is a burning, tingling sensation in the face and chest. He also experienced side effects from Lipitor, which made him feel like an eighty-year-old arthritic man. This scenario didn't bode well for continuing with his very active recreational soccer.

He finally decided to listen to me, his wife. (Sometimes it takes years, folks!) He stopped taking medication and chose to tackle his cardiovascular health by following an anti-inflammatory diet, supplementing with herbs, and exercising regularly. One of my husband's admirable characteristics is that when he sets his mind to something, he commits fully. After three months of strict lifestyle changes, including healthy eating and exercise, he lowered his LDL cholesterol from 260 to 200. Now I had his attention! But the story didn't end there.

After a year of following an excellent anti-inflammatory diet, his numbers had stagnated. He was frustrated. Even though his cholesterol and triglyceride numbers had vastly improved, he wanted them to be optimal. At the time, we both were studying integrative and functional medicine approaches that taught us about how food sensitivities can trigger certain bodily dysfunctions. Our focus had also turned to gut health as we realized its undeniable importance to our overall health.

As my husband's evolution of eating continued, he decided to remove wheat from his diet. He not only wanted to improve his cardiovascular health but also needed to address the recent onset of hereditary arthritis. The results were fast and completely unexpected. After three months of eliminating wheat from his diet, his cholesterol and lipid panels fell to within an optimal range, and the aches in his joints vanished. No disease risk.

Welcome to the undeniable power of food! In our house today, you can just imagine the passion for healthy nourishment that informs our lifestyle. We live it, breathe it, study it, talk about it, and more importantly, enjoy it every day. My husband is now a nutrition science stud, and I remain a faithful card-carrying member of the Nutrition Science Academy for Nerds.

LIFE WITH KIDS

Having kids rocked our world. How could we create such darling little creatures who argue with our sound, intelligent advice? You might think that growing up in a household with a pediatrician and a nutritionist as parents that our kids would be eating sautéed kale with wild-caught smoked sockeye salmon and matcha green tea for breakfast. Although our kids eat much better than most, the reality is we face the same challenges that other American parents encounter. One big difference for our kids may be awareness, because they often hear conversations about honoring their bodies and how food influences body functions.

I believe God gave us two children with opposite taste buds and robust personalities for a reason: to allow us to appreciate the challenge in teaching and influencing different food perspectives. In our house, we have one child with a uniquely broad palate and another who defines the word *caution* when it comes to food. One is an explorer and the other a faithful servant to anything made with white flour, cheese, or meat. As our parental journey has unfolded over the past fifteen years, we have uncovered some wisdom that I am excited to share with you in the pages ahead.

I discuss how and why our food environment at large looks very different than it did sixty years ago and explore what we can—and must—do to improve it. You will learn how we can put an end to chronic childhood conditions, such as obesity and type 2 diabetes, and discover the immeasurable influence food plays on our children's brains, behaviors, digestive and immune functions. Chapter 9 focuses on parent empowerment, strategies for picky eaters, and essential emotional and behavioral tools to help create a healthy *and* happy food tribe.

Food and health are my passions, and sharing knowledge about these with you is my mission. My kids have been my inspiration in writing this book. My motivation has also been fueled by our entire generation of children, those I see as patients, those I teach in schools, those who I love and hug every day, and all those I have yet to meet. This book is my effort to help make their lives better through you, their parents. Teaching our kids to respect, nourish, and love their body begins on day one of parenting and continues indefinitely, just as we never stop teaching kindness, integrity, and good manners throughout their childhood.

We parents play a vital role in shaping the future health of our children. I hope the pages ahead inspire you on this guided journey to nourishing your family's health and vitality. This book is designed to help busy families who want to be proactive participants in their children's health. The forces at play in today's food environment are manipulating our genetic impulses and cultural norms, making us sick. This book highlights key factors involved in helping children grow to their full potential—biologically, physically, and emotionally—through an understanding of how food and nutrients profoundly affect a child's well-being. What parent isn't interested in that?

Here are some highlights of what you will learn by the end:

- How agricultural practices, food marketing, and industrial food products have changed our food landscape.

- How to disengage from cultural food norms and adopt an empowered, nourishing family lifestyle at home.

- How to nurture your family's gut bacteria, the single most essential component for optimal health.

- How food and nourishment link to common childhood conditions like mood swings, ADHD, anxiety, headaches, stomachaches, eczema, asthma, and other developmental problems.

- How to choose the best foods for nutrient density, microbial balance, and a healthy hormonal response.

- Groundbreaking data showing how food can literally turn your genes on and off.

- How to dramatically reduce your exposure to environmental toxins.

- Practical strategies for picky eaters and behavioral tips for helping children grow to their full potential.

- Easy recipes and optimal meal plans.

At the beginning of each chapter, you will find a brief summary that previews the chapter's contents. The summaries are intended to help you choose the chapters that align with your needs first. Or, of course, you can read sequentially.

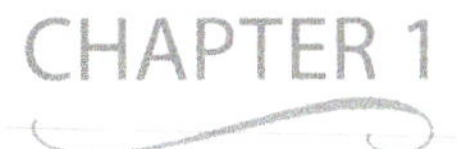

WHY IS NUTRITION SO IMPORTANT?

Any growing, healing, development, and functioning you accomplish must evolve from what you come with, eat, drink, or breathe.

—Kelly Dorfman, MS, LND, *Cure Your Child with Food*

Leading health experts will tell you the one factor responsible for most human disease is lack of nutrition. This issue looks different all around the world, but it's undisputed that good nutrition plays a vital role in the growth and development of children. Many Americans, wealthy and impoverished and at all ages, are malnourished not because of a lack food, but because of a lack of quality food and an overabundance of poorly nourished calories. Most parents are unaware that food and nourishment are linked to common childhood ailments such as ADHD, anxiety, constipation, headaches, irritable bowel syndrome (IBS), eczema, and mood and behavior issues. In fact, the current pace at which chronic diseases are increasing is greater than at any other time in our history. In this chapter, you will learn why our food choices play the most important role in our quest for health. In order for our children to grow to their full potential—biologically, physically, and emotionally—we must teach them good nutrition habits early on and shift our family paradigms at home to support health for life.

We often forget there's no better time for good nourishment than during child-hood—especially puberty—when cells are dividing, replicating, and building new bone and tissue at rapid rates. Nutrition plays a profound role in our children's development and growth and equips them with the energy and strength necessary to maximize their potential and prevent illness. There is a direct relationship between peak performance (both physical and academic) and optimal nourishment. Behavior and mood are also linked to the types of food we eat. Just *how* this happens is often a mystery, so it's time for some demystification.

Generally, people assume that only obese kids have a nourishment problem. Because obese kids *appear* overweight, the assumption is that they eat too much of the "wrong" foods and not enough of the "right" foods. We readily make judgments that *those* children are at risk. I'm going to turn that thinking on its head.

Consider the following scenarios. Imagine a child who looks healthy. You've seen him: he's about nine years old, trim, athletic, always smiling, and he's usually dressed in a matching sporty outfit. He sure doesn't look malnourished. What if I told you that despite his lean physique, his food choices have been slim and nutritionally bankrupt for the past six years? His daily diet, for as long as his mom can remember, has consisted of only bread, pizza, pasta with sauce, crackers, bananas, and sometimes chicken nuggets when the timing is right.

Do you think he's malnourished? I can guarantee he is. The prevailing attitude is that "kids are picky" and "most kids eat this way." Parents expect kids will grow out of such eating habits, hopefully by the time they're eighteen. In fact, it's quite common for parents to discount their children's vulnerability to processed food because of the belief that youth carry a Superman-like resilience.

In another scenario, imagine a child with a broader palate, but who gets the majority of his food energy from highly processed refined-flour products, sugar-laden foods, and processed meats and snack foods. Let's say this child chooses sugar-coated breakfast cereal, chocolate milk, and breakfast pastries to start his day. Lunch is a sub sandwich of processed meats and cheese, with potato chips, and a sports drink. Supper consists of fried chicken nuggets, french fries, cookies, and soda. This child eats "food" as defined by our American culture, but he clearly does not get enough of the quality nutrients to propel him to feel and perform at his best.

Children who have limited palates, like those described above, experience complaints that may not be obviously linked to their diet. Symptoms might not show up in a physical way like obesity but in more subtle ways like headaches, stomachaches, constipation, attention difficulties, and/or mood shifts.

> ## Does your child suffer from any of these chronic issues?
>
> - Acne
> - Autism
> - Aggression
> - Allergies (food and/or seasonal)
> - Anxiety
> - Attention difficulties
> - Behavioral and emotional issues
> - Constipation
> - Depression
> - Developmental delays
> - Diarrhea
> - Ear infections
> - Eczema
> - Failure to thrive
> - Frequent illness
> - Frequent rashes/hives
> - Gas
> - Hyperactivity
> - Joint pain
> - Learning disabilities
> - Mood shifts
>
> Good nutrition plays a vital role in improving each of these common concerns. Removal of irritant foods and/or supplementing missing nutrients can be key to managing many childhood conditions. If your child suffers from a chronic health issue, I recommend keeping a daily food journal along with the status of their daily emotional and physical health. You will be amazed at how daily journaling can bring awareness to your child's health patterns.

It's not uncommon to find deficiencies such as iron, vitamin D, zinc, magnesium, copper, and B vitamins in "normal-looking" children. Unfortunately, many parents express their nutrition and feeding concerns to their pediatricians, only to receive the response, "Kids are picky. You are not alone," or, "He's fine. He's plotting a nice curve on his growth chart." Nutrition should be physicians' first line of defense when talking to parents since it's the most powerful tool in fighting illness, preventing disease, and achieving optimal health in their patients. However, many physicians are not well-versed in nutrition science, so we parents need to become nutrition detectives. Just because children steadily plot on their growth charts does *not* mean they are biologically healthy and nutritionally sound. Growth by itself does not indicate a strong immune system, a well-functioning brain, or a healthy digestive system. For example, a steadily growing child who suffers with anxiety and headaches could be missing out on key nutrients like zinc, iron, and essential fatty acids, or could have sensitivity to foods like wheat or dairy.

In my twenty-year career, I have witnessed an extreme shift in the health of adults and children. In 1996, when I worked in outpatient clinics, it was rare to see a child with type 2 diabetes. Now, type 2 diabetes is so prevalent that we have clinics devoted to only this disorder. The statistics are truly

POSSIBLE LINKS BETWEEN COMMON AILMENTS, NUTRITION DEFICIENCIES, AND FOOD SENSITIVITIES

AILMENT	POSSIBLE DEFICIENCY	POSSIBLE FOOD SENSITIVITY
Anxiety	Magnesium, zinc, iron, vitamin D, essential fatty acids, fiber	Wheat, dairy, egg, soy, corn, sugar
ADHD	B vitamins, zinc, iron, vitamin D, magnesium, selenium, essential fatty acids, fiber	Wheat, dairy, egg, soy, chocolate, corn, citrus, artificial sweeteners, artificial dyes
Constipation	Magnesium, vitamin B12, water, fiber	Dairy
Headache/migraine	B vitamins, vitamin D, coenzyme Q10, magnesium	Dairy, aged cheese, chocolate, artificial sweeteners, sugar, caffeine, MSG, sulfites, nitrites
Inflammatory bowel disease (IBD)	Magnesium, iron, B vitamins, vitamin D, vitamin K, selenium, zinc, fiber	Wheat, dairy, FODMAPs*, disaccharides and polysaccharides (specific carbohydrates)
Recurrent minor viral and/or bacterial infections	Zinc, iron, vitamin D, vitamin C, vitamin B12, vitamin B6, fiber	Dairy, soy
Skin issues, eczema	Vitamin A, zinc, vitamin C, vitamin D, fiber	Dairy, wheat, egg, soy

**FODMAP = Fermentable oligosaccharides, disaccharides, monosaccharides, and polyols. These are types of short-chain carbohydrates that aren't absorbed properly in the gut, which can trigger symptoms in people with irritable bowel syndrome (IBS) and may affect those with IBD as well.*

alarming: type 2 diabetes in children increased 30.5 percent between 2001 and 2009.[2] In adults, the number of diagnosed diabetes cases quadrupled from 1980 through 2012. If these trends continue, one out of three adults in the United States could have diabetes by 2050.[3]

CHRONIC VERSUS ACUTE ILLNESS

The diseases people die from today are much different from those that killed our ancestors. Modern medicine has done a remarkable job at treating *infectious* diseases like pneumonia or gastroenteritis, which are both transmitted through human contact or the air. They are specific *bugs* causing specific *infections*. Historically, these short-term, acute infections have been well treated by antibiotics. In fact, when antibiotics like penicillin were first introduced in the 1940s, the results were revolutionary. Diseases that previously killed thousands of people were suddenly controlled.

Shortly thereafter, physicians and pharmaceutical companies looked beyond antibiotics for acute infections and started to focus on treating chronic conditions like arthritis and heart disease. However, there is a big difference between treating an acute infectious disease and treating a chronic condition: when you treat an infectious disease with drugs, you generally cure the patient. With a chronic disease, the popular medical model only treats the *symptoms*. Here is where the disconnect in our healthcare system began.

Most physicians are trained to treat patient symptoms with drugs rather than try to address the root cause of the illness. Physician education and even our insurance reimbursement model are focused on pharmaceutical treatments and surgery rather than a patient-centered model that focuses on lifestyle choices, environmental exposures, and stress reduction. In the area of chronic illness, our medical model falls short.

Even my personal experiences have left me disenchanted with how the average physician handles chronic illness. Last year, my mother developed IBS, a gastrointestinal disorder that has reached almost epidemic proportions in the US. It is now estimated to affect up to 11 percent of the population at any one time, and four in ten people over their lifetime.[4] She suffered from frequent uncontrollable diarrhea in the mornings, excessive bloating, gas, and stomach pain. Her doctor had recommended a colonoscopy to rule out conditions like diverticulitis, cancer, polyps, and Crohn's disease. After he gave us the good news that the test results appeared "normal," I was curious about what type of diet he recommended for her symptoms. Did he think the herbs Iberogast and peppermint could be useful? Could she possibly have small intestine bacterial overgrowth (SIBO)? He responded with, "Diet doesn't affect IBS," and walked out of the room.

How on earth could a doctor that specializes in colons, the place where all nutrients are absorbed and billions of microorganisms live, be so ignorant about the power of diet? With 70 percent of our entire immune system residing within our gut, surely one must consider what we feed it! Well, the reality is, most average physicians have no clue how diet affects disease. Modern medicine "cares" for patients by writing prescriptions for ailments that mask symptoms rather than cure the problem.

Thankfully, there are many integrative and functional medicine doctors and dietitians/nutritionists (me included) who can confidently say that diet is integral to managing IBS as well as many other chronic illnesses. However, it's not just one food or one vitamin that helps cure a disease. It takes a spectrum of nutrients working together in an intricate web-like fashion to propel our bodies and minds to optimal health. Think of nutrients as interlocking wheels on a grandfather clock; one wheel doesn't turn or function without the other.

As a practitioner who witnesses daily the success of treating illness by addressing the root cause of symptoms, I am convinced we are in the midst of a radical paradigm shift. Change is coming as healthcare practitioners are slowly starting to look at improving our personal bio-chemistry by first addressing nutritional state, exercise habits, and our mental and emotional stress. Once we shift our thinking about chronic conditions, we realize we have a profound influence on our children's basic building blocks of life, which make up and influence every organ system in the body, including the brain as well as the immune and digestive tracts. Without question, the foods we choose to ingest, or better yet, *not* ingest, are among the most powerful tools we have to fight chronic illness and maintain optimal health.

Chronic Illnesses on the Rise

A 2014 report from the Organization for Economic Co-operation and Development (OECD) points out that even though one in three kids in the US is overweight, there are still four countries whose kids are more overweight: Greece, Italy, New Zealand, and Slovenia. In Greece, for instance, 44 percent of boys and 38 percent of girls are either overweight or obese.[5] It's hard to imagine that these countries show worse stats than the US, home to the original golden arches. After all, Italy and Greece are the birthplaces of the renowned Mediterranean diet, which millions around the world follow. But as scientists have discovered, it's not the olive oil and fresh artisan cheeses that are tipping the scales toward obesity for these kids. The trend seems to be the result of three surprising factors: a depressed economy that moves people away from more expensive fresh fruits and vegetables while turning them toward inexpensive processed and pre-packaged meals; a growing departure from their slow food way of life to a new-found love of fast food; and higher rates of inactivity. Sound familiar?

However, let's not let these stats overshadow the grave state Americans' health is in. Our kids may not be the most overweight in the world, but our adults definitely are. As the Centers for Disease Control and Prevention (CDC) graph at right points out, obesity—and diabetes—trends have risen dramatically over the past twenty years.

More than one-third (36.5 percent) of US adults are obese, and approximately 17 percent of children and adolescents from 2 to 19 years are obese; that's almost one in five children and one in three adults. Between 1980 and 2010, the percentage of people living with obesity in the US doubled among adults and tripled among children.[6] Former Food and Drug Administration commissioner Dr. David Kessler said that obesity is "one of the greatest public health epidemics of our time." Something has obviously changed in our environment to create such a drastic shift in just a thirty-year span.

AGE-ADJUSTED PREVALENCE OF OBESITY AND DIAGNOSED DIABETES AMONG US ADULTS

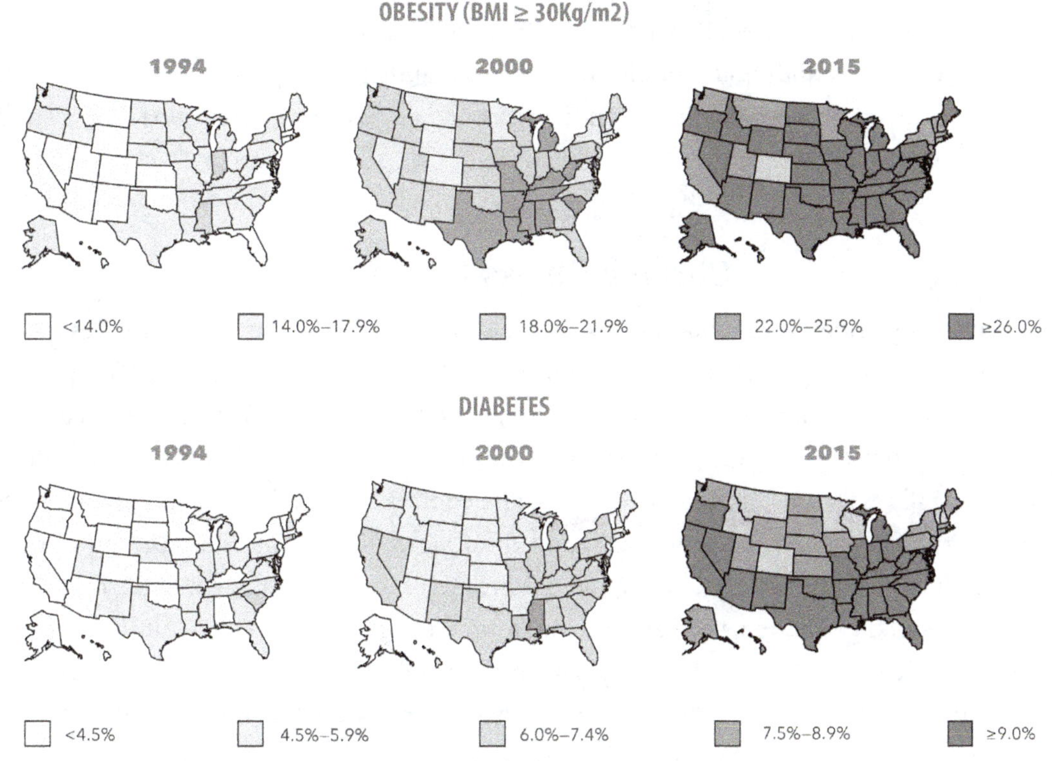

Source: CDC (Centers for Disease Control and Prevention), 2017

Obesity is just one of many chronic conditions that are on the rise. Chronic conditions are defined as lasting longer than a year and can often limit a person's daily activities. These types of illnesses are the most prevalent in our society. In adults, these include heart disease, cancer, Alzheimer's disease, and diabetes. Unfortunately, they are treated mostly by managing the symptoms rather than curing—or better yet, preventing—the disease. The Centers for Disease Control and Prevention (CDC) estimate that chronic conditions account for at least 75 percent of our healthcare costs, and nearly one in two adults in the US live with at least one chronic condition.[7]

The numbers are just as staggering in children. A 2010 study published in the *Journal of the American Medical Association* found that childhood chronic conditions such as obesity, asthma, and learning and behavioral issues more than doubled over a twelve-year period, rising from

12.8 percent in 1994 to 26.6 percent in 2006.[8] The CDC reports that the prevalence of food allergies in children increased by 50 percent between 1997 and 2011. Today, one in 13 children have food allergies, or roughly two per classroom.[9] And from 2003 to 2011, ADHD diagnosed by a healthcare provider increased 42 percent. In 2011, one in 11 children had ADHD.[10]

Other chronic childhood conditions such as autism, asthma, constipation, eczema, migraines, and irritable bowel are also on the rise and can have a negative impact on a child's or an adolescent's quality of life.

Chronic Illness Prevention

The numbers are indeed grim, but there is good news: the increase in chronic diseases is because of lifestyle choices and the changing environment. While it's true that doctors have gotten better at detecting and diagnosing childhood chronic conditions—and this, too, has contributed to the rise in numbers—it's only a small piece of the puzzle. First, it's important to understand that chronic illnesses are "lifestyle" diseases. Daily choices like the food on the end of our forks, the quantity of physical activity we take, and the way we decide to respond to our emotional stressors all contribute to the development of chronic illness. Research confirms that there are many players in the equation, such as poor nutrition during pregnancy and childhood, exposure to chemicals, stress, low physical activity, unhealthy gut flora, as well as increased television and media exposure. But all of these factors can surely be altered based on how we choose to live and interact with our environment—operative word, *choose*.

Take exposure to chemicals in food, for example. Children are actually more at risk to chemicals than adults because children are constantly growing. They breathe more air, consume more food, and drink more water in proportion to their weight. A child's central nervous, immune, reproductive, and digestive systems are all more vulnerable to environmental toxins, which is why we need to be more cognizant of the foods and beverages we offer them. Many parents worry also about the risks of the cocktail of daily chemical exposures that we receive from herbicides, pesticides, food colorings, genetically modified foods, additives, preservatives, and hormones. How can we reduce this exposure in our children's diets?

Nurturing nutritional well-being and health is a lifelong process, with each phase affecting the next. In our current food environment, we can't sit by and wait for our children to "grow out" of their poor eating habits or expect that they are operating at their best potential even though they eat only a limited selection of marginally healthy foods. As kids grow up, their eating habits will either position them to lead a healthy lifestyle or one that will work against them. Well-chosen foods connect children to health and vitality. Teaching children good nutrition empowers them to respect their most precious gifts: their minds and their bodies. I want to empower my children with the wisdom to nourish themselves with healing foods and to be aware of their body's voice. Don't you? What a gift this would be to our next generation of children.

CHAPTER 2

THE CHANGING FACE OF FOOD

*Instead of food, we're consuming "edible foodlike substances"—
no longer the products of nature but of food science.*

—Michael Pollan, *In Defense of Food*

The risks that our food choices pose today are profound, especially for the most vulnerable among us, infants and children. We have unprecedented levels of chronic disease in this country, and for the first time in history we may have a generation of children who have a shorter life expectancy than their parents. Our modern-day agricultural practices and access to food choices have complicated the simplicity of food and eating. The efforts we parents make to find healthy foods have gone far beyond choosing an apple over a cupcake. Now we need to learn about how our food is handled and produced in our pursuit to maximize nutrient intake and avoid harmful contaminants. It's unlikely that industrialized agriculture and governmental ambivalence will change any time soon. Instead, we must educate ourselves about this ever-changing face of food. First, we need to acknowledge the damage modern agricultural practices inflict on our health and the environment that sustains us. Second, we need to be aware that fiscally driven food marketing, which targets unhealthy foods high in sugar, salt, and fat, greatly influences the choices of both children and adolescents. Third, we need to make choices to stop eating foods that harm us and choose foods that nourish us. As parents, it is up to us to set the standard for true nourishment for our children, to help keep them safe and healthy for a long and fruitful life.

We can all agree that food, although naturally simple, has become complicated. Many factors have contributed to our present-day food crisis, in which the nutritional value of our most accessible food is bankrupt. Our acceptance of cultural food norms, our indifference to modern agricultural practices, our unawareness of strategic food marketing, and the lack of government demand for safe, accessible, affordable, and chemical-free food—all put our children's health at great risk. The most significant impact can be attributed to the industrialization of American agriculture and how US food corporations have changed the way we produce, grow, purchase, and think about what we eat.

Here's the good news: we can change what we feed our families. And if we can change what they eat, we can also turn around the rise in chronic diseases, which is influenced by our diet and lifestyle. This book will guide and support that mission. First, we need to examine how these harmful factors have infiltrated our food and our mentality.

INDUSTRIALIZATION OF AGRICULTURE

Before 1950, US agriculture was dominated by family farms, and most farmers relied on healthy soils for productivity. Eating local was the only way of life; people knew where their food came from. After World War II, advanced farming technologies were just coming on the scene, selling farmers on the idea of using commercial fertilizers, pesticides, and farm machinery to make cultivating their land more efficient and thus maximizing profit. Dr. John Ikerd, a leading expert in sustainable agriculture and economics, notes that by the mid-1960s, the public mandate for American agriculture had changed from protecting diversified family farms to providing national food security, which meant making good food cheap. From that point forward, American agriculture has been driven by economic motives of productivity and profits over the interest in maintaining healthy soil, plants, animals, and humans. The focus has been on quantity: acres farmed, heads produced, yields per acre, and economies of scale.

To our detriment, much less value has been placed on quality. Nowadays, emphasis is typically on cosmetic appearance rather than nutritional value. According to Ikerd, "While we have succeeded in making good food cheap, we have failed dismally in providing national food security. A larger percentage of Americans are hungry today than were hungry during the 1960s."[11]

Agriculture is now dominated by large-scale monoculture farms, the practice of intensively growing single crops on a very large scale. Corn, soybeans, wheat, cotton, and rice are the most common crops grown this way in the United States. Industrial farming, which depletes the soil of its nutrients, requires intensive chemical fertilizers and pesticides and goes against the basic principles of nature. In the shift to industrial agriculture, family farms have been transformed into factories, where animals have been removed from pasture and placed in feedlots, mechanized systems with roofs and assembly lines within.

Many of America's health concerns can be connected back to the economic decisions that have governed agricultural practices over the last fifty years. Ikerd remarks, "America's food/health concerns also include carcinogenic chemical residues, endocrine disrupters, growth hormones, antibiotic-resistant bacteria, salmonella, E-Coli 0157:H7, and more recently genetically modified organisms, or GMOs. The health problems associated with these concerns include diminished fertility, various forms of cancers, attention deficit disorder, and a growing variety of food allergies. While we don't know the specific cause and effect relationships for all these health problems we do know all these concerns are linked directly with industrial agricultural technologies."[12] Ultimately, we have traded profit for burdensome healthcare costs.

Today's industrial agriculture is also unsustainable because farming methods are eroding natural resources faster than nature can regenerate them. The gravity and complexities of these problems are beyond the scope of this book, but know that the health of our families and the environment are in peril. Safe, high-quality foods are essential to human health, but our current means of supplying that food is woefully broken: powerful economic interests perpetuate our agricultural systems without concern for soil and nutrient management or, most importantly, consumers' health. Two modern food production practices that most negatively impact the health of our loved ones—especially our kids—involve hormone and antibiotic use.

Industrial Livestock and Dairy Production

We all would like to believe that our meat comes from an idyllic, open pasture. Unfortunately, this is not the case. In fact, most of the pork, beef, poultry, dairy, and eggs produced in the United States come from large-scale Confined Animal Feeding Operations (CAFOs). In CAFOs, livestock and poultry are confined indoors in a single building, crammed into inadequate spaces in order to facilitate feeding and hasten growth for slaughter. The consequences of this farming style are widespread and dire.

Antibiotic Use in Animals

Since 1946, industrial farms have been adding antibiotics to livestock feed to make animals grow faster and to compensate for unsanitary living conditions.[13] In other words, most farmers are not just using antibiotics for their intended use, which is to treat sick animals, but also to prevent infection among animals housed in cramped quarters. *A whopping 80 percent of all antibiotics used in the United States are fed to farm animals.* Let that sink in. Between 1985 and 2001, the use of antibiotics in feed for industrial livestock production rose 50 percent.[14]

This widespread use of antibiotics fosters the evolution of antibiotic-resistant microbes in farm animals. These antibiotic-resistant bacteria eventually reach us through food, water, soil, air, and by direct human-to-animal contact. Antimicrobial resistance thus becomes a biohazard to human and animal health. In the most comprehensive assessment of the problem to date, an expert group including the World Health Organization (WHO), the Food and Agriculture Organization (FAO), and the World Organisation for Animal Health (OIE) concluded: "There is clear evidence of adverse human health consequences due to resistant organisms resulting from non-human usage of antimicrobials. These consequences include infections that would not have otherwise occurred, increased frequency of treatment failures (in some cases death) and increased severity of infections."[15]

What's more, factory-farmed animals are not fed what they are genetically designed to eat. Instead of consuming their natural diets of grass, plants, roots, seeds, grubs, and bugs, they are given genetically modified (GM) soy, corn, grains, and an array of drugs. Why does this matter? First, it significantly lowers the meat's nutritional value. Second, animals that aren't allowed to forage in pastures are at risk for more disease and stress, which results in more antibiotics and other drugs entering the animal, and therefore the meat we eat.

Consider a cow's diet: factory-farmed cows eat milled grains, corn, and soybeans instead of grass. In fact 47 percent of soy and 60 percent of all corn grown in the US is consumed by factory-farmed livestock![16] This diet is a problem for cows because grains create an acidic environment in their stomachs that encourages bacteria growth and other digestive problems. The beef that you find in restaurants or on your grocery store shelves comes mostly from factory-farmed cows that are grain-fed. However, common sense tells us that if a cow eats healthy natural grass and then we eat the cow, our health benefits too. If intuition is not enough, a 2010 study published in *Nutrition Journal* concluded, "Research spanning three decades suggests that grass-based diets can significantly improve the fatty acid composition and antioxidant content of beef."[17]

Poultry also can be strictly vegetarian-fed with corn and soybeans. To be clear, there is absolutely nothing natural about a vegetarian-fed chicken, so don't be fooled when you see this label plastered all over egg cartons and poultry packaging. Chickens and turkeys naturally eat worms, insects, and wild seeds. Raising them on pasture is the best way to ensure their natural diet. Vegetarian-fed chickens result in their meat and eggs having a lower nutrient profile than birds with access to insects and meat scraps.

The noteworthy health benefits of eating meat, dairy, and eggs from grass-fed, pasture-raised animals and poultry include:

- Fewer fat and calories than grain-fed cattle, sheep, and bison.

- Most likely to be free of antibiotics, animal by-products, hormones, or other drugs.

- Contain two to five times more anti-inflammatory omega-3 fatty acids than CAFO cattle and 10 times more than factory hens.[18]

- Contain two to three times more cancer-fighting conjugated linoleic acid (CLA) than CAFO cattle.[19] (CLA is a healthy fatty acid that reduces the risk of cancer, cardiovascular disease, diabetes, and obesity.)

- Higher in vitamins A and E and beta-carotene.

- High in glutathione, a powerful antioxidant that protects all cells from damage.

- Avoid arsenic consumption, a toxin that is added to factory-farmed poultry feed to speed growth.

- Support the environment, the animals, and small farms.

- Lower your risk of food poisoning.

Check out http://www.eatwild.com/ to keep up with pasture-fed research and to find where to source pasture-raised meat, dairy, and eggs in the United States and Canada.

Harmful Hormones in Meat and Dairy Products

Hormone levels in meat and milk have increased dramatically over the last 50 years. Research suggests that elevated levels of these hormones may affect childhood development and increase our cancer risk. Hormone-related chronic diseases such as breast and prostate cancer, thyroid disease, obesity, and diabetes are on the rise, and more and more organizations, such as the American Public Health Association (APHA), are taking formal stances against the use of hormonal growth promoters in beef and dairy cattle.[20]

The US Food and Drug Administration (FDA) currently allows the use of six steroid growth hormones—three natural steroids (estradiol, testosterone, and progesterone) and three synthetic hormones (the estrogen compound zeranol, the progestin melengestrol acetate, and the androgen trenbolone acetate)—in beef cattle and sheep production to promote animal growth and improve feed efficiency. Poultry, veal calves, dairy cows, and pigs are excluded from this practice. At least 80 percent of all US feedlot cattle are implanted with steroid hormones, and it's widely established that residues of these hormones end up in our meat.[21]

Since 1988, the European Union has banned the use of steroid hormones in cattle production and prohibits American milk and meat to cross its borders.[22] The EU Scientific Committee on Veterinary Measures relating to Public Health (SCVPH) concluded that the use of hormones as growth promoters poses a potential health risk to consumers and that even residual amounts in meat may have potentially adverse effects on us.[23] Over 30 countries, including Canada, Australia, and Japan, have banned these hormones, choosing to take a precautionary route to protect their citizens. The US, on the other hand, continues to ignore the threat to our health. Our policy remains outdated, despite our current understanding of inherited changes in gene function, or epigenetics, and the risks associated with hormones originating from outside the body that interfere with our own hormone function.[24]

In 1994, in addition to the synthetic hormones in beef production, the FDA also allowed the use of a genetically engineered protein hormone called rBGH (bovine growth hormone) to increase milk production in dairy cows. Again, Canada, the EU, and developed nations around the world refused to approve rBGH due to its cancer risk. And there are other concerns: Canadian researchers found that rBGH is harmful to cows themselves, causing reproductive disorders along with 25 percent increased risk of mastitis and 55 percent increased risk of clinical lameness.[25] If the impact is that significant in cows, what might it be doing to humans who drink that milk? Even more troubling, rBGH increases as much as tenfold a growth hormone called insulin-like growth factor-1 (IGF-1) in the milk of treated cows.[26] Increased IGF-1 levels are associated with breast, prostate, and colon cancers in humans. Although it's not entirely clear how much we absorb from rBGH-treated cow's milk, do we really want to take that chance?

It's clear that the milk we drink today is quite different from the milk our grandparents drank. Added chemicals aside, even milking practices are detrimental. In the United States, typical dairy cows (organic cows included) are milked for 10 months of the year, which is far more frequently than a pre-industrial dairy herd. Both organic and non-organic cows are often milked while they are pregnant, which could result in a glass of milk with over 50 anabolic hormones in it. In fact, milk from pregnant cows can contain 30 times more estrogen than milk from non-pregnant cows.[27] Perhaps this has something to do with why adolescents in the United States are starting puberty almost two years earlier than they did 40 years ago. Moreover, high estrogen levels in humans are associated with breast and prostate cancer. When external hormones enter our bodies, they have the potential to turn our genes on or off, which can result in abnormal cell signaling. This, in turn, may result in developmental or neurological disorders in children or cancer later in life.

So here's the bottom line: hormones are potent compounds in our dairy foods that pose a significant risk for various cancers in humans. Even low doses of these compounds may have biological effects. We need to pay particular attention to children and pregnant women, who are at the greatest risk given their states of rapid cell development.

Alternative Purchasing Tips for Meat and Dairy Products

So, what can you do to counter the industrial practices that have overtaken our meat and dairy production? Here are some tips to follow when purchasing meat, milk, and other dairy products:

- Try bison, lamb, or elk meat. Wild-caught fish is also a good choice.

- Look for labels that say "100% grass-fed" or "grass-fed and grass-finished" beef. If the label just reads "grass-fed" it does not ensure the animal was "grass-finished," meaning the cow was likely given GMO grain. Both organic and 100 percent grass-fed beef are good options, as both practices represent a dedication to raising healthier, less chemically contaminated cows. Although organic beef ensures that the food is free of antibiotics, pesticides, synthetic hormones, and GMOs, it does not ensure that the animal was strictly grass-fed or pasture-raised. Organic cows may be given organic grains and beans, which will lower their meat's nutritional content compared to 100 percent grass-fed cattle.

- For poultry and egg products, look for labeling that reads "certified organic" and "pasture-raised." There is a caveat with organic poultry. The "good" is that the birds are given organic feed without antibiotics and GMOs. The "bad" is that they still can be raised in inhumane factory-farm warehouses and may never see sunlight. Do not be misled by labels that read "humanely raised," "natural," "no added hormones," "cage-free," or "vegetarian-fed." Instead look for labels that ensure a quality product: "Animal Welfare Approved (AWA)," "Global Animal Partnership," "certified humane," and "certified organic" (with exceptions noted above). Even better, buy your poultry and eggs from local farmers, who you can ask how the birds are fed and raised.

- Choose pasture-raised pork products. In the US, 97 percent of pigs are raised on factory farms, where they have spent most of their lives in unsanitary warehouses crammed in stalls, fed GMO grains and antibiotics. I highly recommend purchasing your pork from a local farmer, who can ensure a pasture-raised product.

- Choose goat, sheep, or buffalo dairy products. They are easier to digest, have fewer allergenic proteins, and cause less inflammation than cow's milk. These options also avoid the risks posed by industrial cow farming.

- If you choose to drink milk from cows, choose organic, grass-fed, whole-milk dairy products. This will ensure no GMOs, antibiotics, pesticides, or hormones were used in production. Additionally, A2 cow's milk, which comes from certain breeds of cattle, is less inflammatory than A1 cow's milk (the vast majority of cow's milk available on store shelves). Labels that read "rBGH free" ensure the product does not come from cows treated with rBGH, but it doesn't mean they haven't been given antibiotics, GMO grains, or weren't milked while pregnant.

- Another good option is to avoid dairy products altogether and replace with coconut, almond, or hemp milk products. Despite the USDA Choose My Plate recommendations, three glasses of cow's milk daily, or any dairy foods for that matter, are unnecessary to obtain optimal health or sufficient amounts of calcium. (Dairy isn't even a required food group.) Bones and calcium balance are better served by monitoring animal protein, exercising regularly, getting adequate sunshine or supplemental vitamin D, and consuming a wide variety of calcium-rich whole foods, such as canned fish with bones (sardines, wild salmon), sesame seeds, broccoli, cabbage, beans, oranges, cinnamon, and leafy green vegetables.[28] Furthermore, if you're lactose intolerant, are sensitive to dairy, or if you suffer from an autoimmune disease, a digestive disorder, allergies, type 2 diabetes, or skin disorders like eczema or acne then you should avoid all dairy completely.

GMOs and Toxic Chemical Cocktails

Genetically modified organisms are living organisms (plants, animals, microorganisms) whose individual genes are artificially manipulated and transferred from one organism into another. Examples include corn with bacteria genes, tomatoes with flounder genes (not yet approved), or salmon with eelpout genes (currently on the market). These GMOs have been rapidly distributed into our food supply since the 1990s. There are currently 10 GMO crops approved in the US today: corn (field and sweet), soybeans, summer squash, cotton, papaya, canola, alfalfa, sugar beets, potato, and apples.[29] Ten crops may not sound like much, but when you begin to understand their ubiquity, you realize how often they are consumed in the foods we eat every day.

Initially, genetic engineering in agriculture showed great promise. We were told that GMOs would make agriculture more sustainable, provide higher yields to feed the world's population, reduce pesticide use, and provide more nutritious foods. Unfortunately, scientific reports have shown us that GM foods have failed on all these fronts.[30] The Union of Concerned Scientists, a nonprofit organization that combines rigorous, independent science with advocacy, agrees that genetic engineering has only worsened the problems of industrial monoculture.[31] In 2016 the *New York Times* released an eye-opening report comparing the United States' and Canada's 20-year use of GMO crops to that of Europe's, a continent that has largely rejected GMO technology. The researchers found no advantages in yield gains of GMO crops over conventionally grown crops and further showed a 21 percent increase in herbicide use in the United States.[32]

There may be a lot of controversy about the benefits of GMO crops, but there is absolutely no question that they lead to higher levels of chemical contamination. More than 80 percent of all GM crops grown worldwide have been engineered for herbicide tolerance.[33] The amount and number of chemical herbicides used on these crops has risen dramatically—the highest in a generation—and further increases are expected in the next few years. Glyphosate, the active ingredient in Monsanto's bestselling weed killer Roundup, has increased by a factor of more than 250, from 0.4 million kilograms in 1974 to 113 million kilograms in 2014.[34] According to Dr. Stephanie Seneff, a research scientist at Massachusetts Institute of Technology (MIT), glyphosate is possibly "the most important factor in the development of multiple chronic diseases and conditions that have become prevalent in Westernized societies."[35] She and her colleagues agree that exposure to glyphosate residues in food can cause nutritional deficiencies and systemic toxicity by destroying beneficial gut bacteria. She asserts that glyphosate can induce diseases such as autism, obesity, depression, infertility, Alzheimer's disease, allergies, cancer, MS, and a number of gastrointestinal diseases, such as IBD, colitis, and Crohn's disease.

Most GM crops are "Roundup ready," meaning they are genetically altered to tolerate Roundup while surrounding weeds perish. This new technology has had one of the most dramatic impacts on modern-day health. The biotech industry, led by Monsanto, has successfully turned our food into poison. Although this may sound extreme, the research on glyphosate reveals it's undoubtedly true. Genetically engineered plants absorb Roundup and as a result deposit a portion of it in the food we eat every day. The International Agency for Research on Cancer (IARC) has classified glyphosate as a "probable human carcinogen" along with four other commonly used insecticides and herbicides.[36] As much as 90 percent of the corn and soy grown in the United States is sprayed with glyphosate.[37] In addition, industrial farmers now routinely apply Roundup as a drying agent to non-GMO crops, making it faster and cheaper to harvest crops like wheat, rye, oats, rice, beans, and potatoes.

To make matters worse, glyphosate-resistant weeds are developing, which now require multiple herbicide treatments. Biotech companies are responding by creating new GM seeds that can resist multiple herbicides. What does this mean for us? Ultimately, we now eat even more pesticide residues soaked up in crops. Of great concern is the Environmental Protection Agency's 2014 approval of Enlist Duo, a new combination herbicide that includes glyphosate and 2,4-D, a component of the Agent Orange defoliant used in the Vietnam War. Both are potential carcinogens and both are capable of causing epigenetic changes, i.e., changes in gene expression, at low doses.

You must be wondering by now how these herbicides keep getting approved. Monsanto, the creator of both GM seeds and the herbicides sprayed on them, is a multibillion dollar agro-giant with strong ties to government. In fact, there has been a "regulatory revolving door" of high-ranking Monsanto associates who have been appointed to key governmental positions that influence federal regulations. They have infiltrated the EPA, the USDA, Congress, and the White House.[40] This has resulted in the exceedingly flawed US pesticide regulation that's persisted for decades. The apparent "approve first and question later" policy that has been shaped by large biotech and industrial agriculture lobbyists has put us all at risk. It also exposes our government's reluctance to accept updated, independently funded science, which has clearly linked GM foods and the herbicides applied to them to cancer risk in humans.

We often don't stop to think about the toxic soup on our crops when we are grocery shopping with a squirmy toddler or cranky kids in tow. Most of us just grab the corn taco shells off the shelf and throw them in the cart. While the idea of GM food might not raise your eyebrows, the chemicals sprayed on them should. If you consume processed foods—soda, soup, crackers, chips, frozen entrees, etc.—you undoubtedly will be exposed to multiple chemicals since *more than 75 percent* of store-bought packaged goods contain GMOs.[41] Challenge yourself to find a package in the snack food aisle without corn, soy, or canola in the ingredient list. I think you'll be surprised.

I write this to help raise critical awareness about the state of our food supply and the toll it's taking on our families' health. According to the WHO, growing children and infants are particularly vulnerable to chemical exposure because their cells are rapidly developing and dividing, creating much higher chemical absorption rates compared to adults. A toddler will

Glyphosate Risks to Human Health

Glyphosate is the most heavily used chemical weed killer in the history of agricultural production. Glyphosate, now labeled as a probable carcinogen, is sprayed on both GMO and non-GMO crops in the United States. Over the past two decades, research has supported findings that chronic low-level exposure to endocrine-disrupting chemicals, such as glyphosate, can result in reproductive problems, obesity, diabetes, behavioral problems, autoimmune diseases, abnormal gut bacteria, ADHD, impaired immune function, and certain types of cancers. Glyphosate residues have been found in food, human urine, breast milk, tap water, rivers, and in 85 percent of tampons.[38]

If you choose to regularly eat processed foods, recognize that you are being exposed to impactful levels of pesticide residue. Chronic low-level exposures between 0.1 and 700 parts per billion (ppb) have shown potential to harm human health.[39] Consider, for instance, the levels in these 10 popular American foods tested for glyphosate by an FDA-registered food safety laboratory.

GLYPHOSATE LEVELS

PRODUCT	MANUFACTURER	GLYPHOSATE LEVELS (PPB)
Cheerios	General Mills	1125 ppb
Honey Nut Cheerios	General Mills	670 ppb
Stacy's Naked Pita Chips	Frito-Lay (PepsiCo)	812 ppb
Lay's Kettle Cooked Chips	PepsiCo	452 ppb
Doritos, Cool Ranch	PepsiCo	481 ppb
Lucy's Gluten-Free Oatmeal Cookies	Westminster Bakers Co.	452 ppb
Oreo Original	Nabisco	289 ppb
Kashi Soft-Baked Cookies, Oatmeal Dark Chocolate	Kellogg	275 ppb
Ritz Crackers	Nabisco	270 ppb

Source: Food Democracy Now! and the Detox Project, Glyphosate: Unsafe on Any Plate: Food Testing Results and Scientific Reasons for Concern (Clear Lake, IA: Food Democracy Now! and the Detox Project, 2016).

absorb between 40 percent and 70 percent of an ingested dose of lead, compared to an adult that absorbs only 5 to 20 percent.[42] Also, an infant's blood-brain barrier is not fully developed until age thirty-six months, which means chemicals can pass into the central nervous system, putting an infant brain at significant risk. This could translate into delayed development, disruptions to the reproductive, endocrine, and immune systems, certain types of cancer, and damage to other organs. Children can be exposed to chemicals not only in food but from all over their environment: air, water, toys, hygiene products, etc.

The point is to evaluate where we might have the largest chemical exposure and to sort out how to minimize risk. This is why it's important to discuss GMOs. While Goliath biotech companies like Monsanto further monopolize the agricultural market and add additional threats to our health, our environment, and the future of our food, we can fight back by educating ourselves to make better, more informed choices and purchase healthier foods for our children.

Tips on Purchasing non-GM Foods

Although 64 countries require labeling of GM foods, the United States is reluctant to enforce this policy, even though proper labeling of GM foods would allow tracking of unusual food allergies and the ability to assess the effects of modern-day herbicides. Since GM foods are now the most heavily treated crops with herbicides—and we know that some pose a cancer risk—labeling should be mandatory. Consumers have the right to know which foods put them at higher risks for chemical exposure. In the meantime, while we continue to lobby for accurate labeling, here are some tips on how to minimize your family's risk of exposure:

- Look for certified organic products. The "USDA ORGANIC" label ensures the product does not include GMO ingredients. Purchasing organic foods also provides the best protection from exposure to Roundup (glyphosate) on both GMO and non-GMO foods like wheat and oats.

- The second best option is to look for food packaging with a rectangular label that reads "NON-GMO Project" to ensure the product is GMO-free.

- Avoid foods with at-risk ingredients. Pay close attention to corn, soy, sugar, cottonseed, and canola, and ingredients derived from these. Your best option is fresh, whole foods without any label.

- Whole papaya, potatoes, squash, and sweet corn are the only GMO foods currently available in the produce aisle. Purchasing organic varieties of these foods will avoid GMOs, as glyphosate and other herbicide residues cannot be washed off.

- Purchasing organic meats and dairy products eliminates our risk of exposure to glyphosate in food, which is sprayed on the GMO grains fed to industrial farm animals.[43]

- Avoid using Roundup around your home, wherever loved ones or family pets reside.

- Go to www.nongmoshoppingguide.com for great GMO-free shopping tips.

- For more information on GM foods and pesticides on produce, visit the Environmental Working Group's website at www.ewg.org.

THE DIVIDE BETWEEN THE US FOOD INDUSTRY AND NUTRITION

As you've seen by now, our American food landscape has been altered in profound ways over the last five decades. We live in a toxic food environment that promotes excessive food intake and the ability to access it at every turn. Today we face a tsunami of lifestyle-related chronic diseases that account for 80 percent of our healthcare costs. So how did we create an environment of too much food, too much eating, and far too many unhealthy choices? The early 1980s, when obesity rates began to rise, is a good place to start. At the time, numerous changes were afoot economically and politically, but a few combined for the most significant impact.

Dual Parents in the Workforce

In the 1980s, women, still the predominant homemakers, were rapidly entering the workforce. This positive shift for women had a negative impact on the nutritional needs of families, partly because of entrenched expectations that women would continue to carry the workload at home. Home-cooked meals swiftly gave way to convenient fast-food or processed meals. The food industry was quick to leverage the perceived daily time crunch. Drive-thru restaurants, frozen processed TV dinners, all-you-can-eat buffets, and "instant" packaged foods all became more appealing as parents' time at home steadily decreased. Today, food consumed outside the home accounts for almost 50 percent of the food budget. This compares to 34 percent in 1970 and 26.3 percent in 1960.[44]

Increased Standard Portions

Over the last four decades, our culture has clearly redefined our portion expectations. Today's American restaurant owners know that most consumers will choose restaurants based on portion sizes, which are mistaken for value. By introducing "Big Gulp" sodas, all-you-can-eat buffets, supersized hamburgers, extra-large pizzas, and kids' meals, convenience store and restaurant owners will continue to keep customers coming back for more. In 1955, a large McDonald's soda was 7 oz. By 1980, the large size had grown to 21 oz., and by 1990 it jumped to a whopping 32 oz. That's 65 g of sugar, which is roughly 16 tsp, in just one drink! We have developed a skewed perception of a "normal" portion size, mistaking overindulgence for value.

The trend of increasing portion sizes has not only affected meals served at restaurants, but it has also influenced food sold at grocery stores and meals prepared at home. The table below shows how our portion sizes have changed over the last twenty years.

PORTION DISTORTION*

FOOD	1993		2013	
	Portion	Calories	Portion	Calories
Bagel	3" diameter	140	6" diameter	350
Cheeseburger	1	333	1	590
Spaghetti and meatballs	1 cup sauce, 3 small meatballs	500	2 cups sauce, 3 large meatballs	1,020
Soda	6.5 oz.	82	20 oz.	250
Blueberry muffin	1.5 oz.	210	5 oz.	500
Coffee	8 oz., whole milk and sugar	45	16 oz., steamed milk and mocha syrup	350
Chicken Caesar salad	1.5 c	390	3.5 c	790
Popcorn	5 c	270	11 c	630
Chicken stir-fry	2 c	435	4.5 c	865

*Source: *NHL BI, We Can! Campaign, September 30, 2013, www.nhlbi.nih.gov/health/educational/wecan/eat-right/distortion.htm.*

Poor Food Choices Abound

Another notable change is the number of food products available to us. In 1980, the average grocery store contained around 15,000 products. Today that number is over 45,000 with the majority of new products being processed goods. Let's face it, we did not invent 35,000 new fruits and vegetables over the past thirty years! You'll find many of these food products on the inside aisles of grocery stores. Ever wonder why we have an entire aisle of breakfast cereals? Of that entire aisle, 99 percent of those cereals are refined flour, low-fiber, high-sugar concoctions that have been fortified (because everything that was once naturally beneficial has been stripped from them) by spraying a few vitamins on them.

In 2006, Hannaford grocery stores implemented the Guiding Stars nutrition guidance program to help shoppers quickly identify more nutritious foods and beverages. A total of 27,466 food products were reviewed by a panel of nutrition and food science experts who rated each food item based on criteria such as vitamins, fiber, trans and saturated fats, cholesterol, added sodium, and sugar. Food items were given one star if they had at least one positive attribute, two stars if they had three to four positive attributes, and three stars (the highest rating) if they received five to seven positive points. The results speak to the poor quality of food contained within the walls of our US grocery stores: only 24 percent of the 27,466 items received stars. That means that over 75 percent of the food tested was junk—zero stars! Only 7 percent of the food items received three stars and almost 80 percent of those were fruits and vegetables.[45]

A recent multi-year study of US grocery purchases revealed that highly processed foods make up more than 60 percent of the consumed calories in food we buy.[46] These items not only tend to have more fat, sugar, and salt but also the majority are made from GM corn and soy. Michael Pollan, author of the blockbuster book *The Omnivore's Dilemma*, discovered that since the 1970s, our industrialized food system has overproduced mountains of cheap, government-subsidized corn and soy, which have made their way into an unimaginable array of products. Since the 1970s, the American corn harvest has grown from 4 billion to 10 billion bushels a year by large-scale monoculture farms.

One of the many negative by-products of the enormous corn surplus has been the invention of high fructose corn syrup (HFCS), a cheap, unnatural, industrial food product made by chemically processing cornstarch into a sugary sweetener. Since the 1980s, HFCS has been pumped into breads, cereals, pastries, candy bars, condiments, cookies, cakes, crackers, drinks, canned fruits and vegetables, ice creams, salad dressings, sauces, snacks, soups, and just about anything with a label. In fact, you would be hard-pressed to find a food product containing HFCS that is also a nutrient-dense, high-quality food. You'd actually find the opposite: food that's been manipulated, overprocessed, genetically modified, and made with other potentially harmful ingredients.

FOOD MARKETING TO KIDS

The food industry is not only leading the conversation about food and nutrition, it has created a harmful cultural norm that begins with manipulative advertising directed at children as young as two years old. Food and beverage companies are well aware that kids are big business. The Federal Trade Commission reported that $1.8 billion a year is spent on food marketing to children, but child advocacy groups claim it's more like $7–8 billion.[47] You may be surprised to learn that 90 percent of these expenditures account for the promotion of fast food, sugary drinks, sugary breakfast cereals, and candy.[48]

With 35 percent of American children now overweight or obese, discussion of how food marketing might play a role in that development seems timely. The apparent causes of our chronic disease and obesity crises are a combination of poor diet choices, genetics, low physical activity, psychosocial variables, and toxic environmental exposures. Food companies deny that food marketing hurts children while spending millions of dollars defending that stance. However, robust science now tells a different story. In 2006, the Institute of Medicine produced a report concluding that food marketing to children and youth contributes to poor diet, childhood obesity, and puts their long-term health at risk.[49]

> *I have a hard time believing that our founding fathers of the United States sat around a table dreaming up the first amendment to protect the right of food marketers to sell junk food to children but that's the way the courts have been interpreting it so the result has been a cacophony of health claims on foods in the market.*
>
> **—Marion Nestle, PhD, MPH,** Institute for Integrative Nutrition Lecture, 2009

As mentioned in chapter 1, childhood obesity rates have tripled since 1980. Coinciding with that period, another major shift marked a pivotal time in US food marketing to kids. In the late 1970s, after hearing from public interest groups, leading experts in health and nutrition, and child psychology experts, the Federal Trade Commission (FTC) proposed sweeping regulations to restrict advertising to children. The food, sugar, candy, and toy industries swiftly fought back, raising record-setting amounts of money to lobby against the regulations. In

1980, even though 6,000 pages of oral testimony from health and child experts said otherwise, Congress sided with commercial industries and stripped the FTC of its advertising regulating authority regarding children. This left companies completely unchecked and free to manipulate kids from any platform. This historic ruling made the US one of the only industrialized countries in the world without strict policies around food marketing to kids.[50]

Over the past thirty-four years since deregulation, we've seen an astounding 852 percent increase in kids' consumer spending: from $4.2 billion in 1984 to $40 billion in 2008.[51] These numbers clearly show that marketing to children works. This unprecedented period has created a new sophisticated obsession with kids and teens within the food marketing world. Marketers have been free to turn kids' most powerful emotional attachments into unheard of profits. Their tactics have been methodical, extensively researched, and play on children's immature biological and psychological vulnerabilities.

Today's youth live in a media-saturated environment. A study from the Rudd Center reported that in 2015, children and adolescents viewed around 13 food-related advertisements a day.[52] Although TV has been the dominant advertising medium to kids in the past, new media platforms such as social media, banner ads, online games, and apps have increased over 50 percent since 2006.[53] In fact, one of the most powerful features of today's advertising to children and teens is that it aims its messages from multiple directions at the same time. Recent estimates from the Kaiser Family Foundation show that the average American child, age eight or older, spends almost eight hours a day devoted to various forms of screen media.[54] This generation of children—as no other generation before—is locked into screens and demands constant gratification. While most of us parents are hyper-focused on protecting our kids from inappropriate adult content or online predators, harmful food marketing is happening beneath our radars.

Becoming Empowered Parents

Food companies have long understood that kids have tremendous influence on their parents' purchasing habits. Their goal is to turn kids into lifelong consumers, which means creating brand loyalty at a young age. Food marketers go to great lengths to understand how children and teens think and act. Believe it or not, there are books, advertising journals, and even conferences dedicated entirely to how to market to children. Marketers study food behaviors, they observe which colors kids like best, they research what characters children are drawn to, and they examine how kids pick up and look at products. They even hire psychologists to help them understand product placement and brand image, because they know that young children do not possess the cognitive ability to understand the persuasive intent of advertising. A 2009 Rudd Center report stated, "By age two, children recognize brand logos on product packages, and by preschool, children recall brand names seen on television." It further stated, "Preschoolers indicated a significantly higher preference for the taste of foods and beverages when such items were placed in McDonald's packaging compared with the same foods presented in plain packaging."[55]

Today's kids have more autonomy and decision-making power within the family than in previous generations, which is why food companies rely on tactics like "pester power," the ability of children, after the bombardment of marketers' messages, to nag their parents to the point of purchase. Instead of marketing directly to parents, marketers let the kids do the work for them: 90 percent of parents say their children demand things when out shopping together. A child's first request for a product starts around twenty-four months of age and continues through adolescence. Food advertisers know that parents honor children's requests for foods like soft drinks, cookies, and candy about 50 to 60 percent of the time, which makes kids a prime target for advertising.[56]

Brand recognition is also part of their profitable formula because it's well established that when a child chooses a brand at a young age, they tend to remain loyal to it into adulthood. As children reach adolescence, food marketers focus on what is called "symbolic advertising," that is, creating social meaning around food products. It is believed that children want products that will make them appear more exciting, fun, or "cool." It's a tactic that plays on a child's desire to be popular. Its message says, "I'm cool because I'm drinking a Coke."

Make no mistake, the food industry's primary goal is to earn large profits and make its shareholders happy. These corporate Goliaths spend billions of dollars each year to undermine parental authority and convince your kids to buy their processed junk. Unfortunately, they do a darn good job. I don't blame food companies for being great marketers; I believe in capitalism and our free market system. I do, however, feel it

According to the aptly titled article "Big Food: Sounds a lot Like Big Tobacco," from the Center for Science in the Public Interest, "The similarities between unhealthy food and tobacco go beyond the health effects. When it comes to corporate responsibility, executives at some of the nation's largest food and beverage companies seem to have learned a lot from their counterparts at Big Tobacco in aggressively promoting consumption and, in the same breath, blaming the consumer."

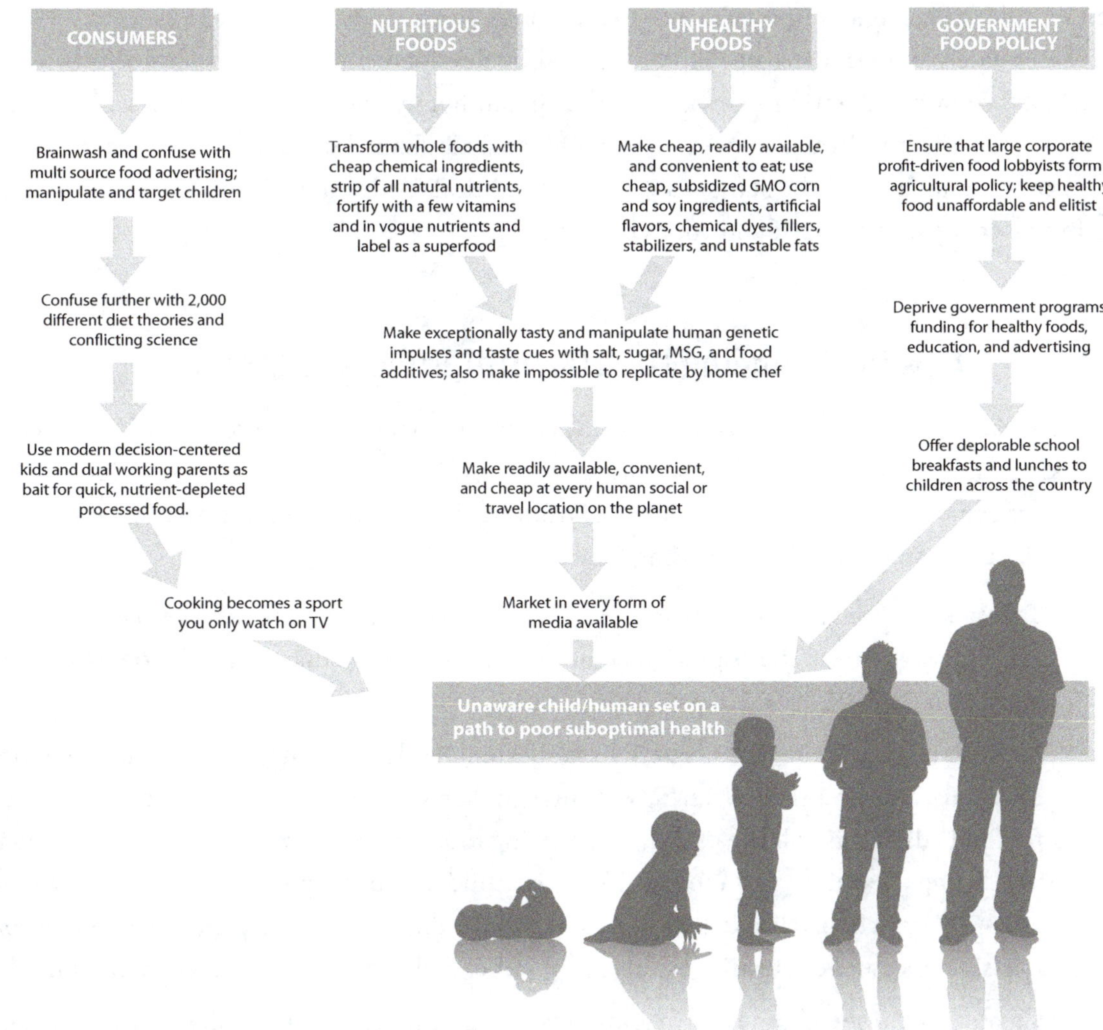

is our societal and parental responsibility to protect the health of children. Both the food industry and the medical community have always preached personal responsibility: stay away from processed junk, eat whole fruits and vegetables, choose high-quality protein, and get some exercise. It seems pretty simple, but public confusion continues about what we are supposed to be eating, how much, and at what time. In our world today, it's not enough to tell people to simply change their diets. We need to understand how we fit into a society that does everything in its power to encourage us to consume vast quantities of prepared foods that harm us.

As parents living in a country without food marketing regulations for kids, we have to fill a tall order of personal responsibility when it comes to our kids' health. It's best that we serve as role models and prioritize our children's healthy development. We accomplish this by going against the grain and setting a new cultural bar in our homes and our communities. I know that choosing the "culturally unaccepted" way of life can be difficult, but going beyond the status quo and refusing to fall into the standard American cultural food trap is by far one of the greatest gifts you can give to yourself and your children.

Tips for Reducing the Harmful Effects of Marketing

We all want our children to grow up healthy, happy, and ready to succeed in life. Many forces working against us have changed the way we view and accept our food and nutrition culture. Here are some ideas to help guard your kids from harmful food marketing and to help foster a healthier understanding of a nourishing food environment.

- Talk to kids about food advertising. While this will only help with kids age eight (roughly) and older who have the cognitive ability to understand media manipulation, it's a good place to start.

- Limit screen time. The benefits here go far beyond food marketing, but limiting cell phone, TV, iPads, etc., after school, during evenings, and on weekends will limit exposure to harmful food ads. TV is still the primary marketing tool for food companies. Eliminate watching during mealtimes and remove TVs from children's bedrooms. In our house, we don't allow TV on school days and we limit screen time on weekends, depending on homework loads. Phones and electronics are also kept out of bedrooms and are "turned in" at night.

- Create ways to spend time away from social media and television and thus advertising. Go on nature walks, create art projects, cook together, play board games, engage in community service, play music, travel to a new place, read together, or try a new form of exercise.

- Set purchasing limits and expectations with your children before entering a store that offers unhealthy food. This can help reduce the "pester or nag" factor.

- Teach your kids how to read nutrition labels and ingredient lists. As they age, this will serve them well to identify bogus food claims and advertisements. Strive to eat only packaged foods that have whole food ingredients you can pronounce and understand.

◆ Create a healthy school culture. This begins with getting food marketing out of schools. In 2009, food and beverage companies spent $149 million on in-school marketing.[57] Work with and educate school leaders to remove the selling or marketing of foods of minimal nutritional value anywhere on school grounds. This includes product sales and fundraisers for unhealthy baked goods and all forms of advertising. Logos and brand names are often featured on curricular materials; signs, scoreboards, vending machines, and incentive programs frequently offer coupons or discounts to fast food or other unhealthy restaurants. Instead, adopt policies that support healthful messages that will strengthen kids' bodies and minds. Rudd Roots Parents is a great resource for building community, gathering information, and proposing policy changes. Find them at https://edibleschoolyard.org.

◆ Assist local school districts by incorporating marketing-related guidelines into district-required school wellness policies. Currently only 10 percent of districts now address marketing in their wellness policies.[58]

◆ Speak out! Parents have enormous power as consumers. Keep demanding healthier products for our kids, and food marketers will have to listen. Like all great change in America, it starts with a grassroots effort to make positive changes that your kids will thank you for down the road.

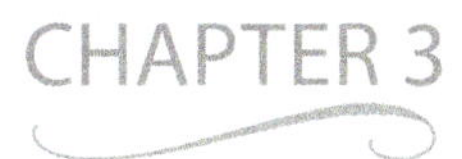

CHAPTER 3

Ancient Answers to Modern Problems:
THE DIET-DISEASE CONNECTION

The more you know about the past, the better prepared you are for the future.

—Theodore Roosevelt

Some of the most important research from early twentieth-century scientists shows that humans suffered disease not from "bad genes" but because modern diets failed to provide optimal nutrition. More specifically, their research showed those civilizations that had adopted modern foods such as pasteurized milk, refined flours, processed foods, and sugar had increased susceptibility to infectious and chronic diseases. In contrast, those civilizations that consumed unadulterated, whole foods as nature intended lived long, quality lives, free of most modern chronic illness. This chapter discusses some of the healthiest cultures on Earth today that practice the same habits: active, family-centered peoples who eat small portions of unprocessed plant foods every day and meat on rare occasions. This is the primer for our children to live with vitality and health.

I am continually amazed at how Americans are obsessed with the next best diet craze or the latest supplement that promises superpowers. Navigating the barrage of speculative information and food industry propaganda has most consumers scratching their heads. Who's telling the truth? Who do we believe? Nutrition advice comes at us from all directions: medical and nutrition professionals, TV commercials, morning news shows, magazine articles, nutrition books, daily wellness blogs, and online health summits. Some so-called experts talk about perfect ratios of macronutrients, others eliminate entire food groups, and some promote diets that have little to no science behind them. Our government also publishes its own nutrition advice through the USDA—advice that's often contradicted by doctors and dietitians. So many concepts have been accepted as valid, only to be exposed as false. A great example is the heart healthy low-fat, high-carbohydrate diet that has been touted by the media, the Academy of Nutrition and Dietetics, and the American Heart Association (AHA) for almost 50 years. We now know that the "fat is bad and will kill you" theory is scientifically disproven.

The truth is, after practicing nutritional medicine for 20 years, I have come to acknowledge that nutrition research is often flawed and misunderstood due to the multitude of variables within studies that vary greatly in design and quality, making comparison difficult at best. Most nutrition research is based on what we call *observational studies*, which show correlation and not causation. These studies run for years and track large numbers of people who are assumed to be eating a certain way based on frequent food surveys. The study subjects are then periodically evaluated to see if patterns emerge, for example, who develops heart disease or cancer. A big problem with this approach is that people often don't report accurate information. Most people underestimate what they eat, forget to record food items, and are unfamiliar with ingredients or don't obtain their food consistently from the same stores.

Another problem with nutrition research is that for years scientists have performed studies focused on single nutrients. Based on these studies, they have drawn broad conclusions about diet and health.[59] For example, in 1971, Linus Pauling declared that high doses of vitamin C would prevent most cancers. In 1994, research results encouraged cardiologists to prescribe vitamin E supplements to prevent heart disease. Unfortunately, these theories were false, as this reductionist approach is unrealistic when studying complex human systems in relation to diet and health. There is no single dietary factor that has been shown to conclusively reduce the risk of developing or delaying the progression of chronic disease. But we do know for certain that overall diet plays a major role in its prevention.

In another example of flawed findings, for years vegetarian diets have been criticized because this diet approach can lead to vitamin B12 deficiency. It seems, though, that we have missed the bigger picture that shows vegetarian diets *as a whole* protect against many chronic diseases like coronary heart disease and type 2 diabetes.[60] Dr. T. Colin Campbell, a brilliant scholar and researcher, said it best:

"We scientists focus on details while ignoring the larger context.…We oversimplify and disregard the infinite complexity of nature. Often, investigating minute biochemical parts of food and trying to reach broad conclusions about diet and health leads to contradictory results. Contradictory results lead to confused scientists and policy makers, and to an increasingly confused public."[61]

We simply can't isolate the metabolism of a food from the whole person. There are an infinite number of variables that play into the functioning of a person's digestive potential. We can't ignore the synergistic properties of food nor the genetic or metabolic differences among individuals. By understanding how diet as a whole impacts each individual's body we can begin to appreciate the power of nutrients. The unique and intricate ways foods interact with each person's genes and extensive gut microbiota are key when evaluating the impact of nutrition on health. Whole food, as Mother Nature intended, still remains the gold standard as we discovered many, many years ago. We have finally come to understand that one nutrient or a single food does not lead to optimal health, but rather it's the synergistic properties of a person's overall diet and their own personal makeup that play major roles in the body's superb function.

RETURNING TO THE HEART OF MOTHER NATURE

The wisdom about complexity of diet that was once handed down from generation to generation seems to have been replaced by a new cultural phenomenon where nutritional truth, as perceived by the general public, is now obtained from misleading science, mass media, and corporate food advertising. This has had a significant influence on our core knowledge and our behavior.

I'd like to offer ways to help reestablish fundamental truths about healthy nutrition. It requires revisiting core concepts from our past generations, specifically two early pioneers in the field of human health and nutrition. Their discoveries provide valuable touchstones for modern nutrition science. In fact, there is a recurring theme when it comes to our modern food climate: abundant historical evidence from all over the world shows a precipitous decline in health once our ancestors abandoned their indigenous diets and embraced modern food. Ignoring this revelation means choosing disease; it says we choose convenience over health and indifference over awareness. Choosing *otherwise* can return us to the path our ancestors benefited from, for health's sake.

Dr. Weston A. Price:
"The Isaac Newton of Nutrition"

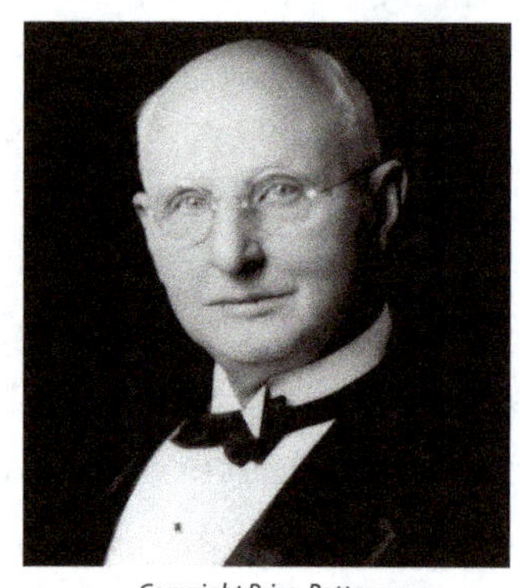

In the 1930s, Dr. Weston A. Price, a Cleveland dentist, traveled the world looking for answers to account for disease. During his journey, he carried out some of the most pivotal nutrition science research that was inspired by a suspicion that tooth decay, crooked teeth, and structural facial deformities (overbites, narrowed faces, lack of well-defined cheekbones) were caused by nutritional deficiencies. He compared the poor dental patterns of his modern patients with the beautiful teeth and excellent health of those in primitive cultures and questioned whether modern diets might be a reason for such differences. His travels led him to discoveries that far exceeded his initial quest for answers pertaining to dentistry. He exposed profound truths linking nutritional deficiencies not just with poor oral health but also with increased occurrences of chronic disease.

For over 10 years, Dr. Price traveled over 100,000 miles studying the health and dietary patterns of numerous isolated societies, untouched by modern civilization. His research took him to mountain villages in Switzerland, the Gaelic islands of the Outer Hebrides, indigenous cultures of North and South America and Alaska, over 30 African tribes, American Indians in the Yukon, eight Polynesian islands of the South Pacific, and numerous tribes in Australia and New Zealand. In each of these remote locations, Dr. Price studied the diets of groups living and eating as their ancestors had done thousands of years before, and he compared these to their counterparts who had chosen (or were forced due to dwindling resources) to introduce modern foods into their lifestyles.

His findings were illuminating. The indigenous societies that remained on their native diets were not afflicted with any of the diseases plaguing their peers who had adopted modern foods into their diets. Not only did he find excellent physical development in indigenous societies, characterized by beautiful facial structures, rare dental crowding, and minimal tooth decay, but he also found an absence of disease.[62] In contrast, children born to parents who had abandoned their traditional diets for the so-called civilized foods—specifically white sugar and flour, pasteurized or skimmed milk, canned foods, and hydrogenated vegetable oils—experienced crowded, crooked teeth, birth defects, poor bone structure, and increased susceptibility to infections and chronic diseases. This pattern prevailed in *every single* location Dr. Price visited.

Seminole Indian Comparison

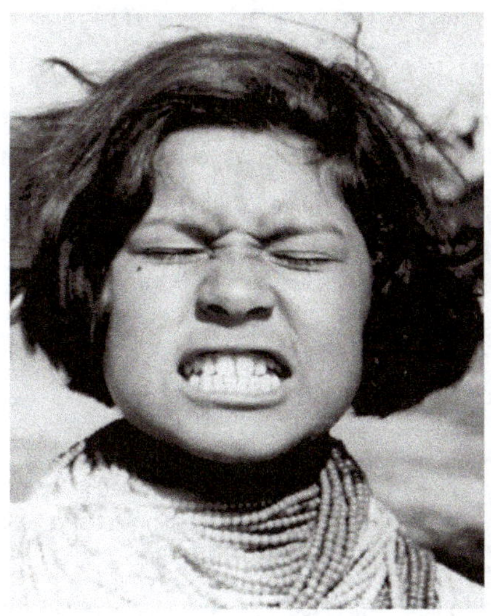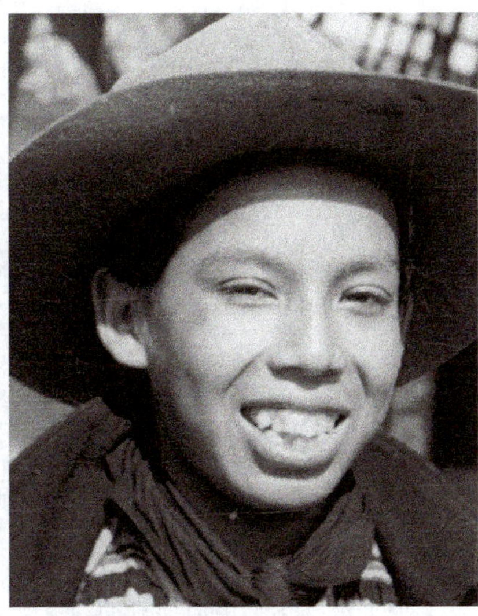

"The 'primitive' Seminole girl (left) has a wide, handsome face with plenty of room for the dental arches. The 'modernized' Seminole girl (right) born to parents who had abandoned their traditional diets, has a narrowed face, crowded teeth, and a reduced immunity to disease."[63]

Interestingly, each of the indigenous diets that Dr. Price studied were vastly different in their macronutrient components. In other words, the ratios of protein, carbohydrate, and fat varied substantially in diets around the world, yet they all provided protection from modern diseases. Some indigenous diets relied entirely on meat and flesh from land animals, while others lived entirely on seafood, fruits, and vegetables (see table on page 38). Even with this variability, the indigenous diets still provided *4 times* the water-soluble vitamin and mineral content and *10 times* the fat-soluble vitamin content of the modernized diets of their native counterparts. This is a very important finding in the context of our conflicting and ever-changing modern dietary recommendations that frequently try to persuade us to eliminate entire food groups or obtain a "perfect" macronutrient ratio. Even more astounding is the superb physical condition and absence of Western chronic diseases that resulted from a diet unadulterated by modern foods.

What really stood out to Dr. Price was that among the healthy civilizations that he visited, they all had diets rich in fat-soluble vitamins, specifically vitamins A, D, and what he referred to then as "Activator X." In fact, he considered this piece of their diets to be the essential ingredient

FOOD SOURCES OF INDIGENOUS AND MODERNIZED GROUPS STUDIED BY DR. PRICE[64]

INDIGENOUS GROUP	NATIVE FOODS EATEN	MODERN FOODS INTRODUCED
Swiss	Whole rye bread, rye cereal, cheese, fresh raw goat's or cow's milk, meat once a week, wine, potatoes	Chocolate milk, white flour products, marmalades, jams, canned vegetables, confections and fruits
Gaelic	Oat products, seafood (fish liver, fish liver oils, organ meats, lobster, crab, oysters, and clams), turnips, potatoes, leek, cabbage, wild nettles, sorrel and garlic, summer berries, no dairy foods	White flour products, canned marmalades, canned vegetables, sweetened fruit juices, jams, confections (sugar, chocolate, cakes), coffee, eggs
Inuit	Fish, organ meat from sea and land animals, oil, blubber, and meat from seals and caribou, summer berries and plant foods, nuts, fish eggs	White flour products, sugar, polished rice, jams, canned goods, and vegetable fats
North American Indians	Wild game (moose and caribou), organ meats, bone marrow, summer plants	White flour products, canned marmalades and jams, canned vegetables, commercial vegetable fats, sweetened goods, syrups, confections
South Pacific Islanders	Shellfish and scale fish, plant roots and leaves, fruits, taro root, coconut	Trade foods (white flour and sugar), canned goods
African Indigenous tribes	Sweet potatoes, beans, cereals (maize, linga, millet), fish, insects (ants and locusts), kefir, corn	White flour products, sugar, polished rice, and canned foods
Native Maori of New Zealand	Large amounts of seafood and shellfish, sea worms, mutton, birds, vegetables, fruits, fern root	White flour, sweetened goods, syrup, and canned goods
Islands North of Australia	Seafood, plant roots, greens, fruits, shellfish, sea cow	White flour, polished rice, canned goods, and sugar
Peruvian Indigenous Tribes	Seafood, angel fish, fish eggs, land plants and fruit, camel, llama, alpacas, vicunas, dried kelp, yucca, potatoes, guinea pigs, corn, beans, quinoa	Refined flour products, sugar, sweetened foods, canned goods, and polished rice
Aboriginal Australian	Kangaroo, wallaby, birds, seafood (fish, shellfish, sea plants), sea cow, plant foods (roots, stems, leaves, berries, seeds of grasses)	White flour and sugar, jams, milk, canned foods, tins of meat and tea

to their robust health and perfect teeth and bone structures. His theory was that these vitamins were fat-soluble "activators" that served as the catalysts for mineral and nutrient absorption. Without them, minerals could not be used by the body no matter how plentiful they may be in the diet.

Today, modern research has validated the findings of Dr. Price. In recent years, "Activator

X" has been discovered to be fat-soluble vitamin K2, a vital nutrient that plays a critical role in building strong bones, preventing heart disease, among many other areas.[65] The "fat-soluble activators" (A, D, and K2) that Dr. Price identified are found as follows:

- Vitamin A: cod liver oil, shrimp, grass-fed butter and cream, pastured egg yolks, fermented fish liver oil, salmon, pastured beef, lamb or chicken liver, and grass-fed dairy products

- Vitamin D: sunlight, fatty fish like salmon, sardines, tuna and mackerel, cod liver oil, and smaller amounts in egg yolks, beef liver, fish eggs, mushrooms, and grass-fed whole-milk cheese

- Vitamin K2: chicken, duck or goose liver, organic beef or lamb liver, grass-fed butter or ghee, pasture-raised poultry, pasture-raised eggs yolks, emu oil, and fermented foods such as sauerkraut, hard or soft cheeses, kefir and natto

It seems that the applications of Dr. Price's studies are as relevant today as they were in 1930s. Although it's without question that Dr. Price's study methods were unconventional and some of his recommendations could use a bit of refining, it is impossible to ignore the connection he discovered between the foods we eat and the health of our entire bodies. He also taught us that the mouth can truly be seen as a natural gateway to the entire body. Like Dr. Price, we need to see how dental disease is an imminent warning sign of other health problems. According to the World Health Organization, 60–90 percent of school-age children living in industrialized countries and the vast majority of adults are affected by tooth decay.[66] This holds true in the United States, where tooth decay remains the most widespread chronic disease in both children and adults. Although largely preventable, a whopping 42 percent of US children develop cavities in their baby teeth.[67] In fact, rotten teeth have become so common in children, that today's parents have grown to accept decay as normal. The same is true for crooked teeth and braces. But the reality is, our children's mouths are simply a reflection of the widespread chronic disease and poor diets among us. In nature, dental problems are rare, and human fossil records have shown us that dental disease, as we know it today, appeared after the Industrial Revolution, when processed foods were introduced to modern societies of the early 1900s.[68] This rapid unnatural degeneration is the result of our change in nourishment. Maybe if we feed our kids the right food, our bones and body systems will develop in the manner in which they were intended to and chronic disease will cease to exist. We know this to be true: the further away we move from an unprocessed, whole food diet, with essential fat-soluble nutrients, the harder it becomes for our bodies to stay healthy and have long, disease-free lives.

Sir Robert McCarrison: Pioneer in Nutrition Research

It's difficult to envision entire populations that have near-perfect health and live free from chronic diseases like heart disease or cancer, even free from the common cold. Can you imagine stepping out of the United States, the land of the sick and medicated, and stepping into a land of strength, stamina, and vitality? During the 1920s, British researcher Sir Robert McCarrison did just that. Dr. McCarrison was a trailblazer in early nutrition research, carrying out the first eye-opening experiments to demonstrate the effects of nutrition on the epidemiology of disease. On one of his research expeditions, he spent seven years in the Himalayan Mountains studying the people of the Hunza Valley, a fairytale-like place located at the northern tip of Pakistan, bordering Afghanistan and China. What made the natives of the Hunza Valley unique was their impeccable health and immunity and their extremely long life-spans. Some Hunza people lived to 110 and occasionally even 140 years of age. It was a land where people did not suffer from common diseases of the West: there were no heart ailments, cancer, arthritis, diabetes, asthma, constipation, or other chronic conditions that seemed prevalent in other areas of the world.

"My own experience," Dr. McCarrison wrote in his book *Studies of Deficiency Disease*, "provides an example of a race unsurpassed in perfection of physique and in freedom from disease in general. Among these people the span of life is extraordinarily long....During the period of my association with these people I never saw a case of asthenic dyspepsia, of gastric or duodenal ulcer, of appendicitis, of mucus colitis, of cancer."[69] So vibrant was the health of the Hunzas that they even appeared to be immune to the common cold.

McCarrison's experience with the Hunza people shifted his conventional medical attitude to quite a revolutionary way of thinking. He no longer viewed health as the prevention of or recovery from disease but rather as a state of "optimal efficiency." After studying the Hunza people, he was determined to discover the answers to what gave them their magnificent physique and health. He found their health was the result of what he called "vital food." Although he also acknowledged other important characteristics such as breast-fed children (for a minimum of two years), abundant amounts of exercise, and abstinence from alcohol, he placed the factor of vital food before all others.

The Hunzas practiced superior forms of agriculture, returning all organic matter back to the soil. Their food consisted primarily of raw fruits and vegetables, sprouted beans, peas and lentils, whole grains, stone-ground flour, nuts, fermented and unpasteurized goat milk products, and occasionally a small portion of meat with bones. Small amounts of fats were consumed, including apricot seed oil, ghee, and butter. The Hunzas' eating frequency was also notable as they didn't eat between meals or before going to bed at night. McCarrison believed so strongly in the link between the Hunzas' diet and their pristine health that he conducted a series of ingenious experiments with albino rats in Coonoor, India, in 1927. He wanted to find out if rats could flourish with the same diet that the Hunzas followed.

For 27 months (equivalent to approximately 45 human years), the rats were fed the Hunza diet from birth. The diet consisted of coarse-ground flatbread with fresh butter, sprouted grains and

> *We often forget the most fundamental of all rules for the physician, that the right kind of food is the most important single factor in the promotion of health and the wrong kind of food the most important single factor in the promotion of disease.*
>
> —Sir Robert McCarrison, The *Transactions of the Far Eastern Association of Tropical Medicine,* 1927

legumes, fresh raw carrots and cabbage, raw whole milk, occasional dried fruit, a single weekly serving of meat and bones, and an abundance of water. The results were amazing: "During the past two and a quarter years, there has been no case of illness in this 'universe' of albino rats, no death from natural causes in the adult stock, and, but for a few accidental deaths, no infantile mortality. Both clinically and at post-mortem examination this stock has been shown to be remarkably free from disease."[70]

McCarrison furthered his experiments by feeding another group of rats the same diet of the Southern India rice-eaters, and a third group of rats the diet of those in England's lower classes, which consisted of white bread, margarine, sweetened tea, boiled milk, cabbage, potatoes, tinned meats, and jams. The results were equally startling. Both sets of rats that ate the Southern Indian and English diets suffered from a wide variety of diseases involving every organ of the body as well as hair loss, anxiety, and aggression. Dr. McCarrison's work showed a clear link between diet and optimal health, which was revolutionary for its time.

In a lecture, Dr. McCarrison noted, "We are passing from a period in which bacteria were held of more surgical importance than diet, to one in which knowledge of diet is to be regarded as more important than knowledge of bacteria. Is it the physician or dietitian who is leading the way? Who would have thought, ten years ago, that an error in diet would render us liable to such diverse conditions as middle-ear disease, duodenal ulcer, renal calculus, or cystitis?"[71] One would think these findings would have turned the heads of Dr. McCarrison's colleagues in the 1930s, but much like the doctors of today, they gave food and nutrition little credit in the world of healing.

Dr. McCarrison was captivated by *health as wholeness* over the medical concept of health, which at the time, was the state reached by recovery from a disease. He looked to displace the traditional way of medical thinking, which focused on individual diseases, and replace it with a focus on optimal health by looking at diets, environments, and lifestyles. He was a revolutionary of his time and compares quite similarly to our twenty-first-century pioneers in functional medicine, such as Dr. Jeffrey S. Bland.

Today's Healthy Hotspots

Other areas around the world have been documented as having cultures in which people live free of diseases that are killing Americans, and they have shown better than three times the chance of reaching 100 years of age than Americans. In Dan Buettner's eye-opening book, *The Blue Zones*, he found five of the healthiest places on Earth, where people live long, *quality* lives free of many major diseases: Ikaria, Greece; Loma Linda, California; Sardinia, Italy; Okinawa, Japan; and Nicoya, Costa Rica, which were all regarded as "longevity hotspots." His team of researchers carefully studied each culture's lifestyle components, and they were able to determine common practices that were distinct in all four populations.

Here's a short list of the fundamental ingredients found in each of those Blue Zones that we can use in our own journey with our families toward healthier living:

- Stop eating when you no longer feel hungry. This is different than eating until you are full. It requires you to be present each moment during mealtimes and eliminates mindless eating. It also encourages and teaches children to listen to their internal cues and eliminates expectations for them to finish every bit of food on their plates.

- Eat small portions of unprocessed whole foods. Eat mostly vegetables, fruits, beans, and nuts every day. Eat at least two vegetables with each meal and eat meat on rare occasions.

- Avoid processed foods altogether.

- Limit alcohol consumption. Enjoy no more than one glass of wine each day with friends.

- Be active. This does not mean running marathons but rather making physical activity part of each day.

- Have a sense of purpose. This looks different for everyone. It may be spending time with family, a job, a hobby, or learning a new instrument. Whatever the engagement, it should elicit feelings of freedom, enjoyment, and fulfillment.

◆ Relieve stress: nap, socialize, practice yoga, meditate. Find ways to slow down.

◆ Surround yourself with people who share your values. Make social connections and try not to be grumpy.

◆ Participate in a spiritual community. The faithful are shown to be healthier and happier people.

◆ Put family first. Take care of all your loved ones, including yourself, and spend time together.[72]

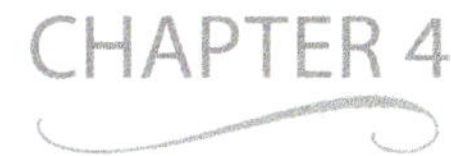

CHAPTER 4

HOW OUR GENES RESPOND TO FOOD

A person's health isn't generally a reflection of genes, but how their environment is influencing them. Genes are the direct cause of less than 1 percent of diseases: 99 percent is how we respond to the world.

—Bruce Lipton

We have been living a lie: genes are not our destiny. The science of epigenetics has flipped the "genes are our destiny" theory upside down. We now know that we are a combination of environmental experiences—some that we can control and some that we cannot. In this chapter you will learn the five pillars of health that we can control: diet, exercise, toxin exposure, sleep, and emotional well-being. They form equal parts of who we are. To optimize these parts, we need to understand the underlying principles of which genes are turned on and off based on our lifestyle choices, a process that's occurring every second of every day. By the end of this chapter, you will know why your choices will allow you and your children to function optimally. And you will recognize the enormous power we have as parents to influence our children's gene expression and, in turn, their health.

It's pretty clear by now that in today's world, our prominent diseases are chronic diseases. In adults, it's high blood pressure, dementia, high cholesterol, arthritis, IBS, and diabetes. In kids, it's ADHD, behavior and mood disorders, obesity, anxiety, acne, depression, type 2 diabetes, tooth decay, asthma, and allergies. What if we could get at the root cause of these illnesses and depend less on medications to treat their symptoms? To do that we need to understand what influences our genes and how our daily choices play a direct role.

Has your doctor ever asked you for your family medical history? And have you ever left your doctor's office feeling like your fate would come down to the answers you gave? I have. My mother's side of the family has been plagued with early onset breast cancer. It's so concerning to my doctors, that I have genetic counselors calling me yearly to consider testing for the BRCA gene, the feared mutation that sends women like Angelina Jolie to undergo preventive mastectomies. This is indeed a serious concern, but the information we don't hear about is that before 1940, women with the BRCA gene had only a 24 percent chance of developing breast cancer compared to today's incidence, which is up to 85 percent.[73] What occurred to cause this enormous change in disease risk over the last 80 years?

To get answers to that million-dollar question we can look to Dr. Jeffrey Bland, a renowned biochemist and leader in the fields of functional medicine, nutritional medicine, and systems biology. In his latest book *The Disease Delusion*, Dr. Bland explains, "Genes can't and don't change." He further explains that what *does* change is how our genes respond to their environment: diet, exercise, chemical exposures, stress, and other lifestyle behaviors. "Alter the environment and you alter the way genes express themselves in response—and the health outcome. It all depends on the message the gene receives."[74]

To better understand this relationship, we need to understand the new field of *epigenetics*, or gene expression. When the human genome project started in 1988, researchers assumed that because the worm had 20,000 genes that humans would have far more to account for our significantly greater complexity. What they found was mind-blowing: our cells only contain roughly 25,000 genes. How can this be? A simple organism, such as a worm, has only 5,000 fewer genes than an elaborate human? Epigenetics holds the answer. The magical expression of these 25,000 genes is environmentally controlled.

We know genes are made up of a chemical called DNA, which carries coded information that determines our inherited traits from our parents. Dr. Bland states, "Your DNA is your DNA, and you can't fight genetic inheritance…but 'inherited' does not mean 'inevitable.'"[75] Genes certainly influence health but not how we once thought. They contain a plethora of information that provides our cells with instructions on how to operate. Recent evidence shows us that our cells can actually choose which genes to express, depending on signals they receive from the environment. And in epigenetic terms, our environment means essentially the world around us and the world within us. It can be our emotional health, amount of exercise, nutrition, toxins (biological, elemental, synthetic), allergens (food, mold, dust, pollen, chemicals), and microbes (bacteria, yeast, parasites). To use a computer analogy, your DNA is your hardware, which is a permanent fixture, but your environmental influences are the variable software that you control and that ultimately determine the hardware's function. This reality is unbelievably profound: we have the *power* to make an impact on our gene expression.

INFLUENCING OUR DNA

A landmark Duke University study published in 2003 by pioneer researcher Dr. Randy Jirtle and his team showed how important a mother's diet is in shaping the gene expression of her offspring.[76] The experiment was performed on mice with the agouti gene, a gene that gives mice yellow coats, a ravenous appetite, and predisposes them to obesity, cardiovascular disease, diabetes, and cancer. Typically, when agouti mice breed, most of their offspring are just like their parents: yellow, plump, and disease prone. Jirtle's team proved the agouti gene could be silenced by altering the diet of the mice. Right before conception, Jirtle's team began to feed one group of fat, yellow agouti mice a diet rich in choline and B vitamins (folic acid and B-12). Surprisingly,

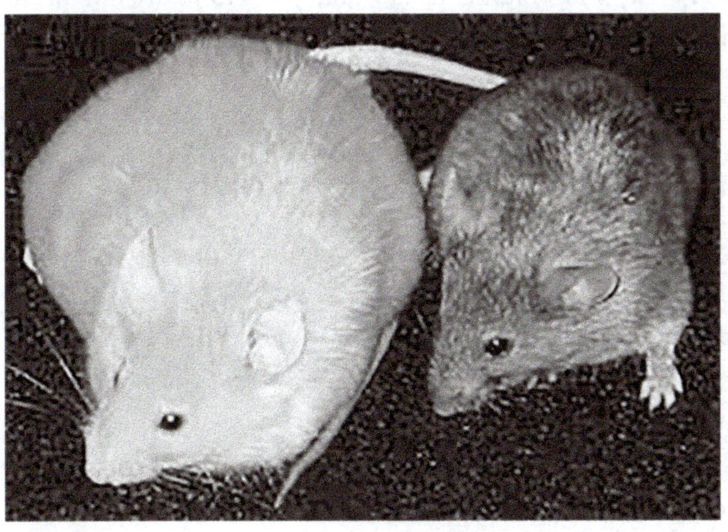

These two mice are genetically identical and the same age. The mother of the mouse on the left was fed a normal mouse diet. The mother of the mouse on the right was fed a diet rich in choline and B-vitamins (folic acid and B-12).

Permission for photos granted from Dr. Jirtle.

the agouti mice produced pups that were brown, thin, and without their parents' susceptibility to disease. The second group of genetically identical pregnant agouti mice were given no prenatal B vitamin supplements. The offspring they produced looked just like their mothers: obese and yellow with a higher risk of developing disease.

These groundbreaking findings showed the power of environment—more specifically nutrition—over gene expression. The B vitamins given to the mice are known as methyl donors, chemical groups that can attach to DNA and turn its expression on or off. Dietary methyl groups are derived from foods that contain methionine and choline such as shrimp, eggs, chicken, dark leafy greens, beans, beets, garlic, and onions.

Researcher Dr. Dana Dolinoy took Dr. Jirtle's study one step further by adding bisphenol A (BPA) to the experiment. BPA is a common hormone-mimicking chemical that frequently shows up in products like plastic water bottles, canned goods, and grocery receipts. It is a known hormone disruptor associated with certain cancers, developmental disorders, and a host of chronic conditions. Dr. Dolinoy exposed Dr. Jirtle's pregnant experimental agouti mice to BPA. The previously improved brown, thin, methylated mothers now produced offspring that were again fat, yellow, and diabetic. The results provided the key understanding that there is a clear push-pull between positive and negative influences on our gene expression.[77]

These studies launched a fundamental shift in our understanding of human disease. We once thought we lived in a world where our DNA determined our fate and our children's fate. Today's science of epigenetics tells us we have the ability to influence our DNA's voice, tinker if you will, with its on/off switch and control its volume. It may take years to figure out all the implications, but one thing is certain: food choices directly affect health outcomes.

Identical Genes Do Not Equal Identical Health

I grew up witnessing the phenomenon of epigenetics firsthand. My father was an identical twin. By definition, identical twins evolve when a single egg is fertilized to form one zygote, which then divides into two separate embryos. The key here is that both eggs contain the *exact same* genetic material. Based on the myth that our genes determine our fate, it may have been reasonable to assume that identical twins should eventually develop similar diseases. This was far from the truth with my father and his twin.

At first glance, you would think their DNA expression was identical because, of course, they looked identical. They were also exceedingly close and did everything in life together. They went to the same college, bunked together in the navy, and started a business together. They were essentially the male version of the Doublemint twins. They ate lunch almost every day together and lived 10 miles away from each other their entire lives. They even had the same social habits. They drank the same gin, drove the same kind of car, played the same sports, and started and stopped smoking cigars at the same time in their lives. Two big differences between the twins were their levels of stress and their food choices.

My father passed away 16 years ago in what I like to call "perfect" health at the age of 71. He had no signs of the most common age-related illnesses such as heart disease, cancer, or diabetes, and his physical form was incredible. He unfortunately had only one problem at 63 years of age: dementia, which doctors labeled as Alzheimer's disease. This disease robbed him of his mind and eventually his life. His twin, on the other hand, lived 10 years longer with *no* signs of Alzheimer's disease. His twin's greatest health challenge over his last 25 years had been heart disease, high cholesterol, and high blood pressure.

The twins were born with the exact same genetic code. How is it possible that they shared not one common symptom of disease? The answer lies in the epigenome. Your epigenome tells your genes to turn on or off, speak loudly or whisper. It's through epigenetic expression that environmental factors like diet, stress, prenatal and childhood nutrition can dictate the activity of genes. This, then, explains how lifestyle factors affected the twins' susceptibility to diseases. The lifetime health of my father and his twin was not predetermined at conception—and neither is yours.

Over the last 10 years, epigenetics has elevated the importance of optimal nutrition to rock star status. It finally proves the profound reality that our diets *can* turn our genes on and off. It teaches us that our cells' DNA responds quite differently to an apple versus a donut, which is why it's so critical to teach our children how to make proper food choices. There truly hasn't been a more exciting time to be in the field of nutrition science. We have finally moved away from singling out and demonizing specific macronutrients like fats and moved toward individualized nutrition. Nourishment looks at what's right for you and your body with regard to your genome and health. We are finally realizing that we are all dynamically evolving beings.

FIVE PILLARS OF HEALTH: THE GENES' ON/OFF SWITCHES

Our children are now predicted to be the first generation in history to have a shorter lifespan than their parents. How can we change this outlook? Chronic diseases are originating in childhood, and poor nutrition during these critical younger years may have consequences that span a lifetime. If we want to make the biggest impact on our gene expression, we must focus on the environmental factors we have the most control over. I've called these the five pillars of health: diet, exercise, toxin exposure, sleep, and emotional well-being. Each of these plays a significant role in gene expression. However, focusing on just one pillar and expecting great outcomes is unrealistic.

For example, a person who consistently exercises and weight trains for two hours a day but eats jelly donuts for breakfast and fast food for lunch is fooling himself if he believes that exercise will protect him from a diet of inflammatory foods that are void of nutrients. Conversely, a person who eats an organic, grass-fed, hormone-free, whole-foods diet rich in vegetables, fruits, and omega-3 fatty acids, but has the enormous unmanaged stress of a failing marriage, a horrible work environment, and/or the responsibility of an ailing parent, will be sending both positive and negative signals to his genes. Genes are constantly responding, minute by minute, to messages received from our external environment, and they respond differently, depending on our personal genetic uniqueness.[78] The bottom line is, the more we do to harness the modifiable areas of our health that influence gene expression, the better we are at living healthy, disease-free lives.

Diet and Nutrition

A person's diet is an exceptionally important source of epigenetic signals. In fact, I'd argue it's the most important. Nutrients in food such as vitamins, minerals, and polyphenols can directly affect enzymes involved in turning on or off specific genes. And this directly affects how our bodies function and how we respond to disease. For example, a diet rich in nutrients such as folate, vitamin B-12, methionine, choline, or betaine can prompt changes in the number of methyl chemical groups attached to a gene, which can silence or modify a gene's activity. Putting this into perspective, let's say a pregnant mother is deficient in the essential nutrient choline during the early stages of fetal development. This may result in an unfavorable expression of genes and thereby negatively alter her baby's fetal brain development.

Numerous epigenetic discoveries just like this one are now being made that are associated with all sorts of health and disease pertaining to embryonic development, cancer, aging, inflammation, obesity, and immune disorders, to name just a few. Recent evidence shows epigenetic disease-fighting potential in compounds like green tea polyphenols or isothiocyanates from plant foods, which may inhibit the development of certain cancers by altering methyl groups attached to DNA. Other food components like resveratrol (found in grapes and blueberries), sulforaphane (found in broccoli), and curcumin (turmeric) have also shown to decrease tumor cell growth by positively altering gene expression.[79] It's vital to understand that these quality foods and many others trigger a domino effect that penetrates all the way to our genetic code.

Even though we are only at the infancy stage of nutritional epigenetics, these examples demonstrate something very powerful: food alters gene expression, and we are in control. This is especially critical in the case of a child whose developing tissues are undergoing a period of rapid cell division. One has to wonder about the long-term gene signals that are occurring in a child who not only is eating a diet depleted of essential nutrients, but one that is also filled with so-called anti-nutrients (sugar, refined grains, additives, preservatives, hormones, pesticides, etc.). The negative impact is likely twice as great. As we continue to uncover the influence of specific nutrients on gene expression, we can take action now by consciously choosing a colorful, plant-based, nutrient-rich diet and avoid harmful contaminants. Not only is it prudent for optimal health but also it will affect a child's likelihood of disease later on in life.

Exercise

Scientists have known that certain genes become more active or quieter as a result of exercise, but now we know why. Epigenetics research has shown that even a small amount of daily exercise promotes positive gene expression in more than 4,000 sites on the genome. Most of these genes are known to play a role in energy metabolism, insulin response, skeletal muscle function, and inflammation. They have also been shown to keep the brain in tip-top shape. A recent study showed that physical exercise keeps the brain healthy by boosting the production of a protein called brain-derived neurotrophic factor, or BDNF, which enhances memory and grows nerve cells.[80] In this context, exercise remains an essential factor for promoting human physiology. We all should aim to include a combination of endurance and strength training exercise most days of the week. It's important to find a type of exercise that you and your family enjoy and try to stick with it. Walk, jog, run, bike, row, swim, hike, climb, play soccer—do anything that gets your heart moving and breaks a sweat.

Toxins

A wide variety of environmental toxins have been proven to modify how our genes get turned on and off in different organ systems. These include metals like cadmium, arsenic, and mercury; air pollutants like particulate matter, black carbon, and benzene; and endocrine (or hormone) disrupting toxicants like BPA, dioxin, and pesticides.[81] Endocrine-disrupting chemicals like BPA in plastics or phthalates in fragrances or cosmetics have been widely studied. The results are quite alarming. They have the ability to turn on or off genes that we don't necessarily want activated. They have been linked to infertility, cancer, obesity, early puberty, heart disease, thyroid problems, and more. Even small doses can lead to devastating health effects.

Taken a step further, studies suggest that the effects of these chemicals create epigenetic changes that are transgenerational. In other words, if your great-grandmother was exposed to a toxic chemical, then you and your children could be at risk for disease. Dr. Michael Skinner at Washington State University has discovered the basic genetic mechanism for how diseases develop in our bodies and how those disease traits get transferred to future generations. For example, if your mother was exposed to a toxic fungicide that alters her gene's biological instructions, it also creates an effect on her ovaries during fetal development, which passes down epigenetic programming to her children and their offspring.[82] Check out chapter 8, where I discuss toxins and their direct impact on our health.

Sleep

It's well accepted that poor sleep is associated with a range of health problems, from poor blood sugar control to depression to poor immune function. We now know that sleep affects our health by altering gene activity. A new study led by a collaborative team of researchers at England's University at Surrey examined the influence of sleep on gene function and found that just a single week of poor sleep altered the activity of over 700 genes.[83] These genes help govern circadian rhythms and metabolic functions, which influence how we respond to stress, inflammation, and how well we fight infection.

Here are some tips to help ensure a good night's sleep: develop a sleep cycle, this means going to bed and waking up at the same time every day; stop drinking caffeine after one p.m.; don't exercise four to five hours before going to bed; regulate your body's melatonin by turning off electronics and bright lights at night and rising with the sun each morning. According to sleep specialist Dr. Michael Breus, an average nightly sleep cycle is 90 minutes long and a typical night's sleep includes five full sleep cycles. This means that an average adult should aim for around seven and a half hours of quality sleep each night. As expected, children's sleep needs are greater and change over time. Sleep guidelines for children are as follows:

Babies: 12–15 hours

Toddlers: 11–14 hours

3–5-year-olds: 10–13 hours

6–13-year-olds: 9–11 hours

14–17-year-olds: 8–10 hours

Emotional Well-Being

When it comes to emotional health, both bad and good habits affect your genes. This includes your relationship with others, daily stress, and even your own thoughts. Addressing social and emotional stress with techniques like yoga, meditation, and mindfulness training are now proven ways to downregulate the expression of pro-inflammatory genes, thus reducing inflammation. In fact, a collaborative team of researchers from Wisconsin, Spain, and France reported in 2013 the first evidence that shows "rapid alterations in gene expression" in people who practice mindfulness meditation.[84] At Harvard Medical School, researchers also found that these same stress-reducing practices turned on genes that protect from disorders like chronic pain, high blood pressure, depression, and even rheumatoid arthritis.[85] You might think that you'd have to meditate for years to change gene expression, but positive changes have been observed in as little as eight hours total of meditation.

All this fantastic news further demonstrates that improving and maintaining great health is within our reach. The power is ours as individuals, and even more crucially, as parents. Even though few nutritional epidemiological studies focus on the role of diet during early childhood, it seems reasonable that we can apply this knowledge to our youth. This genomic revolution in medicine understands that the human genome, otherwise known as our "Book of Life," contains many different stories. It's up to us to determine which of those stories will be read. Let's make it the health-promoting stories, for our kids' sakes.

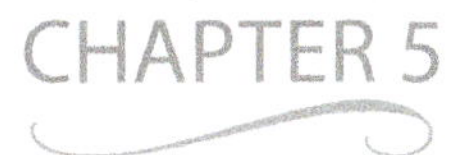

THE MICROBIOME: YOUR BODY'S MVP

All disease begins in the gut.

—Hippocrates

Over the last decade, revolutionary thinking from science's leading experts has revealed groundbreaking discoveries about the importance of optimal digestive function and its connection to our immune system, and thus overall health. We've learned that the assimilation of nutrients, while important, is really only a small part of the greater story. The bigger, more essential piece of our biological puzzle is dependent on a "mini ecosystem" that lives within us, called the gut microbiome, which is made up of many types of microbes (viruses, fungi, and bacteria) that play important roles in health and disease. Properly feeding this ecosystem within our intestines will affect almost every aspect of our health—our immune function, our brain function, nervous and endocrine systems, and how well we digest and extract essential nutrients. It is undoubtedly the number one most powerful treatment we have, not only to prevent disease, but also to attain our highest biological potential. This chapter explores in detail what affects the microbiome, how it affects your tribe's overall health, and what you can do to improve its function.

Most of us don't think about what happens to the food we eat after it's been swallowed. In fact, in terms of vital organs, the thirty-foot-long tube from our mouth to our anus has been underappreciated, even for its traditional role of breaking down food and absorbing nutrients. The most important environmental stimulus to altering our gut health is food, particularly fiber. Eating whole foods like raw or lightly cooked vegetables, fruits, beans, lentils, whole grains, nuts, and seeds will maintain a healthy gut microbiome and by extension a healthier family.

WHAT IS THE MICROBIOME?

All of our biological systems have been primed to predict and respond to microbes. In fact, every plant and animal on earth coexists with microbes that influence its biology, where a microbe provides some critical function that the host cannot do for itself. This is called a symbiotic relationship. For instance, science has proven that plants, such as peas, clover, and peanuts, depend on bacteria that live in their roots to absorb nutrients for survival. These plants need nitrogen to build protein, but are unable to utilize atmospheric nitrogen on their own. They depend entirely on bacteria like the rhizobia that live in the soil and even in the plants' roots themselves to convert atmospheric nitrogen into a usable form. Many insects also have microbial partners. European firebugs, for instance, rely on bacteria that live in their gut to detoxify and digest food, and to provide essential amino acids and vitamins that firebugs don't obtain from their diet. These essential bacteria ensure the firebugs' metabolic stability and survival.[86]

This beautiful coexistence occurs similarly in humans. Living deep within our intestines is a diverse ecosystem collectively referred to as the human gut microbiome. We know that its complexity is so astounding that it has been compared to the Amazon rainforest in density and diversity. The human microbiome is an ecosystem primarily comprised of communities of microbes—bacteria, protozoa, viruses, and fungi—which live all over the body: on our skin, in our gut, mouth, brain, genitals, and other orifices.[87] The groups of microbes from different regions of the body are variously known as microbiota, such as the skin microbiota, the vaginal microbiota, or the gut microbiota, also named "gut flora." These various microbes outnumber our human cells 10 to 1, which is why most scientists would agree that we are more microbe than we are human.[88]

In fact, the trillions of bacterial cells that reside all along the human gastrointestinal tract are made up of about 1,000 different bacterial species that influence almost every aspect of our physiology.[89] This might sound alarming because we have been trained to believe that bacteria are agents of death and disease. After all, in 1900, before the invention of penicillin, the three leading causes of death were from pneumonia, tuberculosis, and diarrhea (enteritis)—all from bacteria.[90] And let's not forget about the bubonic plague that wiped out one-third of Europe's population in 1347. Our former ignorance has given way to understanding the remarkable influence that bacteria and other microbes have on both our physical and emotional health in their life-supporting roles.

Current research and discoveries about the microbiome have shifted modern medicine to explore and understand the gut's delicate balance with nature, which has allowed for new models of optimizing health. In the current era of genomic medicine, scientists are now looking beyond infectious disease, or curing ills with pills, to a path that focuses on a healthy gut microbiome and stable human ecosystems. Their research is changing our potential to heal and thrive.

> *Up to 90 percent of all known human illness can be traced back to an unhealthy gut. And we can say for sure that just as disease begins in the gut, so too does health and vitality.*
>
> —Dr. David Perlmutter, *Brain Maker*

A Society of Heroes: Roles of the Gut Microbiome

The majority of bacteria that line our intestinal walls are not invaders but healthy colonizers that have a profound influence on human development, immunity, and nutrition. In fact, I can't stress enough how these bacteria are in fact our lifeline to thriving health and longevity. Here's a glimpse of some of the astounding ways these healthy gut bacteria work for us:

- **Digest your food**. Bacteria provide enzymes needed for the digestion of complex carbohydrates. The fermentation of plant polysaccharides, most commonly found in fruits, vegetables, and whole grains, produce short-chain fatty acids (SCFA), which are the critical food source for the cells that make up our intestinal wall.

- **Regulate your immune system.** Of the entire immune system, 70 percent resides in the gut.[91] Bacterial cells generate signals that communicate with your gut's immune system, which boost the body's ability to deal with toxins and control local and systemic inflammation, and ultimately teach us which objects are foods, benign entities, or threats.

- **Regulate fat storage, obesity, and insulin resistance.** Obese and lean people have different microbiota. Western diets high in unhealthy fats and sugar have been shown to promote pathogenic bacteria that release harmful substances like lipopolysaccharides (LPS), which promote inflammation and metabolic disease.

- **Influence brain health.** Bacteria in our gut stimulate intestinal nerve cells to produce important chemicals for brain health, including neurotransmitters like serotonin, glutamate, and GABA.

- **Support detoxification.** Beneficial gut bacteria neutralize many toxins found in food, decreasing the liver's workload. They also help degrade toxic metabolites found in bile, allowing for safe elimination.

- **Prevent growth of harmful microbes.** Beneficial gut bacteria produce SCFAs like butyrate that enhance the immune response by promoting the growth of mucus membranes, which protect the intestine walls. Gut bacteria also slightly increase acidity of the gut, creating an unfavorable environment for pathogens like salmonella and E. coli to grow. Some bacteria have hair-like threads (known as flagella) that can stop a dangerous rotavirus dead in its tracks.[92]

- **Synthesize and regulate vitamins and nutrients.** Gut bacteria aid in the production of certain vitamins, including biotin, vitamin K, vitamin B12, among others.

- **Complement and support genetic weakness.** Often referred to as the "second" human genome, the gut microbiome complements the human genome with 100-fold more genes.[93]

I know, it sounds unlikely that your gut microbiome can influence so many aspects of your bodily functions, but it does! Your microbiome also affects everyday ailments—like your low energy and mood swings, your daughter's allergies, your son's ADHD, your sister's irritable bowel, your mother's poor bone density, and your father's obesity—because all of these conditions, and many, many more, begin in the gut.

Our First Introduction to Microbes

Microbial colonization of the human gut begins at birth, when a baby's immune system is first introduced to the mom's microbes. In the womb, a baby's intestines are relatively sterile, but as soon as he slides through the vaginal canal and is put to the breast to feed, the intestines, lungs, and skin immediately get colonized with bacteria.[94] After first receiving healthy microbes from the birth canal, a newborn then receives bacteria along with his preferential food source from his mother's breast milk. After months of nursing, a newborn is exposed to microbes from the immediate environment and solid food sources. The quality of both the environment and the food will have a major impact on which bacteria proliferate, good or bad. These observations are bringing us back to long-honored birthing traditions, which supply infants' intestines with beneficial bacteria that set up and promote a healthy gut ecosystem. Nature has a plan. We just have to listen!

Because the immune system undergoes profound development during infancy, it seems the microbes that first take hold may have significant effects on future immune development and subsequent health and disease.[95] An infant's first exposure to microbes, which depends on his mode of delivery and exposure to breast milk, plays a vital role in determining his long-term health, such as development of asthma, obesity, diabetes, autoimmunity, and many other chronic conditions.[96] In fact, the increasing rates of allergies, autoimmunity, anxiety, and depression in children today are significantly influenced by impaired gut health that most likely begins at birth.

A recent study found that infants delivered by C-section and fed formula had lower bacterial diversity and higher representation of "bad" or problematic bacteria.[97] We now have a convincing body of evidence that shows that breast milk is the best nourishment for growing babies. One study comparing breast milk and formula found that only breast milk fosters healthy colonization of beneficial biofilms—colonies of healthy bacteria that protect against pathogens, aid in nutrient absorption, and foster immune system development.[98] Infant nutrition affects how bacteria grow, which is profound in terms of infant and child health.

It's crystal clear that the links between mode of delivery (vaginal birth versus C-section), diet (breast milk versus formula), microbial diversity, and childhood disease are important. More mothers need to be made aware of this relationship so that they can best prepare for healthy deliveries and nurture strong, disease-free kids. I recognize that mothers don't always have control of the mode of birth for their children, but if choice is available, the route of Mother Nature will always offer more protection from illness and a stronger, more robust immune system. For those moms whose babies were born by C-section or weren't breast fed, it's not the end of the world. In time, their microbiome can be rebalanced with a proper diet, probiotics, exposure to animals and nature, and stress management techniques.[99]

Beneficial Microbes Evolve as We Age

We know that throughout the natural progression of life, our bodies' microbes change and evolve with life events that impact both the type and quantity of microbial species living in us. Just as our nutritional needs are different as infants, so too are the needs of the microbial communities that exist within us. Major life events such as puberty, pregnancy, and menopause, as well as gender, climate, age, and occupation also influence different microbial patterns among individuals.[100]

Modern living and evolving hygiene practices have played a role in separating us from a myriad of microorganisms that we have co-evolved with over thousands of years. To put it simply, we are too clean. The lack of early childhood exposure to both symbiotic and parasitic agents disrupts the natural development of the immune system, which in turn increases susceptibility to allergic disease, autoimmunity issues, and excessive inflammation. Evidence for the biome depletion theory—the idea that allergies and autoimmune disease are associated with our abnormal over-reactive immune response, which in turn is caused by a loss of critical microbes that normally train and interact with our immune system[101]—can be found in studies that compare the incidence of allergies in industrialized and developing countries and rural environments.

Researchers have found that in populations where hygiene standards are lower, the inhabitants experience much lower rates of asthma and allergies. Children from large families or those that go to daycare early in life are also less likely to have allergic disease. It may seem counterintuitive, but growing up on a farm, owning a pet, biting your nails, sucking your thumb all show supportive evidence of long-term benefit in preventing allergies and benefiting immune function. A recent study of ethnically and genetically similar Amish and Hutterite communities has proven that children exposed to animal farm dust have decreased prevalence of asthma and allergies. The house dust from the Amish community's homes was laden with bacteria from the animals that lived on the family farm. The Hutterite community had shifted to a centralized mechanized farm, separating the children from the farm animals, which was shown in the lack of bacteria in their house dust. The authors of the study proved causation by exposing mice predisposed to asthma at birth to dust from both communities. The mice exposed to the Hutterite dust developed disease while those exposed to the Amish dust did not! This again demonstrates the protective effect of early exposure to an environment rich in microbes to build a robust immune system.[102]

There's no doubt that hand-washing and cleaning are important to prevent harmful pathogenic bacterial exposure. A more practical approach would be to rethink your habits if you are a hyper-obsessed hand sanitizer or someone who bleaches everything in sight. On the flip side, it would also be wise to start living more in nature. According to internationally renowned microbiome researcher Dr. Jeff Leach, "For 99.99 percent of human history, the outside was always part of the inside, and at no moment during our day were we ever really separated from nature.

Today, a National Activity Survey found that between enclosed buildings and vehicles, modern humans spend a whopping 90 percent of their lives indoors."[103] More to the point, open your windows, get your hands dirty, start to garden, let your kids play in the dirt, own a pet, visit a farm, and encourage your kids to play with lots of other children.

The biome depletion theory still needs more research to unravel which microbes and at what period of exposure might offer protection against development of disease. In the meantime, don't be afraid of a little dirt on your carrots or a kiss from your dog.

HEALTHY BACTERIA CREATE A THRIVING HUMAN ECOSYSTEM

Now that we have established how the microbiome comes into existence and its critical roles, let's explore how to keep it healthy. The large intestine contains the largest ecosystem in the human body. It is here that trillions of gut microbiota reside and perform countless functions that influence your health. They are made up of symbionts (good bacteria), pathogens (bad bacteria), and commensals (the neutrals that just exist). This dynamic ecosystem is set up for competition, with each group trying to force out the other to win control. What constitutes a "normal" distribution of species in the gut microbiome, if that exists at all, is yet to be determined by scientists. What is clear is that the overall balance and diversity directly affect the development of disease. In other words, more species diversity equals less disease, as more diversity has been proven to protect against disturbances that harm the gut environment and, ultimately, your health.

Imagine that your GI tract houses an ecosystem that is populated by humans (bacteria) and animals (viruses, fungi, and protists). For the ecosystem to survive—or better yet thrive—the inhabitants must work together to build a society. The humans (bacteria) make up most of the inhabitants and thus have the greatest effect. Now, some of the humans work together to build a society, while others work to destroy it. The balance of power of these players dictates the vitality of the society. For example, if the beneficial humans far outnumber the harmful types, then society flourishes. Reverse this ratio and destruction occurs. In the case of the gut's ecosystem (microbiome), too many bad bacteria cause disease.

It makes sense then, that we would want to make lifestyle decisions that best support the growth and stability of good, or symbiotic, bacteria so that potentially harmful pathogens cannot gain a foothold and proliferate. In growing children and in adults, there are a lot of ways the microbiome can become out of balance or lose diversity, but certain lifestyle factors are more impactful than others, such as our exposure to chemicals, our overuse of drugs (especially antibiotics), and most importantly, our unhealthy diets, with refined sugar and processed foods being major culprits.

Exposure to Environmental Chemicals

An increasing body of evidence has shown that environmental chemicals, including heavy metals, air pollution, and endocrine-disrupting chemicals (EDCs) can significantly affect the balance of the gut microbiome. Arsenic (found in water, soil, and rice) and lead (found in old paint, dust, food, and drinking water) have been shown to disrupt metabolic pathways and shift gut microbiota populations from beneficial societies to the harmful types. Endocrine disruptors like bisphenol A (BPA), an industrial chemical often leached through plastic water bottles, canned goods, and retail receipts, has also been found to greatly reduce bacteria diversity and create a proliferation of damaging pathogens.[104] And don't be fooled by the "BPA-free" label that is now advertised all over water bottles and plastic products. Recent research has revealed that a common BPA replacement, bisphenol S (BPS), may be just as harmful.[105] In fact, there are many types of bisphenol out there, and there is no federal agency that tests the toxicity of these new materials before they are allowed on the market.

Some of the most disturbing research points once again at glyphosate, the most heavily used herbicide in the world. Three hundred million pounds of this chemical are applied to crops each year in the US alone, which makes it quite hard to avoid consumption unless you eat 100 percent organic, avoid all processed foods, and consume non-GMO meat and dairy products. [106] Multiple studies have shown that glyphosate may preferentially kill off beneficial bacteria species, like enterococcus, bacillus, and lactobacillus, while leaving potential pathogens like salmonella and clostridium to run wild.[107] As it turns out, many of the most dangerous bacterial pathogens are resistant to glyphosate, yet some of the healthiest bacteria are quite sensitive to it.

This really is bad news for both humans and animals. In fact, this glyphosate-induced bacteria imbalance is causing salmonella outbreaks in commercial chicken facilities and botulism in industrially raised beef from the glyphosate in animal feed.[108] Frequently consuming glyphosate-sprayed crops will add to the harmful bacterial societies, on par with handing machine guns over to your bad bacteria—their killing power against the good bacteria will be *that* much greater. And remember, if the bad bacteria outcompete the beneficial sorts, our healthy ecosystem starts to crumble. All bacteria produce waste. The good bacteria produce short-chain fatty acids, which are like trees that nurture the environment around them. The bad pathogens release lipopolysaccharides, which create inflammatory fires all over town.

Another problem with glyphosate is that it binds together important minerals like iron, manganese, cobalt, molybdenum, and copper so that the beneficial microbes do not have access to them. This leads to chronic inflammatory states and impaired gut lining, which is at the root of many chronic diseases, including IBS, thyroid disease, depression, and autoimmune disease (a condition where the immune system attacks the body, such as diabetes, IBD, arthritis, etc.) While most of the research done to date focuses on interactions with single chemicals like glyphosate, it's important to note that in the real world we are bombarded by more than just one chemical at a time. So we have to wonder what the effects are of multiple chemical challenges to the gut microbiome over time.

Overuse of Antibiotics

Antibiotics play a disturbing role in destabilizing the human gut microbiome. In today's world, we are so accustomed to leaving the doctor's office with an antibiotic prescription in hand, that these drugs seem safe and somewhat habitual. There's no doubt they are necessary for serious harmful bacteria, but not for viral colds or stomach infections. Unfortunately, antibiotics have been prescribed for infections that they do not fight, particularly viral colds, flu, sore throats, and pediatric ear infections.[109] This enormous overuse is the result of misguided ignorance about the truth behind the risks and benefits of these medications and where they are truly needed. (Other overprescribed drugs that significantly impact the gut microbiome are non-steroidal anti-inflammatory drugs such as Motrin and Advil, birth control pills, and proton pump inhibitors, i.e., heartburn drugs like Prilosec, Prevacid, Nexium, Pepcid, and Zantac.)[110]

So why are antibiotics so bad for our gut microbiome? An antibiotic goes to work killing off unwanted pathogens. The downside is that it also kills sensitive beneficial bacteria, weakening the critical balance and thus the overall function of the gut microbiome.[111] The average child in the United States receives 10–20 courses of antibiotics by the time he or she is 18 years old.[112] I know this was the case for me. I recently reviewed my pediatric medical records from the '70s and '80s and was shocked to find that I had been given antibiotics 15 times from birth to age 18. That's almost one antibiotic prescription each year.

According to gastroenterologist Dr. Gerard Mullin, "Even a short five-day course of a common antibiotic like ciprofloxacin has been shown to kill up to one-third of the gut microbiome, resulting in an unbalanced and reduced biodiversity of the gut microflora."[113] While some of the beneficial bacteria recover once the patient goes off an antibiotic, scientists have found that many bacterial species may never fully recover.[114] When the beneficial bacteria die off and do not recover, the bad bacteria take their place, which has a direct and significant role in the dramatic increase of chronic diseases such as obesity, diabetes, allergies, asthma, irritable bowel, arthritis, and many others.[115] The bottom line is that we need antibiotics to kill deadly pathogens, but judicious use is the only way to preserve the sensitive microbiome.

Food: Friend or Foe to the Microbiome

The foods we choose to eat have a profound impact on our health because those decisions are instantly altering our bacterial composition. A sudden shift in dietary patterns, say from an American-style diet to a Mediterranean-type diet, can alter our microbial makeup in just 24 hours; that's how quickly our ecosystem responds. It makes sense though, because our gut microbes eat what we eat. Depending on which foods we choose, some microbes will go hungry while others will thrive. The vast majority of foods in the Western diet have little to no benefit to the microbiota residing in the large colon. If you and your children consume what most Americans eat, chances are you're feeding the wrong microbes, because most Americans' diets include highly processed, refined-carbohydrate foods, small amounts of vegetables and fruits, minimal whole grains, and low fiber. In addition, they are consuming high volumes of sugar, inflammatory fats, and conventionally raised corn-fed meat.

This cocktail is destructive to our beneficial bacteria because it quickly cuts off their natural fiber supply that they rely on for food. As a result, bacteria begin eating the very important mucus layer that lines our intestines to a point where dangerous bad bacteria can infect the colon wall,[116] inviting a perfect storm for bacterial imbalance. Lack of fiber with a sprinkle of sugar, a dollop of inflammatory fats, and a side of processed starchy foods gives a belly filled with inflammation, blood sugar bombs, and angry bacteria set up to hurt us.

Repeated studies consistently show that diets low in fiber and high in certain fats and sugar lead to overgrowth of the wrong type of bacteria while low-fat, high–plant carbohydrate diets produce the opposite.[117] And fiber makes the most difference. Fiber fuels our beneficial bacteria, keeps our intestinal mucus layer healthy, and prevents systemic inflammation. Without it, our ecosystems fail. The standard American diet, which consists mainly of fat, animal meat, and starch, is woefully depleted of fiber—and most kids' diets follow suit as they barely reach 12 grams a day. Another problem is the lack of variety that exists in most Americans' diets. Many people assume they consume a wide range of foods given the plethora of foods available to us at every turn, but it's not the case.

Let's take 12-year-old Tom for example. Before school on Monday he ate toaster waffles with syrup and orange juice, for lunch he ate a sub sandwich with turkey, an apple and chocolate milk, and for dinner, which was on the run due to soccer practice, he stopped at a fast-food restaurant and ordered a fried chicken sandwich with fries and a soda. He also ate cheese and crackers and a squeezable yogurt as snacks during school. If you stop to think about it, his diet consists of refined flour at every meal, lots of sugar, meat, and inflammatory fats. No fibrous plant food anywhere except for the modest apple at lunch.

The idea that processed food is bad for you is not new, but if you think about it in terms of diet diversification, it's quite alarming. Dr. Tim Spector, professor of genetic epidemiology at King's College London, believes the restrictive nature of highly processed diets is reducing our microbial diversity and is making us ill. He states, "Each species of microbe has a preference for certain food sources which allows them to feed and reproduce."[118] If the majority of your diet is made up of refined carbohydrates and processed foods, then it's likely that over 80 percent of your diet consists of corn, wheat, soy, and meat. Chances are your gut's microbial richness is quite poor to say the least. And if you continue to crave junk food, Spector says it's because bad bacteria in your gut have their own "evolutionary drive" to stay alive.[119] They are manipulative in a way that scientists believe can alter our physiology and behavioral responses to food. Because the gut is linked to our immune, endocrine, and nervous systems, it is thought they release signaling molecules that make us crave certain foods like pizza or cookies.[120] It's our own personal bacterial brainwashing! Thus, we crave sugar all the time.

It just so happens that harmful bacteria such as clostridium and enterococcus *love* sugar in all its forms: breads, cereals, cookies, chips, cakes, candy, etc.[121] What about artificial sweeteners, you ask? Turns out they are just as noxious. Invented by chemists, aspartame, sucralose, and saccharin have been ingested for years in diet sodas and many sports drinks, fruit juices, ice cream, baked goods, and candy. Current research has shown that artificial sweeteners actually stimulate our appetite, making us crave more food and increase fat storage in the body. They have been linked repeatedly to obesity and diabetes, and finally we know why: the bad bacteria love them! Israeli scientists found that certain bacteria thrive on artificial sweeteners. These specific microbes appear to be more efficient at pulling calories from food and turning them into fat. Even more disturbing, these bacteria appear to impact the balance of hormones, such as leptin which controls our hunger signals.[122] My advice: stay far, far away from artificial sweeteners.

So here's the bottom line: you and your kids need to eat a high-fiber diet every day to maintain a healthy gut microbiome and thus a well-functioning body. You achieve this by eating vegetables like artichokes, leeks, split peas, and Brussels sprouts; fruits like avocados, berries, Asian pears, and coconut; legumes like black beans, chickpeas, and lentils; whole grains like quinoa and raw oats; and seeds like flax and chia. A diet low in fermentable fibers and high in certain fats, proteins, and sugars will foster a whole cascade of unwanted conditions brought on by the proliferation of unfriendly bacteria.[123] Reduced intestinal mucus, poor absorption, systemic inflammation, food reactions, and blood sugar imbalance are the beginning of what leads to chronic disease, intestinal permeability (or leaky gut, which we're getting to shortly), and microbiome dysfunction.

Archenemy: Refined Sugar

Excessive sugar consumption, due to such culprits such as HFCS, is a public health disaster. Our bodies can generally handle moderate amounts of sugars like those naturally occurring in fruits and vegetables. But there is a limit, and if it's exceeded, a cascade of toxic events ensues. Many of our leading health experts, such as Dr. David Ludwig, Dr. Mark Hyman, and Dr. Bruce Ames, agree that our unnatural overconsumption of both HCFS and sugar are significant contributors to our epidemic of obesity and other metabolic disorders. Dr. Hyman stated recently, "We are consuming HFCS and sugar in pharmacologic quantities never before experienced in human history—140 pounds a year versus 20 teaspoons a year 10,000 years ago."[124] But it's really only been in the last century or so that we've seen such a marked increase in sugar consumption, and the trends show an unquestionable parallel with our obesity epidemic.[125] In fact, recent trends over the 1980s, 1990s, and 2000s, show sugar consumption increased by more than 30 percent in just those three decades.[126]

Our societal shift in sugar consumption is problematic but few of us are listening. Picture me, standing on a mountaintop waving my arms, trying to get your attention. *This is critical folks!* And I'm not talking about just table sugar. There are many types of sugars, apart from the man-made ones, that occur naturally in a wide variety of fruits, vegetables, and dairy foods. But no matter what the source of the sugar you eat—fruit sugar, table sugar, HFCS, maple syrup, or milk sugar—your body will try to break it down into a usable form of glucose or fructose. As far as your body is concerned, there is a huge difference in how these two simple sugars are metabolized: in short, glucose gives you fuel and fructose gives you fat.

In his insightful presentation titled "Sugar: The Bitter Truth" (available on YouTube), Dr. Robert Lustig, a professor of pediatrics in the Department of Endocrinology at UCSF, shows clear differences in how fructose and glucose are metabolized by the body.[127] He points out that not just HFCS but all added sugars are detrimental to our health due primarily to the increase in fructose consumption. Sweeteners like HFCS, table sugar, honey, and even sweeteners made from concentrated fruit juices all contain glucose *and* fructose in roughly equal amounts. HFCS contains about 55 percent fructose and 45 percent glucose, compared to table sugars, which have a 50/50 fructose-glucose ratio.

While every cell in our body can use glucose for energy, fructose gets shipped straight to the liver. Fructose, although a simple sugar, is not life-sustaining. On the contrary, it creates fat in the liver and arteries and forms damaging free radicals that wreak havoc on our cells and even our genes, increasing metabolic conditions such as diabetes, weight gain, heart disease, and dementia. Also unique to fructose is that it doesn't suppress our hunger hormones that help regulate food intake. Fruit that contains a natural form of fructose is unique, simply because it's consumed in a package of fiber and nutrients so that digestion is slowed and the impact on the liver is reduced. But this clearly is a volume issue: today, Americans are averaging upwards of 22 tsp a day (equivalent to about 350 calories and 25 percent of their daily calories) from added sugar.[128] This sugar intake, and particularly of fructose, is by far one of the greatest destroyers of our health.

I first learned about this fructose phenomenon when I worked as a clinical nutritionist in the hospital, taking care of critically ill patients. We were often required to feed patients intravenously. The carbohydrate portion of the IV solution consisted of glucose, which is the primary source of energy for all our cells. If we gave our patients IV fructose, not only could their cells not readily use it, but they would end up with deranged liver metabolism. And in addition to liver dysfunction, chronic fructose exposure creates hypertension, obesity, high cholesterol and high triglycerides.

All that said, sugar is not *entirely* evil. It is best consumed in its natural forms, such as in dairy, vegetables, or in small amounts of fresh fruit. The problem arises with the indulgent amounts of *refined* sugar that greatly affect how food is metabolized, our cravings, our hormonal response, fat and triglyceride formation, and the health and integrity of cells at their core. Although fructose produces more metabolic harm than glucose, in excess they both fuel disease. Learning ways to eliminate refined sugar or judiciously use small amounts of natural alternatives will be

Hidden Names for Sugar on Food Labels

In our food system today, sugar has over 60 different names and sneaks into our food in ways we are completely unaware of. We must read labels in order to identify added sugars on ingredient lists. You can start by looking for words that end in "-ose" like "fructose," "dextrose," or the word "syrup." Also don't be fooled by manufacturers' labels that say "no added sugar," which is often their stealthy way of marketing sweetened foods with "fruit juice" or "fruit juice concentrate."

Those many identities of sugar include:

- anhydrous dextrose
- barley malt
- beet sugar
- buttered syrup
- brown sugar
- cane juice crystals
- cane sugar
- caramel
- carob syrup
- castor sugar
- confectioner's powdered sugar
- corn syrup
- corn syrup solids
- date sugar
- Demerara sugar
- dextran
- dextrose
- diastatic malt
- diastase
- fructose
- fruit juice
- fruit juice concentrate
- galactose
- glucose
- golden sugar
- grape sugar
- high fructose corn syrup (HFCS)
- honey
- invert sugar
- lactose
- malt syrup
- maltose
- maltodextrin
- maple syrup
- molasses
- nectars
- raw cane sugar
- refiner's syrup
- sorghum syrup
- sucrose
- treacle
- turbinado sugar
- white granulated sugar

one of the best changes you and your family can make to improve your health. If you are looking for the best natural alternatives to sweeten something, I recommend using real grade B maple syrup or local raw honey because they are a bit sweeter than table sugar and you typically don't need as much, plus they contain some minerals and phytonutrients. Remember to use them sparingly.

Here's the tricky part: not only is sugar addictive but also we are hardwired to crave it. Back in the Stone Age, our bodies recognized sugar as an instant good energy source, which instinctually made us want more. Even as early humans, we were trained to crave sugar because it meant getting energy for our cells without needing to work very hard. In today's world, our bodies respond to sugar the same way, but now it's vastly easier to come by, and as a consequence we are consuming truckloads of it.

How much sugar do you think you consume in a day? Few people know because it's in virtually all processed foods. Another problem is that sugar is reported in grams on nutrition labels, and grams are not a familiar measurement to most of us. Teaspoons are much easier to visualize. So learning that 4 g of sugar equals approximately 1 tsp of sugar makes reading a nutrition label more accessible. For example, your favorite 4-oz. serving of fruit-flavored yogurt can contain upwards of 20 g or 5 tsp of sugar (20 g divided by 4 g = 5 tsp). That translates to about 1 tsp of sugar per bite of yogurt!

Once you start to read and decipher nutrition labels, you will start to look at food differently. Even if you don't use table sugar, you may be surprised at the quantity of sugar you're

How Refined Sugar Harms Kids

1. **Creates intense cravings.** Repeated consumption of sugar leads to prolonged dopamine signaling, which over-activates the brain's reward pathway. Sugar has addictive effects on the brain and increases cravings.[129] In fact, studies have shown that refined sugars increase dopamine and reward pathways in the brain in a manner that is not unlike drugs such as cocaine, tobacco, or morphine.

2. **Impairs memory and learning skills.** A 2012 UCLA study in rats found that a diet high in fructose and low in DHA impaired cognitive abilities by reducing synaptic activity in brain cells.[130] This means that high sugar intake literally slows down the brain and affects learning.

3. **May contribute to depression and anxiety.** High consumption of sugar disrupts the brain's hormone messengers that help keep moods stable. You may have even experienced a sugar high and subsequent crash, which can cause irritability, tension, and feelings of panic. Moreover, sugar actually changes the way the brain processes stress. According to new animal research, adolescents who consume a diet high in fructose can worsen their depression or anxiety.[131] Sugar is also at the root of chronic inflammation, which impacts the brain.

4. **Changes the structure of neurons in the brain.** New evidence suggests that children and young adults who consume high-sugar diets end up with the same brain deficits we see in children with significant early-life stress. In other words, just as early-life adversity increases risk of psychiatric disorders, researchers also found that high consumption of sugar early in life exerts the same long-lasting molecular changes in the brain.[132] An effective way to help prevent psychiatric disorders in our kids is to greatly limit their consumption of refined sugar in all its forms. Sweetened beverages, desserts, and packaged foods are good places to start.

consuming in everyday convenience foods. In fact, half of all American sugar consumption is in the form of sugar-sweetened beverages like soda, sports drinks, and fruit juice. Here's a list of some common high-sugar foods that both kids and adults consume, paired with suggestions for healthier alternatives.

HEALTHY ALTERNATIVES TO REFINED SUGAR

HIGH SUGAR	HEALTHY ALTERNATIVE
Milk chocolate	70%+ dark chocolate or dark chocolate sweetened with stevia
Agave	Monk fruit
Brown sugar	Coconut palm sugar
Processed molasses	Blackstrap molasses
Maple syrup	Chicory syrup
Processed honey	Raw local honey
Chocolate chips	Chocolate nibs
Table sugar	Stevia or monk fruit
Frozen yogurt or ice cream	Low-sugar smoothie
Fruit-flavored yogurt	Plain full-fat Greek-style yogurt
Sweetened soy or almond milk	Unsweetened coconut, almond, or cashew milk
Dried fruit snacks	Whole fruit
Fat-free or low-fat baked goods	Full-fat baked goods made with coconut, oat, or almond flour sweetened with fruits like banana, dates, pumpkin, or apples
Soda	Club soda with a squeeze of lemon/lime and couple drops of liquid stevia
Energy drinks	Coffee or green tea
Fruit juice	Green vegetable juice or fruit water
Sweet tea	Unsweetened tea with lemon
Vitamin water	Unsweetened coconut water
Jelly or jam	Nut butter
Salad dressings	Champagne vinegar, extra virgin olive oil, and herbs
BBQ beans	Pinto beans
Canned fruit	Whole fresh fruit
Dried fruit	Freeze-dried berries

Leaky Gut Syndrome

Many of us have impaired gut health. Our gastrointestinal system (or simply "the gut") has surprising exposure to the outside world—more than our skin and lungs combined. This exposed surface area is why 75 percent of our immune system is situated right around this long tube. In fact, the gut is intimately connected to the immune system, the nervous system, and the hormone-producing endocrine system. In order for the gut to function seamlessly, all of these systems need to work in unison. In today's modern world, our digestive system undergoes daily assaults that are a direct consequence of our lifestyle choices and our environment. As you've just read, these attacks come in the form of agricultural and industrial chemicals, antibiotic and drug exposure, unhealthy diets, high stress, and many other factors that degrade digestive performance.

It's amazing to think that while our intestines are selectively breaking down and absorbing life-sustaining nutrients, they also have the important role of keeping foreign invaders, toxins, and undigested food proteins from entering our bloodstream. Even more amazing is that the epithelial cells that line our gut are only one-cell-layer thick. This means there is only one thin line of cells, like soldiers in a line locking arms, separating our external world from 75 percent of our immune system. You can appreciate now why the health and integrity of the intestinal lining is so critical. In fact, leading scientists say it's the key to our health.

As discussed, when negative assaults like antibiotic use or a poor diet are chronic, microbial balance becomes upended. The healthy mix of microbes starts to diminish and the quantity of pathogenic microbes takes over more intestinal real estate. At this point, the integrity of the gut lining is compromised. All bacteria produce end products that either help or hinder the host's gut environment. Whatever gets produced goes directly into the gut's absorptive organ. For example, good bacteria produce compounds like short-chain fatty acids that help to nourish intestinal cells, decrease inflammation, and improve immune function. They also make the gut environment more acidic, which inhibits the growth of pathogenic bacteria.

The bad bacteria, if allowed to flourish, will produce endotoxins (toxins produced inside your body) that, if absorbed in the bloodstream, can cause systemic inflammation and chronic disease. For example, lipopolysaccharides (LPS), cell wall components of bad bacteria, have been shown to be among the most potent substances causing intestinal inflammation. As more unfriendly bacteria proliferate, more toxic by-products are released that directly damage and weaken the cells' protective lining.

When the intestinal barrier becomes permeable we have a condition known as *leaky gut syndrome.* You may have heard of the condition; it gets quite a bit of attention these days. The thin, snug wall of the intestine, known as the epithelium, should only absorb small nutrient molecules of proteins, fats, carbohydrates, vitamins, and minerals. But when small gaps in this thin wall occur, it causes the intestinal barrier to "leak," allowing large undigested food particles, microbes, and toxins like gluten, glyphosate, or BPA to escape through the epithelium into the bloodstream. This is where disease and inflammation begin. The immune system, which sits on the receiving side of the intestinal lining, becomes activated as abnormally large foreign particles cross over, triggering a war in a perceived safe zone.

Scientists have discovered that there are many genetically susceptible people whose bodies are incapable of handling these foreign particles correctly once they have leaked through a weakened intestinal barrier. Instead of killing and eliminating the foreign substance, their immune cells respond by inappropriately producing inflammation and attacking the body itself. This, in simple terms, is what we call *autoimmunity.* Unfortunately, what happens in the gut doesn't stay in the gut. These inflammatory messengers travel all over the body attacking, inflaming, and damaging tissues they shouldn't. Some go to the joints (arthritis); some to the thyroid (Hashimoto's thyroiditis); some to the skin (eczema, acne); some to the pancreas (type 1 diabetes); and others to the brain (anxiety, depression).

The end result of this inflammation can present in adults and children as brain fog, autism spectrum disorder, irritable bowel syndrome, allergies, and ADHD. The good news is that because of the pioneering work of Dr. Alessio Fasano, we now know that the epidemic of chronic autoimmune diseases can be improved, if not halted, by reestablishing intestinal barrier function in genetically susceptible people.[133] It starts by reestablishing a healthy balance of gut bacteria by eating a good diet, limiting environmental toxin exposures, avoiding drugs, and managing stress.

So let's break this down. The key to having and keeping excellent health is to maintain a diverse and balanced gut microbiome, also known as biodiversity, and a strong well-functioning gut lining. The right foods achieve both goals. The question is, does your diet contain foods that encourage the growth of microbes that reduce inflammation, strengthen immune function, prevent chronic medical problems, and improve almost all physiologic functions? Or does your diet reduce biodiversity and weaken gut barrier function? To reverse the unprecedented rise in chronic conditions discussed throughout this book, we must take care of our guts.

Once you start to see yourself as a walking human ecosystem, your view can't help but shift your thinking regarding food. This opens a new door to exploring how we can protect and

Signs of an Imbalanced Microbiome

- Acne
- ADHD
- Adrenal fatigue
- Allergies
- Anxiety
- Arthritis
- Asthma
- Autism
- Autoimmune disorders
- Bloating and gas
- Brain fog
- Candida
- Chronic fatigue
- Chronic pain in joints and muscles
- Constipation
- Depression
- Diabetes
- Eczema
- Fibromyalgia
- Food allergies/food sensitivities
- Frequent colds or infections
- Hashimoto's disease
- Headaches
- Heartburn
- Nutrient malabsorption
- Hypothyroidism
- Inflammatory bowel disease
- Loose stool
- Lupus
- Memory problems
- Mood disorders
- Obesity
- Poor concentration
- Poor digestion
- Psoriasis
- Rosacea
- Slow metabolism
- Weight gain

optimize our own health and our children's health. There are proactive steps we all can take to increase our chances of maintaining a healthy mix of microbes, especially for those of us who didn't grown up on farms, weren't breast fed, or like me, were exposed to a lot of antibiotics early in life. The next chapter explains in detail the best nourishing foods for a thriving gut.

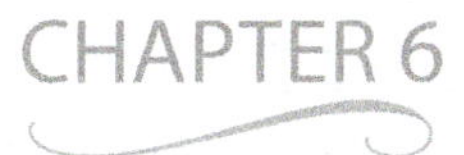

CHAPTER 6

FOODS FOR A HAPPY GUT

Every aspect of our health and physiologic function is dependent upon the health of the organisms that live upon us and within us.

—Dr. David Perlmutter

Learning to care for your gut's community of interacting organisms is mission critical to long-term health and vitality. In this chapter, you will find details on how to improve and maintain a proper microbial balance in your gut. The best way to achieve this is to consume both prebiotics and probiotics. Prebiotics, in the form of fibrous plant foods, are the gut bacteria's preferable food source, such as raw or lightly cooked veggies, fresh and dried fruits, whole grains, beans, roots, leaves, fibrous skins, nuts, and seeds. Probiotics, on the other hand, are live bacteria or yeasts naturally found in fermented foods, dietary supplements, and sometimes in processed foods. Aim for one or two servings per day of foods like sauerkraut, kombucha, kimchi, kefir, raw cheese, pickles, and miso. Probiotics in capsule form can also be a great way to improve your gut microflora. We need to take care of our gut bugs so they, in turn, can take care of us.

By now you have come to understand the profound connection between chronic disease, optimal health, and the little critters that live within us. Our individual microbiomes are in many ways our genetic fingerprint, constantly interacting between "us" and our environment as they send chemical messages all over the body that have enormous influence on its functions. Our gut bacteria play a large role in shaping our immune system, determining whether our kids have an allergic reaction to a peanut, or how well they fight off a cold virus, or even protect their brains from depression. How mind-boggling is it that they also contribute to our appetite, weight gain, blood lipid levels, nutrient absorption, and much more!

FEED THE GOOD BACTERIA

Your decisions at the dinner table—or the drive-through—tweak your microbial balance with every meal. In as little as 24 hours, we can change the functionality and abundance of bacteria, depending on what we choose to feed them. Remember, they eat what we eat. If we choose foods that the beneficial gut bacteria thrive and multiply on, we in turn produce an environment that promotes health and fights disease. To accomplish this we must eat their food of choice: fiber. Dietary fiber is known to help bulk up stool, reduce hunger, increase colonic movement, reduce cardiovascular disease and metabolic syndrome, improve diabetes, reduce cancer and inflammation, improve blood sugar levels, and so on.

Okay, there I said it, the "f" word. Dietary fiber is undoubtedly the chief operating substance of our digestive system. Also known as *roughage*, fiber is the indigestible portion of plant foods. You may be surprised to know that American children and adults consume woefully inadequate quantities of fiber in their diets. The average American consumes about 15 g of fiber each day, and most of it is eaten in the form of refined flours, grains, and potatoes.[134] The Institute of Medicine recommends 25 g of fiber per day for women and 38 g for men. For my patients and clients, I often recommend trying to consume at least 40–50 g of fiber per day, which may sound like a lot, but when compared to the 100 g our ancestors ate, it's really a drop in the bucket. Historically, humans consumed large volumes of fiber as vegetables, fruits, whole grains, roots, and tubers. The advent of refined and processed foods has dramatically reduced our fiber intake to less than 10 percent of historical norms for many Americans; It's no surprise that our gut ecosystems have changed in concert.

For years, we have broadly categorized fiber on a nutrition label as *insoluble*, meaning it does not dissolve in water and *soluble*, meaning that it does. Almost all plant foods have both soluble and insoluble fibers but in different proportions. For instance, the fiber in kidney beans is 30 percent insoluble and 70 percent soluble, while wheat is about 90 percent insoluble, and oats are 5%/50. But it wasn't until 1995 that nutrition researchers discovered something quite remarkable about certain soluble fibers: while all fiber remains unchanged until it reaches the large intestine, only some fibers are fermented by our beneficial gut bacteria as a food source. We call these fibers *prebiotics*.

The human gastrointestinal tract allows us to extract and absorb nutrients from protein, fats, and simple sugars in the small intestine, which resides between the stomach and the large intestine. Complex carbohydrates like fiber and some starches, however, take a different route. When we eat carbohydrates, the body passes the indigestible fibers through to the large intestine, where trillions of microbes live. It is here that fiber is fermented and devoured by friendly gut bacteria, stimulating their growth, improving the gut barrier function, and enhancing SCFAs production, which are critical for health. If we starve our microbes of fermentable prebiotic fibers the consequences can be toxic. Not only will our friendly bacteria stop producing the multitude of beneficial functions required for our survival, but their resulting death will pave the way for harmful bacteria to break down our intestinal wall and create low-grade inflammation that can lead to a host of chronic diseases.

It has long been established that societies that eat large amounts of whole plant foods tend to be healthier with less occurrence of disease, but we didn't necessarily know why. Now we do, and fiber plays a starring role. Some of the most fascinating research comes from Dr. Patrice Cani, a Belgium-based microbiologist who studies the connection between inflammation and gut microbes. He found that feeding a high-fat, "junk food" diet to mice resulted in weakened gut barriers, which led to leaky guts and low-grade inflammation. Even more intriguing, when he fed gut-friendly prebiotic plant fibers to mice on a high-fat diet, he was able to stop the inflammation cascade associated with obesity, insulin resistance, and a host of other metabolic diseases.[135] In my opinion, the single most important strategy for improving the diversity and health of our gut microbiome is to consume large quantities of whole plant foods loaded with fiber.

Currently, the best studied prebiotic fibers are carbohydrate compounds such as polysaccharides, oligosaccharides, inulin, oligofructose, lactulose, resistant starch, and other isolated carbohydrates. These different prebiotic types feed different species of gut bacteria, which offer us different health benefits. A diet that includes these fermentable fibers is one that includes various fruits, vegetables, nuts, seeds, and whole grains. In addition, many of these foods also contain special antioxidants called *phenols* that inhibit the growth of harmful bacteria and help beneficial bacteria tame inflammation.[136]

Below is a list of the top foods that contain the best prebiotic fibers and gut-supporting dietary phenols. The list also includes herbs and spices that have been reported to kill pathogenic bacteria such as H. pylori.[137]

TOP PREBIOTIC FOODS

VEGETABLES	FRUITS	OTHER SOURCES	BEST DIETARY PHENOLS	HERBS AND SPICES
Jicama	Tomatoes	Raw honey	Beans	Cloves
Leeks	Apples, with skin	Dark chocolate	Lentils	Star anise
Onions	Berries	Coconut flour	Black currant	Peppermint, dried
Globe artichoke	Green bananas	Green banana flour	Blueberry	Celery seed
Jerusalem artichoke	Green mango	Unmodified potato starch	Black elderberry	Sage, dried
Daikon radishes	Kiwifruit	Flaxseeds	Black chokeberry	Rosemary, dried
Celery		Hempseeds	Sweet cherry	Thyme, dried
Cucumbers		Pumpkin seeds	BlackberryPlum	Turmeric
Green and snow peas		Chia seeds	Chestnut	Cumin
Asparagus		Legumes	Hazelnut	Ginger
Bell peppers		Quinoa	Pecan nut	Borage
Beets and beet greens		Wild rice	Olives	Black caraway
Yams		Raw oats	Globe artichoke heads	Mexican oregano, dried
Garlic (raw and dried)		Psyllium	Juices of dark berries	Licorice
Dandelion greens		Almonds	Tea (green and black)	
Chicory root		Cashews	Red wine	
Sweet potatoes		Pistachio nuts	Red wine vinegar	
Cabbage		Acacia gum	Dark chocolate	
Ginger root		Cassava starch	Cocoa powder	
Fermented veggies & legumes		Human breast milk	Coffee, filtered	
Cooked and cooled potatoes			Flaxseed meal	

Source: Monash University, FAQs, last updated 2017, http://www.med.monash.edu.au/cecs/gastro/prebiotic/faq/#6.

How a prebiotic food is prepared is important when trying to obtain maximum benefit. Because heat breaks down fiber, it's better to consume foods for their prebiotic benefit in a raw or lightly cooked state. Think of fiber like a string of beads on a necklace. The length of the fiber "necklace" varies widely, but the longer the better so that it reaches the large intestine. For example, the fructan fiber in an onion has an average bead length of 26. Once it's lightly cooked it drops to 8–10 beads. If you keep cooking to caramelization, all of its starch is converted to sugar, and you obtain very little prebiotic benefit.[138] It's also important to eat more of the whole plant. In other words, eat the stalk and the leaves of the broccoli, not just the crown, and consume all the greens on top of the leek, not just the white bulb. These harder-to-digest portions are great fuel for your microbiome.

Naturally occurring resistant starches are also great prebiotic fibers that have distinctive benefits when consumed. They are named "resistant" because they resist digestion in the small intestine and pass into the large intestine where they are happily fermented by bacteria. Resistant starches produce less gas than other fibers and have been shown to improve blood glucose control, insulin sensitivity, obesity, and weight management. One very important property of resistant starch is that it produces high yields of SCFAs like butyrate, acetate, and propionate, which perform a plethora of functions that strengthen our gut lining and protect us from disease.[140] Butyrate's functions in particular go far and wide throughout the human body. It not only is intestinal cells' primary energy source, but also has potent anti-inflammatory and anti-cancer effects.

Underripe green bananas are very high in resistant starch, but the longer they ripen, the more the resistant starch gets turned to sugar and the less benefit it provides to the bacteria in your colon. Other starches like potatoes start off resistant to enzyme digestion in their raw state. But who eats raw potato? What's unique about potatoes and other starchy foods like rice and pasta, is that if you cool them after you heat them, their chemical structure changes back toward a more indigestible starch. It seems complicated, but it really just comes down to food chemistry.

Most Americans consume about 5 g of resistant starch per day, which is well below the current recommendation of at least 6 g *per meal* for health benefits.[141] Instead of consuming foods such as cooked potatoes, refined flour products, and breakfast cereals, which are all low in resistant starch, Americans are better off choosing foods such as beans, legumes, peas, nuts, and cooked and chilled potatoes.

Just as I was describing earlier, the preparation method of resistant starches has a major effect on the ultimate amount of resistant starch in food. The foods high in resistant starch that

MOST COMMON FOODS CONTAINING DECENT AMOUNTS OF RESISTANT STARCHES.[139]

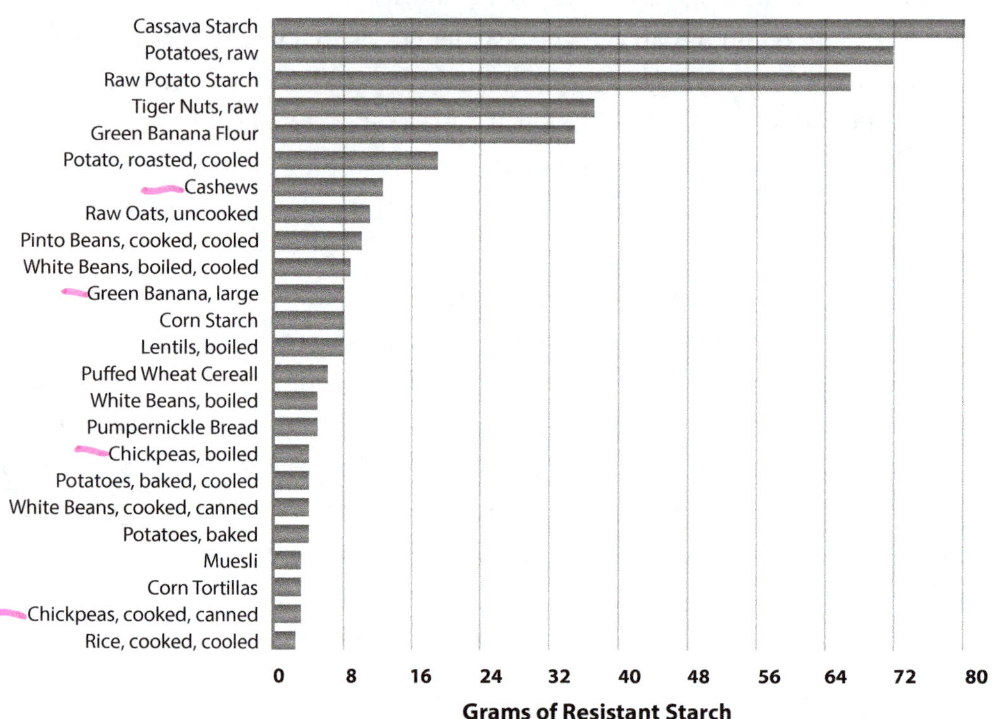

I personally enjoy are green bananas (in smoothies), beans, chickpeas, cashews, raw tiger nuts, and potato starch. I like that with these whole foods I'm getting not just resistant starch, but other important prebiotic fibers like inulin. I also particularly like Bob's Red Mill raw unmodified potato starch because it can be added to any diet without adding a large glycemic load of carbohydrates. It contains about 8 grams of resistant starch per tablespoon and is very inexpensive. I like to add it to my morning smoothies or creamy concoctions I make with kefir or coconut milk. I recommend starting slowly at around ½ tsp and working your way up to 2–3 tbsp over a two-to-four-week period to avoid any stomach discomfort or flatulence.

PROBIOTICS: EAT BACTERIA ITSELF

Live beneficial bacteria called *probiotics* provide positive health benefits when consumed in adequate amounts. Probiotics normally live in our digestive tracts, but they also naturally occur in fermented foods, are found in dietary supplements, and are sometimes added to processed foods. The microflora that naturally live in fermented foods are excellent for gut health because they help outcompete harmful gut microbes as well as produce bioactive compounds that offer a large list of health benefits. Probiotics are being used to treat and prevent a broad range of human diseases and conditions, ranging from gastrointestinal disorders to depression to cancer.

How probiotics exert their maximum benefit likely depends on what strains are used and what specific ailment they are treating. Although scientists are only at the early stage in determining these links, there is enough data to strongly suggest that we should include probiotic-rich foods as part of our daily diet. Thousands of studies have shown how probiotics benefit the gut microbiome and influence health conditions in the following ways:

◆ Improve digestion and absorption of food and nutrients

◆ Reduce antibiotic-induced diarrhea and fight food-borne illnesses

◆ Heal inflammatory bowel conditions

◆ Promote intestinal healing and help with overall digestive management

◆ Offset bacterial imbalance caused by taking antibiotics

◆ Reduce anxiety and depression

◆ Reduce long-term memory loss

◆ Reduce the risk of colon cancer and hypertension

◆ Improve insulin resistance and liver function

◆ Reduce the risk of allergies and manage eczema in children

◆ Support and strengthen the immune system

The goal with probiotics is not only to increase the diversity of healthy gut microorganisms but also to crowd out the potentially harmful bugs. Each strain of microbiota is uniquely prepared to influence different biological systems. Some help with energy storage and nutrient absorption while others help fight infection and calm inflammation. As Dr. Gerard Mullin reminds us, "There's no single strain of bacteria, fungi or yeast that works as a magic bullet to completely rebalance your inner garden and permanently shift you toward a lean metabolism. There are a few favorable species that seem to enhance overall health. But the data are varied, and the benefits are often strain-specific."[142] We have over 500 different species of bacteria residing in our colon, each influencing our health from head to toe. The most ideal way to support our existing beneficial bacterial populations is to eat traditionally fermented foods rich in probiotic bacteria.

Fermented Foods

Whether you are trying to maintain optimal health or healing your gut lining, balancing gut bacteria is achieved with foods that inoculate and feed the gut, that is, fermented foods. Before the advent of industrialized food and the invention of refrigeration, our ancestors fermented all kinds of foods: cereals, dairy products, vegetables, fish, seafood, and meats. They recognized the obvious benefits of this ancient preservation technique that enhanced the digestibility and the shelf life of food. What they weren't aware of at the time was the vast proliferation of good bacteria as the food fermented. Today, we fully understand the potential of these microorganisms.

When we ingest fermented foods, we eat thousands of different strains of live probiotics that outcompete the harmful microbes as well as produce bioactive compounds that offer a wide range of health benefits. Friendly bacteria immediately go to work releasing enzymes that improve digestion, making it easier for our bodies to extract and absorb nutrients from the food we eat. For example, sauerkraut (fermented cabbage) contains 20 times the available amount of vitamin C of raw cabbage. Fermented foods have also been shown to improve weight loss, reduce inflammation, produce antioxidant activity, and protect against chronic illnesses such as cardiovascular disease, Alzheimer's disease, diabetes, and cancer.[143]

Another important benefit of fermented foods is that they degrade anti-nutritive compounds, that is, they break down potentially harmful compounds like phytic acid found in beans and cereals and flatulent-causing carbohydrates in soy foods. A recent study has also shown that a combination of charcoal, sauerkraut juice, and humid acid (organic acid from soil) can reverse the toxic effects of glyphosate.

The thought of fermenting your own foods may be daunting, but it really can be quite fun. After all, it's the same process that changes grapes into wine, barley seeds into beer, and milk into cheese. No store-bought product is going to compare to what you can create at home, plus it's much more cost-effective. Foods like yogurt, kefir, kombucha, sauerkraut, kimchi, and pickles are a good place to start. Two great books that will tell you everything you need to know are Donna Schwenk's *Cultured Food for Life: How to Make and Serve Delicious Probiotic Foods for Better Health and Wellness* and Sandor Ellix Katz's *The Art of Fermentation*. A great online resource for in-home fermentation can be found at www.culturesforhealth.com.

But if cooking is not your thing, you can purchase fermented foods at your local health-food store or farmers' market. However, a word of caution when you purchase commercially processed fermented foods. Manufacturers often use methods with vinegar and high-heat pasteurization that damage all the health-promoting probiotics and beneficial enzymes of traditionally fermented foods. Read labels to make sure you are getting the real deal.

BEST FERMENTED FOODS AND PURCHASING TIPS

FERMENTED FOOD	PURCHASING TIPS	BRANDS	WAYS TO EAT	BENEFITS**
Coconut water kefir and other probiotic beverages†	Look for organic products that are actually fermented with a kefir culture, rather than drinks that simply have bacteria strains added.	**Best** Body Ecology Coco Biotic Inner-eco Kevita	Drink as a refreshing beverage Add to a smoothie or juice recipe	Provides vitamin K2, which is cancer protective and helps absorb vitamin D
Kefir†	Look for organic full-fat milk with live cultures. Buy plain varieties with less than 10 g sugar per serving. Avoid preservatives, sweeteners, thickeners.	**Best** Maple Hill Organic Kefir Forager Dairy-free, organic cashew milk Amasai **Good** Green Valley Organic Plain Whole-Milk Kefir **Avoid** Lifeway	Add to a smoothie In place of milk on cereal Pour over fresh fruit As a replacement for milk in recipes (that aren't heated)	Contains high levels of B12, calcium, magnesium, vitamin K2, biotin, and folate Boosts immunity Heals irritable bowel disease Builds bone density Fights allergies Kills candida Improves digestion
Kimchi†‡	Look for naturally fermented, raw, organic, refrigerated products.	**Best** Sunja's Granny Choe's Original Kimchi Mrs. Kim's Kimchi Wildbrine **Avoid** Nongshim Kimchi Noodle Soup Bowl Tobagi Assi	Add to stir-fries and sandwiches As a condiment Mix with eggs Eat with sushi Combine with brown rice and meat	Potent antioxidative activity Supports immune system Anti-obesity effects Antimicrobial affects agents' pathogens

FERMENTED FOOD	PURCHASING TIPS	BRANDS	WAYS TO EAT	BENEFITS**
Kombucha	Look for raw or unpasteurized products in dark bottles made of glass. Look for low-sugar varieties and organic. Some people (like those with candida) are sensitive to wild, airborne yeast in kombucha.	**Best** GT's KombuchaDog Brew Dr. **Good** Kombucha Wonder Drink Kevita	As a cold drink instead of soda, sports drinks, or sweet tea As a detox beverage after too much alcohol	Improves digestion Helps with weight loss Increases energy Detoxes the body Supports the immune system, and reduces joint pain and prevents cancer
Miso	Look for organic, raw, or unpasteurized. Darker miso is stronger in flavor.	**Best** Miso Master South River Chickpea Miso **Good** Eden Foods **Avoid** Kikkoman	Make salad dressing Make miso soup Consume as hot beverage Make miso hummus As seasoning to replace salt in recipes	Anti-aging properties Helps maintain healthy skin Boosts immune system Lowers risk of cancer Improves bone health Promotes healthy nervous system
Natto	Look for organic, non-GMO. Avoid MSG varieties.	**Best** Organic Megumi Natto Rhapsody **Avoid** Hoshi Dried Natto Osato Umai Ichiban Natto	Eat with rice, broth, mustard, soy sauce, vegetables, or eggs Eat with sushi	Supports the immune system Supports cardiovascular health Enhances digestion of vitamin K2
Pickles	Look for naturally fermented, raw products made with brine. Avoid vinegar and preservatives. Organic is best.	**Best** REAL Pickles **Good** Bubbies **Avoid** Vlasic Claussen	Eat by itself or with a sandwich Make pickle rolls with sliced turkey Add, chopped, to salads Drink the juice	High in vitamins and minerals, vitamin K and antioxidants

FERMENTED FOOD	PURCHASING TIPS	BRANDS	WAYS TO EAT	BENEFITS**
Raw cheese	Look for raw, unpasteurized, organic, grass-fed, sheep, or goat whole-milk cheese made with rennet. Imported European or New Zealand cheese is a great choice. Aged cheeses have more probiotics. Avoid pasteurized processed cheese. Avoid heat-treated or pasteurized after the cheese-making process.	**Best** Imported European or Local Raw Pasture-Raised (Gouda, Brie, Edam, Cheddar, Colby, Goat, Parmigiano Reggiano, Swiss, and Gruyere) **Avoid** American Velveeta Cheese Whiz Spray Cheese Most US mozzarella, cottage cheese, and ricotta are prepared without fermentation (culturing), and instead treated with vinegar or citric acid	By itself or in a sandwich Melt over vegetables Pair with figs and raw honey or wine Mix with pasta dishes Add to salads Avoid heating above 100°F to retain probiotic benefits	Heals digestive issues Helps neurological disorders Helps mental health problems Boosts immune system Destroys harmful bacteria
Sauerkraut	Look for "unpasteurized", "live cultures," and "raw" on labels. Avoid products with vinegar and refined salt (mineral depleted).	**Best** Wildbrine Jacob's Raw Farmhouse Culture Kraut Rejuvenative Foods **Good** Bubbies **Avoid** Boar's Head Silver Floss Del Monte All other canned varieties	As a condiment for sandwich or sausage With scrambled eggs As a targeted gut therapy eat two forkfuls with each meal. Don't forget to drink the juice!	Boosts digestive health Aids circulation Fights inflammation Strengthens bones Reduces cholesterol levels
Tempeh	Look for organic, non-GMO varieties.	**Best** Lightlife Organic, Rhapsody Organic **Avoid** Tofurky	Marinate and roast, bake, or grill to add to sandwich Cube and add to stir-fries or soups Make into burger Substitute for meat in meatballs	Reduces cholesterol Increases bone density Reduces menopausal symptoms Promotes muscle recovery High in vitamins B5, B6, B3, and B2

FERMENTED FOOD	PURCHASING TIPS	BRANDS	WAYS TO EAT	BENEFITS**
Yogurt*†	Look for "live active cultures," whole or full-fat milk, plain, grass-fed, organic versions. Look for goat or sheep milk varieties. Avoid flavored yogurts, preservatives like carrageenan, colorings, thickeners, and sweeteners.	**Best** Redwood Hill Farm White Mountain Bulgarian Maple Hill Creamery Traders Point Creamery Butterworks Seven Stars Farm Forager Dairy-free Organic cashew milk yogurt Kite Hill (dairy-free almond milk yogurt) **Good** Straus Nancy's Organic Whole-Milk Plain Yogurt So Delicious Cultured Coconut Milk Wallaby Organic **Avoid** Yoplait Dannon Activia	By itself or mix with fresh fruit Add to a smoothie Mix with granola Mix with ¼ tsp raw honey, chia seeds, and berries	Improves metabolic profiles Improves blood pressure Improves triglyceride levels

Sources: *Cornucopia Institute, "New Report Criticizes Yogurt Industry," November 19, 2014, http://www.cornucopia.org/yogurt/

† Lucy Shewell, "Everything You Always Wanted to Know about Fermented Foods," October 30, 2015, https://www.sciencebasedmedicine.org/everything-you-always-wanted-to-know-about-fermented-foods/#h.tyjcwt

‡ Annie-Rose Harrison Dunn, "4 Probiotic Strains Found in Kimchi," Nutraingredients.com, April 15, 2016, http://www.nutraingredients.com/Research/Kimchi-probiotic-strains-investigated

**Dr. Axe Food is Medicine, "10 Healthiest Fermented Foods & Vegetables," n.d., https://draxe.com/fermented-foods/ and S. Parvez et al., "Probiotics and their Fermented Food Products Are Beneficial for Health," Journal of Applied Microbiology vol. 100, no. 6 (April 2006): 1171–1185, https://doi.org/10.1111/j.1365-2672.2006.02963.x

Probiotic Supplements

The very best way to support digestive health is to eat more prebiotic and probiotic foods together like overnight raw oats with kefir, sauerkraut with beans, or my favorite, very lightly sautéed garlic, onion, leek, and asparagus washed down with homemade kombucha! However, if you don't care for the taste of fermented foods, then the next best alternative is to take a probiotic supplement. The main probiotic supplements on the market today typically contain lactobacilli, streptococci, and bifidobacteria strains, but there are many others that contain microbes, such as yeast, that are also used in formulations. Specific guidelines have yet to be determined for optimal probiotic doses, but most current recommendations are based on existing peer-reviewed research that has proven their safety and efficacy. Today, we base dosing suggestions on the collective experience of scientists and practicing physicians that have confirmed results in study subjects and patients across the globe.

Probiotic supplements can be a great addition to a healthy diet and have proven beneficial in many conditions; however, oral probiotic supplementation does not appear to alter or replace the existing resident species of the gut. Instead, they appear to leave their mark on existing beneficial communities by helping them populate, and thus calming inflammation and changing the gene expression of permanent strains while they live.

Health Tip: If you or your child are prescribed an antibiotic for a bacterial infection, the antibiotic will most likely kill both good and bad bacteria in your gut. It is best to re-inoculate your intestines with beneficial bacteria by eating fermented foods like kefir, kombucha, or sauerkraut and take a broad spectrum probiotic supplement with at least 25 billion CFU, two hours after each dose of antibiotic, and continue at least two weeks after the prescription is finished.

Probiotics are measured in colony-forming units, or CFUs, which is typically in the billions. A dose of 20 billion CFU may be prescribed to maintain good health, whereas a dose of 50 billion CFU may be used to treat eczema or even a dose as high as 2–3 trillion CFU to treat severe bowel diseases like Crohn's. If you are considering targeted supplementation as treatment for a specific condition, it is wise to consult an integrative or functional medicine practitioner who can guide you in the best choice.

Probiotics are not regulated the way drugs are. They are not tested or analyzed by the FDA or any other governmental agency for that matter. The responsibility is left to the consumer to ensure they are buying an effective product with the expected number of live microbes. In my 13 years of researching and using probiotics to optimize health, I have found there are specific criteria to pay attention to when buying probiotic supplements in capsule form:

◆ **Strain Diversity**: Look for a supplement that contains multiple different strains of bacteria. While many people think the total number of bacteria is most important in a product, the research to date has taught us that the number of different strains is equally, if not more, important. Look for products that contain members from both the *Lactobacillus* and *Bifidobacterium* groups such as *L. acidophilus, L. plantarum, B. longum, L. brevis, B. bifidum, B. lactis, L. fermentum*, and *L. rhamnosus*. Soil-based probiotics, which are also getting a lot of attention these days, are spores that come from the soil. They are thought to be beneficial due to the reduced exposure that humans now have to soil-based organisms in dirt. They are also more robust organisms than food-based bacteria, don't require refrigeration, and are more resistant to stomach acid. They are often prescribed when a different approach is needed from the traditional lactic acid–forming type of probiotics. They appear to be helpful in people with SIBO and constipation.[144]

- **Well-Respected Brands**: Studies from independent laboratories have shown that there are a lot of ineffective products out there. Check independent laboratories like www.ConsumerLab.com that perform quality testing and publish supplement reviews that confirm if probiotic brands contain the live amounts of organisms contained on the label. I also look for brands that have been used in peer-reviewed scientific studies, which proves their efficacy.

- **"Best By" Date**: Look for an expiration date on the bottle which is the manufacturer's promise that the bacteria will remain alive in the bottle to that date. Many companies alternately provide a "date of manufacture" stamp, which seems useless. Most of us want a guarantee that bacteria in the bottles we purchase will last at least three to four months. Purchase bottles well within their expiration or "Best By" date. It's also important to store your bottle of probiotics away from light, heat, and moisture.

- **Good Delivery System**: The best probiotic supplement ensures a large percentage of bacteria will reach your intestines and colon alive. After all, what good are dead bacteria to your body? It's important to research the delivery system to make sure the probiotics can survive the stomach's acidic environment. Recently, there have been a lot of advances in delivery systems, but my current favorite is a controlled-release enteric coated tablet or beadlet.[145] To ensure bacteria's survival of stomach acid, it's also wise to take your probiotic supplement with a meal.

- **Consider Specific Strains**: Research continues to expand in the area of strain-specific treatment. If you have a specific aliment you are treating, it would be wise to investigate if there is evidence that supports using certain strains. For example, certain strains have been shown to help with allergy symptoms and irritable bowel syndrome while others are more supportive for diarrhea and weight loss.

Recommended Probiotic Supplement Brands

As a quick reference, here are some brands that I currently like for general use:

Align

BioGaia L. Reuteri (for young children)

Biokult

Culturelle with Lactobacillus GG (studies show 10 billion CFU helpful for viral diarrhea in infants and children)

If you choose to consume probiotic supplements, it would be wise to rotate different strains every few months to encourage diversity and avoid single species proliferation.

Garden of Life Primal Defense Ultra

Garden of Life Raw Probiotics Kids

Garden of Life Doctor Formulated Probiotics

Genestra HFM Neuro Probiotic Supplement

Jarrow-dophilus

Klaire Labs Ther-Biotic Complete

Metagenics Ultra Flora Acute Care and Ultra Flora IB

Nature's Way Primadophilus Kids

Prescript Assist and MegaSporeBiotic for those interested in a soil-based option.

Pure Encapsulations Probiotic 50B

Ther-Biotic Infant Formula

Ther-Biotic Children's Chewable

VSL#3 (US formulation) (Use under a physician's supervision.)

In Appendix B you will find a complete Supplement Buying Guide to give you more information on how to purchase the best supplements.

As you've now learned, there are a number of things you can do to optimize your family's microbiome.[146] I've summarized some key recommendations from the last two chapters for you to consider:

Tips to Support an Optimal Microbiome

- Consume prebiotic foods daily in raw or lightly cooked states, such as Jerusalem artichoke, asparagus, onion, leek, garlic, raw oats, unmodified potato starch, greenish bananas, psyllium, chia seeds, and sweet potatoes.

- Increase all types of fiber foods. Work up to 40–50 g a day. Especially good sources are beans, lentils, peas, artichoke, broccoli, avocado, chia seeds, berries, pears, apples and oats.

- When eating meat, always consume with fiber to help sop up secondary bile salts that make it to the colon.

- Limit meat portions to 4-oz. or less.

- Eat as many species of plants as you can in a week. Your family's dinner plates should be at least 50 percent vegetable.

- Eat fermented foods such as grass-fed organic kefir, kombucha, and fermented veggies.

- Take a probiotic supplement if you don't eat fermented foods.

- Reacquaint your immune system with microbes: work with soil, garden, play on a farm, go camping, open your windows, own a dog or cat, and get out in nature.

- Diversify your plant intake. Don't ignore the more fibrous parts of plants; eat the asparagus ends, the broccoli stalks and leaves, and the leek's green parts.

- Breastfeed your baby, if possible.

- Consume prebiotics and probiotics together.

- Seek out ways to reduce stress: yoga, meditation, prayer, exercise, and breathing techniques are a few examples.

- Drink eight glasses of water per day and exercise for increased bowel movement.

- Have your child's gut microbiome analyzed for a risk assessment with a functional medicine practitioner if a chronic ailment presents.

- Adults aim for at least 7.5 of sleep each night. Toddlers and preschoolers need around 10–14 hours of sleep, and school-aged kids and teens need between 8 and 11 hours.

- Learn to modify high-stress lifestyles. It's important to find relaxed states each day, especially when eating. Your gut is your second brain and responds to your consciousness and mood. High-stress states have been shown to impact intestinal barrier function, gut permeability, and microbiome composition.[147]

◆ Avoid processed foods as much as possible. This includes refined carbohydrate foods, inflammatory fats, and all forms of sugar, which promote the growth of bad bacteria in the gut.

◆ Avoid refined grains of all kinds. Eat grains in their whole intact form. Organic, soaked, and sprouted is best.

◆ Avoid antibiotics, non-steroidal anti-inflammatory drugs (Motrin, Advil), and proton pump inhibitors (heartburn drugs like Prilosec, Prevacid, Nexium, Pepcid, Zantac) unless absolutely necessary. If you do take any of these drugs re-inoculate your gut with fermented foods or a high-quality probiotic supplement. A good alternative to non-steroidal drugs is a natural anti-inflammatory herb called *curcumin*.

◆ Avoid conventionally raised meats; CAFO animals are routinely given hormones and anti-biotics and are fed genetically modified feed with pesticides.

◆ Avoid food additives and emulsifiers such as polysorbate 80, lecithin, carrageenan, and polyglycerols and commercial food dyes like Red 40 and Yellow 5&6.

◆ Avoid GMOs and agrochemicals like glyphosate (Roundup) and atrazine. The foods with most genetic modification are corn, soy, canola, sugar beets, Hawaiian papaya, alfalfa, and zucchini and yellow squash. They likely have been grown with heavy pesticides.

◆ Avoid artificial sweeteners: aspartame (Equal, NutriaSweet), saccharine (Sweet 'N Low, Sweet Twin), sucralose (Splenda), acesulfamepotassium (Ace K, Sunette, Equal Spoonful, Sweet One, Sweet 'n Safe,) sorbitol, and xylitol (Nutrinova).

◆ If possible, avoid C-section deliveries. If given a choice, opt for a natural birth.

◆ Avoid hyper-sterilizing your environment with chemical antibacterial disinfectants. Simple soap and water or vinegar and hydrogen peroxide can be used for most hand or home cleaning. Reserve antibacterial soaps for only higher risk exposures such as handling raw chicken or animal feces.

The food choices we make for our family directly affect every aspect of their biology. Our children's bodies are put under enormous demands as they develop and grow: their cells are constantly dividing, their brains are continually maturing, their hormones are ebbing and flowing, all while they cope with life's daily stresses. The bacteria that reside within our children are interpreting and responding to all of it. As parents, we can help them immensely by priming their microbiomes to set them up for lifelong thriving—mentally, physically, emotionally, and metabolically. I encourage you to shift away from processed, refined convenience foods and move toward an anti-inflammatory, microbe-friendly diet. While we are still at the beginning stages of understanding the human gut microbiome in health and disease, it's safe to say the writing is on the wall: we ignore it at our children's peril.

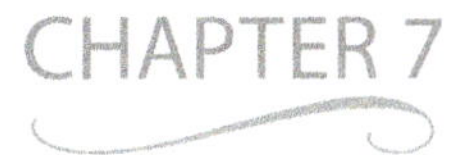

FOOD FOR YOUR TRIBE

The doctor of the future will no longer treat the human frame with drugs, but rather will cure and prevent disease with nutrition.

—Thomas Edison

Food provides instructions for every single cell in our bodies. So ask yourself, are you feeding your kids calories or nutrients? It is imperative that we, as parents, learn how to help our children develop awareness of the impact food has on their bodies. Not only is food affecting their well-being, it may be preventing them from functioning at their best. As mentioned, food is the most powerful tool to keep them performing well in all aspects of their lives. What most parents want to know is simple: what foods does my family need to eat to stay healthy, function at our best, and prevent chronic disease? This chapter pieces together the often confusing world of carbohydrate, fat, and protein to explain the importance of each macronutrient and how to make the best choices for your family's health. The recommendations are designed to support a healthy microbiome, keep hormones balanced, and reduce inflammation.

How did nourishing our kids become so complicated? It's easy to get discouraged when trying to decide what to feed your family for breakfast, lunch, and dinner every day. For some parents, a trip to the supermarket has become one of their least favorite tasks, right up there with cleaning toilets. Let the games begin as you enter through those sliding glass doors into the land of too many choices and ingredient trickery at your local grocery store. If I were to put an imaginary speech bubble above the head of a savvy parent shopper trying her very best to choose the right foods for her family, it might go something like this:

Which foods should I buy organic? Do these tortilla chips contain GMO corn? How much fiber does this granola bar have? Are there trans fats in these crackers? Is stone-ground flour or sprouted wheat flour better in my bread? What is azodicarbonamide? Will it give us cancer? This kids' cereal has 15 grams of sugar per serving; is that too much? Which kind of canned tuna has less mercury? Is that lunch meat nitrate free? I don't have $12.95 to spend on two pieces of organic hormone-free chicken! If it's just hormone-free, is it good enough? Is the salmon wild-caught or farm-raised? How many pesticides are used on blueberries from Mexico? Are the cans of black beans BPA free? Whoa, is that Starbucks? I'm getting a soy milk latte on my way out...but then again, I really shouldn't eat soy products, right?

Two hours later, the "savvy parent" leaves the store throwing caution to the wind, hoping and praying that the potpourri of foods in her bags will appeal to the tastes of her family and at the same time won't give her loved ones some form of life-altering disease.

MEETING INDIVIDUAL NUTRITION NEEDS

I am very aware that food shopping invokes fear and frustration in many American parents. You'd think that with the bombardment of health information we receive from media, "experts," and friends that we'd all be well informed when it comes to food knowledge. But nowadays, it seems that making intelligent choices only gets more challenging. Food manufacturers don't necessarily make our choices easier; on the contrary, they intentionally try to hide the often glaring negatives and promote the minor positives.

Indeed, food shopping became complicated when we started eating foods that needed labels. Understanding a label is important, but sometimes even more important is knowing where our food comes from and how it has been treated, as chapter 2 attests. We spend so much time arguing about which diet is superior and what foods to eliminate that we often lose sight of the end goal: our own *personal* health. Each and every one of us responds *differently* to food, so we should all be exploring how nourishment makes us feel and how it connects us to a well-functioning metabolism and thriving inner ecosystem. In our modern age, we are constantly looking for the golden ticket to health. Should we eat like a caveman and go the Paleo route or stick strictly to plants and eat like a rabbit? Both diets clearly have merit.

Ancestral eating is probably the biggest trend happening right now, and for good reason. Many people who have followed the Paleo, Mediterranean, or Blue Zone diet approaches have reported fabulous health, touting increased energy, weight loss, and the reversal of many chronic diseases. So what is ancestral eating? It really depends on what part of the world you live in. As Dr. Weston Price's research showed us, ancestral diets in Alaska look very different from those in sub-Saharan Africa and different again from those in Japan. Throughout human history, diet has been dictated by geography. In the pre-industrialized world, you ate foods that were available to you. Some ate a lot of plant foods and beans, others a lot of fat and organ meats, while others ate seafood and aquatic vegetables. People over generations adapted to tolerate very different nutrient thresholds contained within their specific regional diets.

We are layered with recent and ancient adaptations, making each one of us unique, genetically and microbially. For thousands of centuries, humans have evolved and adapted with their gut microbes changing within various nutritional and cultural landscapes. Suddenly (and yes, 100 years compared to the past 2000+ years is "suddenly"), we have drastically changed the playing field for our human ecosystems, with artificial shelf-stable food, hyper-sanitized environments, overuse of antibiotics, sugar at every turn, chemical contamination of our food supply, increased numbers of C-sections and formula-fed babies, and sedentary lifestyles. When we get at the foundation of what makes us sick and what makes us thrive, we find that food is at the core. We should focus on the parts of ancestral eating that are more intuitive, such as the quality of ingredients, local culture, and the time-honored process in which food is locally grown and prepared. If you think about it, nobody tells a gorilla how to eat. Why do we no longer understand what human food is best to eat?

My healthy food prescription for adults and children could be called ancestral, more because it's about simplifying and going back to what's historical, natural, and intuitive. Eat a variety of whole, unprocessed real foods, made up of mostly colorful plants free from as many food additives and chemicals as possible. This approach was backed up in 2014 by two Yale physicians who reviewed the supporting evidence of every major diet plan in the *Annual Review of Public Health*. They concluded that "a diet of minimally processed foods close to nature, predominantly plants, is decisively associated with health promotion and disease prevention."[148]

Count Nutrients Not Calories

Foods we eat fall into one of three major categories: carbohydrates, fats, and proteins. If I told you to eat 40 percent of your food as carbohydrates, 30 percent as protein, and 30 percent as healthy fat, you'd probably glaze over those numbers because, frankly, we don't think in percentages when we sit down to eat. We think in terms of taste, health, and fulfillment. My philosophy is not about counting carbohydrates, fat, or protein grams. It's about food quality and hormonal response. If you want to count something, count the quality of nutrients in each meal. Learn how carbohydrates, protein, and fat combine to maximize nutrient absorption and a healthy insulin response. It's much more practical (and realistic) to teach people the types of foods to eat and how to cook them. The rest will take care of itself.

As you well know, there are thousands of diet approaches out there. And while many have sound principles, there is no "one diet" that works for everyone. Success depends on identifying the underlying mechanisms for each individual and understanding how environment influences well-being. There are many factors that influence metabolism, such as age, sex, toxin exposure, hormonal imbalances, and the composition of your own microbiome, just to name a few. I would not necessarily prescribe the same exact diet for a pubescent 15-year-old boy as I would for a perimenopausal, sleep-deprived mom or a body-building dad looking to reduce his body fat from 14 percent to 10 percent. Some of us may need to heal our gut and eliminate inflammatory foods in order to heal an autoimmune condition, others may just want to lose a few pounds of body fat, while others may be training for competitive endurance sports and are searching for ways to maximize performance. It's beyond the scope of this book to provide specific diets for each of these scenarios. I am going to offer a set of principles that can actually make the biggest difference to the majority of those reading this book—sound wisdom based on centuries of science, historical intelligence, and proven strategies that are true for basic human physiology.

Food-Body Connections

So many of us are out of touch with connecting food to our well-being that we often blame stress or aging as the culprit of our adult ailments. For example, a headache suddenly arises in the afternoon and you quickly blame it on your stressful workday or your screaming children. Instead, think back to what you ate for lunch two hours prior, and maybe your symptoms were caused by the sixteen-ounce soda you consumed or the MSG in your Chinese food or the high levels of gluten in your pizza. The same goes for kids. I often watch kids at school consume lunches filled with high volumes of sugar, unhealthy fats, and processed flour: think chocolate milk and fish-shaped crackers (which they eat in volumes!).

Let's dispel the myth that all calories are created equal. One serving of popular fish-shaped crackers will provide your child with 140 calories, 5 g of fat, 230 mg of sodium, 0 fiber, genetically modified canola and soybean oils, and close to zero vitamins and minerals. It will also spike blood sugar and contains autolyzed yeast, an MSG flavor-enhancer that stimulates taste receptors. Compare that to 140 calories of red peppers and the nourishment factor gets knocked out of the park. Instead, your child's body would receive 9 g of fiber, no sodium, his daily requirement of vitamins A and C, as well as a plentiful amount of naturally occurring vitamins K, B1, B2, B3, B6, folate, potassium, manganese, vitamin E, and a whole host of cancer-fighting phytonutrients. Blood sugar is minimally affected. His cells know exactly how to use these nutrients in every organ of the body, whereas the cells that receive the processed crackers remain undernourished.

Moreover, if calories are all that matter when it comes to food, why don't we tell pregnant women to eat 2,000 calories of donuts every day? Or how about if we fed patients in the hospital preparing for surgery 1,700 calories of bread, butter, and packaged juice—do you think it would get them optimally prepared for successful outcomes? The answer is, obviously, no. And why not feed our kids 350 calories of breakfast pastries and soda on their final exam days when they need four hours of optimal brain function and focus? The answer: because we know food is powerful. We make specific nutrient recommendations for all these different scenarios because we know our bodies don't work like a calculator. It's not just calories in that equals optimal growth or optimal brain function. This thinking simply undermines the complexity of our powerful biological systems; it does not work and our bodies tell us as much.

The point is, there are high-quality food calories that make us thrive and low-quality food calories that make us crash, crave, and crumble. Our bodies obtain energy or calories from three main macronutrients: carbohydrate, protein, and fat. Most foods contain a combination of these macronutrients, but we often designate a food as a protein, fat, or carbohydrate based on whichever macro it contains the most of.

CARBOHYDRATES: FUEL OR FIRE

Carbohydrates are the sugars, starches, and fibers found in fruits, vegetables, grains, legumes, and milk products. Your body breaks down these foods into small units of glucose, which is a universal fuel source for all cells in the body. Carbohydrates or "carbs" have received a bad name over the past decade, which has scared people away from this nutritious macronutrient. The problem hasn't been carbs, per se; it's what we've done to them that's made them unhealthy. We've refined them, processed them, stripped them of their nutrients, and added lots of sugar to them. The result has translated into foods like bread, white rice, juice, cereal, pasta, cookies, bars, pastries, and crackers. While tasty, these are not the kind of carbs that will promote optimal health for your family. In fact, they do the opposite.

Vegetables and whole plant foods are the true carbohydrate powerhouses. They are packed with nutrients like vitamins, minerals, and fiber that support growth and development and aid in cellular repair. They also contain tens of thousands of special chemicals called *phytonutrients* that function as antioxidants, phytoestrogens, and anti-inflammatory agents, which go to work repairing damage from free radicals and preventing disease.

Figuring out which kinds of carbs are best to eat is not so difficult. Healthy carbs are whole intact foods that are packaged as Mother Nature intended. To evaluate whether you're choosing a good carb, simply ask yourself two questions: 1) Does the food contain a good source of fiber and phytonutrients? 2) Is it whole and unprocessed? If the answer is yes to these two questions you are on the right track.

EXAMPLES OF GOOD AND BAD CARBOHYDRATE CHOICES

NON-STARCHY VEGGIES	STARCHY VEGGIES AND LEGUMES	FRUIT, NUTS, AND SEEDS	WHOLE GRAINS	CONDIMENTS AND EXTRAS	POOR CARB FOOD CHOICES	POOR CARB BEVERAGE CHOICES
Broccoli	Sweet potato	Berries	Quinoa	Vinegar	Bread/Bagel	Soda
Cauliflower	Beets	Orange	Millet	Mustard	Crackers	Fruit Juice
Onion	Butternut squash	Kiwi	Buckwheat	Tahini	Cakes / cookies / pastries	Sweet tea
Leek	Rutabaga	Lemon	Wild rice	Hummus	Cereal	Lemonade
Asparagus	Turnip	Pear	Amaranth	Kimchi	Chips / Pretzels	Frappuccino
Celery	Yam	Almond	Sorghum	Pesto	Instant oatmeal	Chocolate milk
Garlic	Green Pea	Walnut	Teff	Horseradish	Refined grains and flour	Sweetened nut milks
Cucumber	Beans	Chia Seed	Oat	Salsa	White rice	Sport drinks
Peppers	Lentils	Pumpkin seeds	Brown rice	Hot Sauce	Sugar	Energy drinks

Carbs and Glycemic Response

When we eat carbohydrate-rich foods, our body releases specific hormones called *insulin* and *glucagon* that are responsible for regulating our blood sugar levels and maintaining a healthy equilibrium. All foods that contain carbohydrates, including grains, fruit, vegetables, legumes, and dairy products, are converted to simple sugars that are absorbed from our intestines into the bloodstream. This is a good thing, because the body can use sugar or glucose as a quick energy source to fuel the majority of its many functions.

You may be surprised to learn that different carbohydrate foods, because of their composition and complexity, will raise blood sugar at different rates. A ½ cup of buttered broccoli, for example, has only 3 g of carbohydrate. It will have minimal effect on blood sugar and its digestion will be slowed due to the fat from the butter and the 6 g of fiber in the broccoli stalks. A breakfast pastry, on the other hand, which consists of refined flour and sugar, has 40 g of carbohydrate and 0 g of fiber, is rapidly digested, and spikes blood sugars quickly. As a general rule, processed carbohydrates that are quickly digested are often the worst for us. These include foods made with refined flours (bread, cereals, pretzels, pasta), liquid carbohydrates (soda, fruit juice, lemonade, sweet tea), and sweet snacks (pastries, cookies, candy, fruit bars).

When we eat a serving of quick-digesting carbohydrate food, in the short term we might feel a little high from the quick blood sugar rise. The feeling is short-lived because our pancreas responds quickly by secreting insulin, a hormone that carries blood sugar into the cells to be used for energy or stored as fat for later use. This works until we start consuming large, sustained doses of refined flours and sugar, causing our pancreases to be perpetually stimulated by the presence of glucose in the bloodstream, thus releasing ever-increasing amounts of insulin. This pattern of high levels of glucose and insulin in the bloodstream will cause glucose to be stored as fat. Over time, the chronic overstimulation causes your body to develop resistance to insulin and an inflammatory response begins. This affects appetite regulation, energy metabolism, cardiovascular health, and can also lead to type 2 diabetes. It also creates fat accumulation in the liver, making it difficult for your body to detoxify your blood, resulting in disease.

> *Insulin in the bloodstream is primarily determined by the carbohydrates we consume. When insulin levels go up we store fat. When insulin levels go down we use that fat for fuel. It's the quantity and quality of carbohydrates that determine how much fat we accumulate.*
>
> —Gary Taubes, "Why We Get Fat," Food and Agriculture Association

Ideally, we want the foods we eat to create a slow, steady rise in blood sugar. One of the ways we achieve this goal is by learning how carbohydrate foods affect our blood sugar, in other words, the glycemic response. A concept known as *glycemic load* (GL) was developed to give a numerical value to the amount of carbohydrate in a portion of food, together with how quickly it raises blood glucose levels. Foods with a high GL are easily digested and cause a quick rise in blood sugar, and foods with a lower GL get digested more slowly. A low GL is considered 10 or less; medium is 11–19; and 20 or greater is considered high. It's best to try to stick with foods that have a glycemic load of 11 or less. For example, $\frac{1}{2}$ cup of strawberries has a low GL of 1, while a bagel has a high GL of 33.

Although this is a helpful guide, it isn't entirely accurate since glycemic load changes with a food's cooking preparation, its variety, its ripeness, its processing, or when other foods are eaten with carbohydrates. Fat, protein, or fiber mixed with carbohydrates will slow digestion, which in turn slows the body's uptake of glucose into the bloodstream. For example, a cooked sweet potato by itself has an average GL of 19, which is pretty high, but if it's eaten with some fat (butter), fiber (broccoli), or lean protein (chicken), then the meal gets digested much more slowly and has a lower GL.

Another thing to think about is the quantity of starchy, high-glycemic foods at each meal. For example, choosing a meal consisting of fish, baked potato, a side of baked beans, and a dinner roll with butter will send your blood sugar on a roller coaster ride from the sugary baked beans, the starchy baked potato, and the refined flour roll. A much better choice would be fish with Brussel sprouts, a small sweet potato with grass-fed butter and an unsweet tea. In this meal, the only choice that affects blood sugar is the sweet potato, and it's packed with nutrients and lots of fiber in the skin that helps stabilize blood sugars.

Each macronutrient combination essentially creates its own hormonal response depending on the amount of carbohydrate you eat, its quality, and whether it's eaten in isolation. Since carbohydrates have the greatest effect on raising blood sugar, I always recommend consuming them with healthy fat, quality protein, and fiber.

Although glycemic load is not perfect, it does provide a fundamental guide for us that proves the carbohydrates present in different foods affect post-meal blood sugar differently. This ultimately affects all aspects of our health, from cravings and energy to weight and concentration. The best approach is to maximize your plate with whole plant foods—fruits, vegetables, whole grains, and legumes. They are naturally packed with fiber and will digest and absorb carbohydrate the way your body prefers.

Discussions about blood sugar are usually paired with concerns about diabetes, metabolic syndrome, or other forms of insulin resistance that are plaguing Americans in epidemic proportions. We all should be managing our blood sugars, even if we don't have diabetes. Here's why: poorly managed blood sugar can lead to fatigue, weight gain, sugar cravings, insomnia, mood swings, brain fog, and more. It's also a key factor in the development of disease and encourages inflammatory activity.

While blood sugar is directly linked to the quality and quantity of carbohydrate foods consumed, it can also be influenced by other lifestyle factors such as sleep, exercise, and stress. Insulin and glucagon are not the only hormones that impact the rise and fall of blood sugar. Stress hormones like cortisol, growth hormone, and epinephrine further impact your own internal chemistry, which makes it even more important to make healthy lifestyle choices. In fact, we know now that glycemic response to food is much more personalized. Researchers at the Weizmann Institute have shown us that food affects people in different ways and that lifestyle factors along with our individual microbiome composition also influence our blood sugar response.[149] This comes as no surprise, given the variability of gut microbiota from person to person and how it uniquely affects the body's metabolism, energy, and inflammation.

The future holds a lot of promise in terms of individualized diet plans that can optimize blood sugar responses, but we are not quite there yet. There will come a day when we can identify our own personal hormonal response to food and modify specific lifestyle factors to achieve optimal results. But until then, we can use our current knowledge of metabolism and nutrition science to reduce our risk of chronic diseases, lose body fat, manage healthy blood sugar levels, and maintain sustained energy for optimal mental and physical performance.

Although these concepts might seem complex, putting them into practice is quite straightforward. Let's look at some of the best proven ways to maintain healthy, normal blood sugar levels for your whole family.

Tips to Maintain Normal Blood Sugar Levels

♦ Eat in balance by incorporating quality protein, healthy fat, nutrient-dense whole carbohydrate foods and fiber with all your meals. This helps slow the absorption of glucose (carbohydrate) into the bloodstream.

♦ Aim for half of your plate to be made up of colorful non-starchy vegetables like lettuce, leafy greens, broccoli, spinach, onion, and green beans. Most of these foods don't even register on the glycemic load scale and can be eaten in unlimited amounts.

- Starchy vegetables like sweet potatoes, winter squash, peas or corn are healthy too, but have bigger impacts on blood sugar and should be consumed in smaller amounts.

- Consume fruits in their whole forms and avoid fruit juice. The average serving is $\frac{1}{2}$ cup or one piece of fruit. Dried fruits like dates, figs, raisins, prunes, and cranberries are highest in sugar and should be limited.

- Eat snacks that are balanced with protein, healthy fat, and whole-food carbohydrates such as apple with nut butter or cucumbers and hummus.

- Avoid refined-flour products like bread, processed breakfast cereals, pretzels, crackers, cookies, cakes, or desserts. If flour is absolutely needed, try coconut or almond flour.

- Reduce or avoid sugar in all its forms: table sugar, cane sugar, HFCS, agave, etc. If a sweetener is needed, use small amounts of natural sweeteners such as 1 tsp of raw local honey or maple syrup, dates, blackstrap molasses, or organic stevia.

- Always try to consume grains in their whole form, such as buckwheat, amaranth, quinoa, teff, or steel-cut oats, but consume them in smaller amounts. A $\frac{1}{2}$ cup serving a day is adequate.

- Remove sweetened drinks from your diet, such as fruit juice, soda, sweet teas, and lemonades. Instead choose water, seltzer, herbal or green teas, lemon water, or black coffee.

- Acidic foods like apple cider vinegar, lemon juice, or fermented yogurt help lower the glycemic response to food by slowing stomach emptying to the small intestine. Incorporate these ingredients in salad dressings or combine directly on foods.

- Incorporate herbs and spices that help maintain your cells' sensitivity to insulin and slow the uptake of glucose into the bloodstream: turmeric, ginger, and cinnamon are excellent choices.

- Strive for exercise most days of the week. When exercising, muscle cells use glucose in your bloodstream for fuel thereby reducing blood sugar levels. A brisk walk after meals is excellent for blood sugar control. Resistance training is also excellent for keeping blood sugar levels regulated.

- Manage stress. Hormonal cycles can get disrupted with high stress, contributing to high blood sugar and food cravings. Studies have found yoga, exercise, deep breathing, and meditation are helpful.

◆ Get restful sleep each night. Adults need 7–8 hours; teens need 8–10 hours; children ages 6–12 need 9–12 hours; children under age 6 need between 10 and 14 hours. Poor sleep has been proven to disrupt appetite hormones that encourage sugar cravings and promote unbalanced eating.

◆ Digestion is best performed in a relaxed state. Our parasympathetic nervous system plays a big role in processing and using the food we eat by increasing blood flow to the digestive tract, regulating stomach acid, and supporting the immune system. Deep breathing exercises before and after eating improve digestion, improve elimination, and help with brain functioning after you've finished eating.

◆ Do not eat three hours before bedtime.

PROTEIN: THE OVERHYPED MACRONUTRIENT

We are a little obsessed with protein in this country. The thought of not having a grilled rib eye steak or roast chicken as the centerpiece of a meal seems unnatural to many Americans. The debate over animal versus plant protein is never-ending, and I could provide science to back up both camps. I believe one person can be healthy as a vegetarian and another can be healthy as an omnivore. If we can accept that we are all biologically and metabolically unique, then we can begin to understand that some thrive on mostly veggies, beans, and whole grains while others feel much more energized when animal protein is included in that mix. Hall of Fame football player Joe Namath, legendary tennis star Martina Navratilova, Ironman record holder Dave Scott, and world-famous track star Carl Lewis were all vegetarians at their respective peaks.

However, there are many different variations of vegetarianism, which have a big impact on nutrient intake. Most vegetarians do not eat meat, but still consume some dairy and eggs and occasionally some fish. Vegans on the other hand, do not eat meat, dairy, eggs, or anything that comes from an animal. I'm not a big fan of vegan diets simply because they often make humans vulnerable to certain nutrient deficiencies like B12, vitamin D, trace minerals, iron, zinc, calcium, and omega-3 fatty acids.[150] If one chooses this path, you need to carefully monitor your nutrient stores and pay very close attention to your dietary choices. I have found that many who choose the vegan lifestyle feel great at first, but start to decline after a few months.

Meat versus vegetarian debate aside, protein is a sensationalized macronutrient that is consumed in great proportions. In general, an average 140 lb. woman should get 65–70 g of protein a day, and an average 180 lb. man should get 90–110 g a day. In kids, the requirements vary greatly, but start between 20–35 g for children ages 4–12 and 45–55 g for teens. These numbers will vary depending on weight and body composition. Your protein requirements also shift if you are under stress, healing from an injury, or if you perform heavy resistance training. For example, a 140 lb. woman can reach her daily protein goal just by eating 6 oz. of beef (44 g), 5 oz. of yogurt (14 g), and 1 egg (7 g). That's not including all the other animal and plant sources she eats in a day. The truth is that most of us could cut way back on the quantity of animal protein we eat and replace it with good-quality plant sources. In fact, meat is better viewed as a condiment and vegetables as the main course.

PROTEIN AMOUNTS FROM ANIMAL AND PLANT SOURCES

ANIMAL SOURCES	AMOUNT (G)	PLANT SOURCES	AMOUNT (G)
Beef (6 oz.)	44 g	Almond Butter (2 tbsp)	7 g
Chicken, breast (6 oz.)	52 g	Almonds (¼ c)	8 g
Egg (1 large)	6 g	Black Beans (1 c)	15 g
Greek yogurt, cow (5 oz.)	15 g	Hempseed (2 tbsp)	11 g
Salmon (6 oz.)	34 g	Lentils (1 c)	18 g
Shrimp (3 oz.)	19 g	Quinoa (1 c)	8 g

The lesson for all of us is learning to listen to your body's voice and figuring out what makes you thrive inside and out. No matter which type of protein you choose, quality is the absolute key. If you focus on good-quality protein that makes up about 25 percent of your plate with every meal, you are on the right track. The following guide will provide you with insight on choosing the best protein sources to include in your diet.

Red Meat

Choose: Grass-fed, hormone- and antibiotic-free varieties of beef, bison, elk, lamb, pork, or venison. Although grass-fed, pasture-raised meat may cost more, it provides a much better nutrient profile with lower saturated fat and higher content of healthy omega-3 fatty acids, vitamins A and E, and CLA. It also avoids supporting the horrific inhumane conditions of factory-farmed animals. The term "organic" guarantees the animal has had at least 30 percent of their nutrition from pasture but most likely has consumed some organic grain prior to slaughter. Labels that say

"100% grass-fed and hormone-free" are therefore best. Look for "American Grass-fed" or "PCO Certified 100% Grass-Fed" labels for assurance that the claim was verified.

Avoid: Factory-farmed meat, grain-fed animals that have received hormones and antibiotics. Avoid processed deli meats, conventional hot dogs, bacon, and sausage with preservatives, added sugar, artificial ingredients and nitrates. Also avoid meat replacements that are typically made with soy protein isolates, chemicals, and GMOs.

Tip: Consider leaner cuts of red meat and eat no more than 3-oz. portions once per week. Consider buying directly from local farms to ensure you know exactly what you are buying and how the animal was raised. Farmers will often sell you a whole or half animal that you can freeze to reduce your per pound cost. Sharing or splitting with family members or friends is another great option. Go to www.eatwild.com to find a comprehensive directory of pasture-based farms.

Poultry

Choose: Certified organic and humane, pasture-raised, and antibiotic-free when possible. Chicken and turkey are often good lean alternatives to red meat and are often less expensive than other protein options. Pastured, organic duck is also a good choice.

Avoid: Conventionally farmed chickens and turkeys raised in cages or sheds, fed GMO soy and corn, and administered antibiotics. It's common practice to feed arsenic, a known carcinogen, to conventionally raised chickens to speed up weight gain, fight disease, and make their meat pinker. Some of the arsenic ends up in the chicken meat that we in turn eat. A Johns Hopkins study found that conventional chicken has twice the amount of inorganic arsenic compared to antibiotic-free or organic chickens.[151] Researchers believe that those who regularly consume conventional chicken might be at an increased risk of lung and bladder cancer. The only way to reduce your exposure is to purchase organic poultry whenever possible.

In 1920, a chicken took nearly 16 weeks to reach 2.2 pounds. Today they can reach 5 pounds in 7 weeks due to specially formulated feeds and animal pharmaceuticals.

—Mercola's Egg Infographic

Tip: Avoid misleading labels like "all natural," "Kosher," "cage-free," "free-range," "hormone-free," or "vegetarian-fed." Instead look for certified "organic" labels. The next best label is a "raised without antibiotics" or "no antibiotics ever." Do not trust claims that say "no medically important antibiotics," "no critically important antibiotics," or "no growth-promoting antibiotics" as they do not ensure the product was raised entirely without drugs. Two of my favorite websites for finding local pastured poultry are www.localharvest.org and www.eatwild.com.

Dairy

Choose: Goat, sheep, or buffalo dairy products are easier to digest, have fewer allergenic proteins, and cause less inflammation than cow's milk. These options also avoid the dangers of industrial cow farming. Fermented organic goat kefir is my preferred choice along with grass-fed butter or ghee, raw goat cheese, and plain whole-milk yogurt.

Avoid: Non-organic industrial cow's milk products. If you choose to drink milk from cows, choose organic, grass-fed, whole-milk dairy products. This will ensure no GMOs, antibiotics, pesticides, or hormones were used in production. Avoid reduced-fat dairy products of all kinds and stick with full-fat versions. Since dairy is an inflammatory food that causes problems for many, I recommend consuming it in small amounts or eliminate it. Avoid it completely if you are someone with lactose intolerance or dairy sensitivity. In addition, if you suffer from an auto-immune disease, have skin issues like eczema or acne, struggle with weight, have hormonal challenges, digestive distress, or any chronic disease for that matter, I strongly suggest you consider eliminating dairy for at least three weeks and see how your body reacts. It often helps reduce symptoms associated with these conditions.

Tip: There is very little evidence to support drinking dairy to promote stronger bones.[152] In fact, countries with the highest dairy consumption face the highest rates of osteoporosis and vice versa.[153] Coconut, almond, or hemp milk products are great alternatives to dairy. Let's also debunk the notion that dairy is a required food group. Your kids do not need to consume three glasses of cow's milk a day, or any dairy foods for that matter, to obtain optimal health or sufficient amounts of calcium. Bone health and calcium balance are better served by focusing on monitoring animal protein, exercising regularly, getting adequate sunshine or supplemental vitamin D, and consuming a wide variety of calcium-rich whole foods such as canned fish with bones (sardines, wild salmon), sesame seeds, broccoli, cabbage, beans, oranges, cinnamon, and leafy green vegetables.[154]

Seafood

Choose: Fish and shellfish in general are low in fat, high in protein, and can be one of the best sources of omega-3 fats. Wild-caught fish and shellfish are the best choices as they are higher in nutrients and have lower levels of toxins. Smaller fish lower on the food chain are better choices to avoid high mercury contents. Good seafood choices are wild-caught salmon, black cod, tilapia, flounder, sole, sardines, anchovies, herring, Atlantic haddock, farmed rainbow trout (farmed exception), scallops, mussels, shad, and crab. If you buy fish in cans, stick to salmon, herring, anchovies, sardines, trout, and mackerel and make sure the cans aren't lined with BPA.

Avoid: Farm-raised fish and shellfish which are commonly sold include salmon, shrimp, tilapia, catfish, and scallops. Farmed fish are less nutritious (little or no omega-3s), are fed GMO corn and soy, and are regularly given antibiotics to fend off disease and parasites from their tight living quarters. It's also wise to avoid large predatory fish with high mercury content, such as tuna (canned and fresh), tilefish, orange roughy, freshwater trout, grouper, walleye, king mackerel, Chilean seabass, shark, marlin, and swordfish.

Tip: Check out Environmental Working Group (ewg.org), Seafood Watch (seafoodwatch.org), or CleanFish (cleanfish.com) to find the most sustainable fish with the lowest toxin contamination.

Eggs

Choose: Organic pastured eggs from your local farmer or grocery store are of the highest quality. Look for eggs raised from pastured, free-roaming hens on certified organic feed without exposure to pesticides, antibiotics, or GMO corn or soy. Eggs from hens raised on pasture contain two-thirds more vitamin A, two times more omega-3, three times more vitamin E, and seven times more beta-carotene than commercially raised eggs.[155] That's because they are allowed to eat a natural outdoor diet that includes worms, insects, and various plants found from foraging in the ground.

Avoid: Eggs that come from conventional hens given antibiotics and raised indoors in inhumane conditions. Be careful of terms like "all natural," "Kosher," "cage-free," "free-range," "hormone-free," or "vegetarian-fed." Egg cartons are notorious for using many of these confusing and mostly meaningless labels. Your best bet is to look for a certified "organic" label on an egg carton. If you can also find a "Certified Humane" or "Pastured" label, even better.

Tip: Eggs are one of the best sources of protein you can find packed with healthy lutein, zeaxanthin, choline, and vitamin B12. They do *not* raise your cholesterol as previously thought,[156] so go ahead and eat an egg every day—and don't forget to eat the yolk (it's where most of the nutrients are). Don't be afraid to branch out and try duck or quail eggs. They often can provide an even richer nutrient profile. Go to www.cornucopia.org to get your organic egg scorecard that rates egg suppliers all over the country based on 27 criteria for optimal egg production.

Nuts

Choose: Pretty much all nuts are fabulous due to their healthy blend of monounsaturated and omega-3 fatty acids, vitamin E, protein, and fiber. Choose raw or dry roasted with the skins on (skins contain disease-fighting polyphenols). If you are eating them for protein and nutrient density choose almonds, black walnuts, cashews, and pistachios, which have about 6 g of protein per oz. But don't forget about Brazil nuts, hazelnuts, pecans, and macadamias that also offer an array of health benefits. Nut butters made from almonds or cashews are also good choices, provided they don't contain added oils or sugar. The ingredients should list the nut and maybe some salt, that's it.

Avoid: Avoid nuts covered in sugar, paired with sugary candy mixes, or those roasted in inflammatory oils. Dry roasting nuts above 170°F can damage the nuts' polyunsaturated fats and cause unhealthy free radicals to form (which is the case with most store-bought roasted nuts). Some nuts contain tannins and phytates that can cause digestive issues as well as block the absorption of some minerals contained in the nuts. Soaking nuts in filtered water for eight hours overnight and then roasting in a 160°F oven can improve digestibility. Also, use caution when eating peanuts (which are really a legume) due to potential aflatoxin contamination. Organic peanuts do not ensure safety from this mold but will avoid pesticides.

Tip: Because nuts are naturally calorically dense, it's wise to eat no more than a handful or about 10–12 nuts at a time. Same goes for nut butters. It's easy to get carried away with the portion size but try to keep it to 2 tbsp or less. Studies have shown that those who eat nuts on a regular basis have lower blood pressure, greater longevity, and a reduced risk of cardiovascular disease.[157]

Seeds

Choose: Like nuts, seeds in their whole form offer an array of life-enhancing nutrients. Hemp is a particular favorite due to its impressive range of nutrients including iron, zinc, vitamin E, calcium, and a balanced supply of anti-inflammatory essential fatty acids. Most plants don't offer much of a protein punch, but hemp offers a whopping 10 g of protein per oz. and is complete with all nine essential amino acids. Other powerhouse seeds like pumpkin, chia, flax, sesame, and sunflower contain around 5 g of protein per oz. along with an abundant supply of fiber, minerals, and disease-fighting phytosterols. Choose organic, raw seeds if possible and add them to smoothies, blend them into pudding, use them as a topping, mix them into baked goods, spoon them into yogurt, or sprinkle on top of veggies, fish, or meat.

Avoid: Roasted seeds (pumpkin, sunflower) in inflammatory vegetable oils. Instead, try dry roasting yourself but do not set your oven higher than 170°F, and do not roast seeds longer than 15–20 minutes, as it changes the structure of their fats.

Tip: In order to get the maximum benefit from flaxseed, purchase it whole to ensure freshness and grind yourself. Store in the refrigerator after grinding to prevent its fragile oils from going rancid.

Beans and Legumes

Choose: Beans and legumes contain a unique blend of nutrients unlike any other food. They contain meat-like benefits such as protein (15–19 g in 1 cup), iron, and zinc; yet they also contain concentrated sources of vegetable attributes like fiber, folate, copper, zinc, potassium, and antioxidants. They are also low in fat, sodium, and contain zero cholesterol. Beans also contain resistant starch, which is a preferred food for your good gut bacteria. The one caveat to beans is that unlike meat, they are not a complete protein source, meaning they lack some important amino acids—particularly leucine and methionine. So if you are a vegetarian, make sure you consume a varied diet that includes foods like cheese, yogurt, eggs, tempeh, nuts, and seeds to fill in the gaps. Some of the most nutritious varieties of legumes are lentils, black beans, garbanzo beans, adzuki beans, black-eyed peas, mung beans, and pinto beans. If you purchase precooked canned beans, look for those in BPA-free cans (I like Eden Foods). One ½ cup serving of beans each day, along with a varied diet, can be a great addition to your health.

Avoid: Red kidney beans have the highest lectin content of all beans. Those with autoimmune conditions should be particularly careful with lectin-containing foods which are found in beans, legumes, grains, and nightshade vegetables. If you have IBS or any other digestive distress or have difficulty managing blood sugar, avoiding beans is a good idea until symptoms are under control. Baked beans should also be avoided due to their high-sugar content.

Tip: Beans and legumes contain a moderate amount of anti-nutrients such as phytic acid and lectins, which are pro-inflammatory and can disrupt our immune systems. Essential to reduce anti-nutrient content is proper cooking techniques, such as soaking, sprouting, and fermenting, which will greatly improve their nutrient availability. For all legumes, it's best to cook them well with high heat. Pressure cooking (I love my InstaPot!) is the best method to destroy lectins and phytic acid.[158] (Canned beans are thoroughly pressure cooked and are not a concern.) Avoid slow cookers and crock pots, they will actually increase lectin content due to the low temperature used. Also, studies have shown that when lentils and chickpeas are sprouted, their antioxidant power doubles and quadruples respectively.[159] Nutrient availability can also be improved when consuming beans and lentils with mineral absorption enhancers like garlic and onions.

For some, beans can be difficult to digest because they contain starches called oligosaccharides. To improve digestibility of canned beans, drain and rinse them well prior to eating. If you prepare dry beans, soak them 24–48 hours before cooking (rinsing twice per day) and then cook with a strip of kombu (a seaweed), fennel seeds, fresh minced gingerroot, or turmeric. Digestive enzyme supplements can also improve bean digestibility.

Soy Foods

Choose: Organic, fermented, whole soy foods like tempeh, natto, tofu, tamari soy sauce, and miso. These foods have been consumed by Asian cultures for centuries and can be added to a healthy diet in small portions. Contrary to popular belief, Asian cultures consume soy as a condiment rather than a staple food and generally eat no more than 10–20 g of soy protein per day.

Avoid: Soybeans are the number one genetically modified crop in the United States. GMO soybeans have been engineered to resist the herbicide Roundup, which allows farmers to spray toxic weed killers on the soybeans without the soybeans themselves being affected.[160] Studies have shown that these pesticides found on GMO soybeans interfere with embryonic development, disrupt hormones, and have a toxic effect on human tissue.[161] I advise completely avoiding unfermented, processed soy foods, such as soybean oil, soy protein isolates, textured soy protein, soy supplements, soy infant formula, and imitation soy foods like soy cheese, soy burgers, soy milk, soy ice cream, and soy "meat" alternatives.

Tip: Until we have more conclusive evidence on soy toxicity, for individuals with thyroid or autoimmune disease, or those with a cancer history, all soy products should be avoided. Also keep in mind that soy is one of the most common immune-triggering foods, which cause gut sensitivities and provoke symptoms like acne, skin rashes, congestion, gut disturbances, fatigue, and more. Overconsumption of soy is a huge problem in United States. Once you start reading food labels, you will find that soy is found in most packaged foods and is commonplace in most restaurants. If you do choose to consume soy, make sure it's whole, organic, and fermented, and in small quantities.

Ancient Pseudograins

Not technically grains, pseudograins are the seeds of broadleaf plants, unlike cereal grains such as wheat and oats that are the seeds of grasses. Like all seeds, nuts, grains, and legumes, pseudograins contain anti-nutrients such as saponins, lectins, phytates, and protease inhibitors that can be difficult to digest. Proper cooking methods, such as rinsing, soaking, sprouting, or fermenting, are recommended to reduce some of the anti-nutrients that can interfere with nutrient absorption and potentially damage your gut. When preparing the three pseudograins below, rinse and soak prior to cooking. To soak, simply add 1 cup of pseudo grain, 2 c of warm filtered water, and 1–2 tbsp of an acid like apple cider vinegar or lemon juice to a glass bowl and let soak in a warm spot for 12–24 hours. Pour off soaking liquid and add fresh water and stir to remove foam. Drain, rinse, and then cook as usual.

While we don't typically think of them as protein sources, there are three pseudograins worth mentioning that pack quite a protein punch:

- **Teff:** This nutty, molasses-tasting, gluten-free, grain-like seed contains a whopping 7 g of protein in just ¼ cup! One serving also includes 20 percent of your daily iron needs, 25 percent of your magnesium requirements, and 4 g of fiber. Teff is also high in resistant starch and is the only ancient pseudo grain to contain vitamin C. It's great eaten as a breakfast porridge but can also be used in baking or added as a grain alternative to dishes.

- **Quinoa:** This gluten-free, grain-like seed is a member of the spinach and chard family. It contains 8 g of protein per cup, along with providing a great source of magnesium, antioxidants, and fiber. Eat it in place of rice, mix it in stir-fry dishes, combine with zucchini to make veggie meatballs, or bake with it. Rinsing and soaking as described above will also remove the bitterness often found in cooked quinoa.

- **Amaranth:** This gluten-free, grain-like seed is also a member of the spinach and chard family. It contains 7 g of protein per cup cooked. Like the other pseudograins above, it is a great source of iron, B vitamins, and magnesium. Use it in burger recipes, as an alternative to rice, or pop it like popcorn.

Nutritional Yeast

Mostly known for its abundant stores of B vitamins, nutritional yeast is a fantastic protein and fiber source with 8 g of protein and 4 g of fiber in just 2 tbsp. It's also a complete protein source, meaning that it contains all the essential amino acids that the body cannot produce on its own. This is an affordable go-to food not just for people on a plant-based diet. It imparts a cheese-like flavor and is used in all kinds of dishes from salads to sauces or any dish that you would typically use cheese in.

Spirulina

Don't be afraid of this blue-green algae powder that was once harvested by ancient Aztecs and is still harvested in parts of West Africa. It was made famous by NASA as a dietary supplement for astronauts on space missions due to its many health benefits and rich source of nutrients. It packs 80 percent of your daily iron needs and 4 g of protein in just 1 tbsp and contains a very high amount of vitamin A. Spirulina was previously thought to be a good source of vitamin B12 for vegans, but recent studies show its format is not readily absorbed in humans.[162] Spirulina is probably best taken in supplement form as it's not an "eat off the spoon" kind of food. However, one or two teaspoons masked in a fruit and cacao smoothie will never be noticed, except for maybe its green color. It is a more costly source of protein but is clearly a nutritious option.

Tip: It's essential to buy spirulina from a reputable manufacturer to ensure proper processing to remove potential toxic metals like lead or mercury, harmful bacteria, or other toxins like microcystin and anatoxin. I would also avoid spirulina if you have an autoimmune condition, are on blood-thinning medication, or if you have phenylketonuria.

FAT: EAT FACTS, NOT FICTION

Over the past 40 years, we've been told to eat low-fat diets, which coincided with the largest rise in obesity and disease rates in history. Americans consume by far the most low-fat diet foods in the world, yet they lead the world in obesity rates. I grew up in the "low-fat," "non-fat," "cholesterol-free" period of the '70s, '80s, and '90s. In fact, I bet if you are reading this book, chances are at some point you, too, were consumed by the same societal health recommendations that steered you away from butter and cheese, and encouraged you to choose low-fat alternatives.

We've all been scared of fat for quite some time now. The idea that "fat makes us fat" has been branded in our collective consciousness. We were told liquid vegetable oils, being plant-based, were good for us, and animal fats like butter and eggs were scary, artery-clogging solid fats that would lead us all to heart attacks. Saturated fat and cholesterol have particularly been vilified as the big instigators of disease, especially heart disease. Think of all those people ordering egg white omelets! For years, the well-known diet-heart hypothesis scientists touted was that the saturated fat we ate raised the saturated fat in our blood. And the same goes for cholesterol: too many eggs would elevate your cholesterol level. Decades of research and billions of dollars have been invested to encourage us to eat low-fat diets. In truth, the direct relationship between the amount of saturated fat and cholesterol in our diets and the incidence of heart disease is highly contradictory, and there is very little evidence supporting it.

The most current available evidence shows no correlation between saturated fat and heart disease.[163] Is this surprising? In 2010, the *American Journal of Clinical Nutrition* published a remarkable study that revealed the shocking truth about the long-standing belief linking dietary saturated fat to heart disease.[164] The study, a retrospective evaluation of 21 previous medical reports conducted between 1981 and 2007, concluded that there was insufficient statistical evidence to support the association of dietary saturated fat with increased risk of heart disease.

Then in 2016, a randomized controlled trial in the *American Journal of Clinical Nutrition* studied 38 men and compared a low-saturated fat, high-carbohydrate diet versus a high-saturated fat, low-carbohydrate diet. Not only did the high-fat diets not cause heart disease, but they also led to improved triglycerides, blood sugar sensitivity, blood pressure, and reduced fat storage in both the liver and heart.[165]

Another big shake-up came in 2017, when the largest prospective observational study was published in the *Lancet* assessing the association of nutrients with cardiovascular disease and mortality in low-income and middle-income populations from 18 countries across 5 continents. The researchers found that there was no association between total fat, saturated fat, or unsaturated fat with the risk of heart attack or dying from heart disease. It further showed that higher fat intake was associated with lower risk of total mortality and higher saturated fat was associated with a lower risk of stroke. The data continues to pile up, effectively putting an end to the "fat causes heart attacks" rationale.[166]

If you are wondering by now how we missed all these findings in the '70s, '80s, and '90s, there are many reasons, including poor science, weak correlations, corporate agendas, government oversight, and a mistaken belief that humans could improve health by manipulating nature in ways that were superior to its authentic form.

The point is, the past 40 years of fat recommendations set forth by the AHA and the Dietary Guidelines for Americans have been *completely* misguided. So here we are today in a world of confusing marketing and medical professionals still promoting outdated science. If this long, painful journey has taught us anything, it is to understand that not everything reported in a medical journal is always true. More importantly, we cannot make broad conclusions about any macronutrient being "bad" or "good" until we completely understand how each of its different forms are managed in the body.

Evidence-based medicine has its limitations. Our predecessors deserve credit, but science is the process of reevaluating. The tools we have now tell us so much more than those of the past. And an important piece of what we've learned is that not all fats are created equal. Indeed, unhealthy fats create inflammation all over the body, and eating them contributes to chronic health issues. We must learn to distinguish between the healthy and unhealthy fats, for the sake of our families.

We need to completely change our relationship with fat. If we want the truth, then we need to look to nature and evolution. If we want cutting-edge medical advice on fats, then we need to look to lipid scientists not influenced by industry, rather than organizations like the American Heart Association, the American Diabetes Association, the Academy of Nutrition, and even the FDA, who all receive heavy lobbying and financial support from the food industry. We need to seek out medical professionals who can judiciously review research data, rather than believing the recommendations of TV doctors, local news channels, or even worse, the food industry. We also need to take into account our clinical experiences, the science of metabolism, our individuality, and our evolutionary perspective. We've lived far too long on this industrial, artificial, low-fat, carb-loving journey. It needs to stop now!

Fat Can Be Your Friend

From an evolutionary perspective, we are hardwired to crave fat, as it makes us feel safe and secure. A meal with fat actually heightens the taste of foods and helps us absorb essential fat-soluble nutrients. Think of a sweet potato with butter and strawberries with cream. For centuries, populations all over the globe have been eating different quantities and types of fat without the damaging disease risks that humans in the United States now face. In fact, in 1900 heart disease barely existed, and up until the Industrial Revolution, all of our ancestors ate whole, grass-fed animal foods that were naturally rich in fat.[167] But, as discussed, our diets are much different today. Whole foods are no longer whole. Our food has been manipulated and changed more in the last 75 years than it has in the previous 1000. Years of inaccurate links between saturated fat and cardiac disease led us to replace saturated fats with carbohydrates, sugars, and even worse, trans fats.

> *There are wide differences in diets in different populations. For example, the Japanese consume 15 percent of calories from fat, the Mediterranean cultures consume 40 percent of calories as fat, and the Pacific Islanders and the Masai warriors consume mostly saturated fats. Yet none of these populations have the high rates of modern civilization diseases such as obesity, heart disease, diabetes, cancer, and dementia that we have in America.*
>
> —Dr. Mark Hyman, Eat Fat, Get Thin

The diversity among diets of various populations teaches us that varying quantities and types of fat can be consumed without leading to modern diseases such as obesity, heart disease, and cancer. For example, many Pacific Islanders consume up to 65 percent of their calories as fat with no evidence of ill effects from saturated fat.[168] Among European populations, France and Switzerland eat the most saturated fats and have the lowest rate of heart disease deaths in all of Europe.[169] In 1968, the northern population of India consumed 17 times more animal fat than the mostly vegetarian southern population and had 7 times less prevalence of coronary artery disease.[170] Today however, cardiovascular diseases have assumed epidemic proportions in India which is in large part due to the increased consumption of Western-style processed foods and trans fats.[171]

Contrary to what we've been hearing in the West, studies from all over the world show populations that eat large amounts of animal fat also have low rates of heart disease. The Masai tribes in Africa, inhabitants of Crete, the Inuit, Soviet Georgians, and Okinawans from Japan all have shown this example.[172] An equally important piece of the puzzle is recognizing what they are *not* eating: refined vegetable oils, hydrogenated fats, white flour, sugar, and processed foods.[173]

It may seem difficult at first to shift deeply engrained beliefs about fat; I know it was for me. But as I began changing my own eating habits and my recommendations to my clients, I noticed changes in my own health as well as in my clients' health. In order to obtain an optimal human diet, we must understand the enormously vital role fat plays in our survival.

Before we begin to consider the types of fats that support our health as well as the types of fats that damage it, let's review some of the basics about fats. Although the functions are too many to count, here are some key roles:

✔ Helps slow digestion and aids in the absorption of fat-soluble vitamins A, D, E, and K.

✔ Serves as an energy reserve after your body runs out of carbohydrate stores.

✔ Serves as building blocks for cell membranes (specifically cholesterol—yes, it's good) to allow transport of nutrients in and out of the cell.

✔ Provides energy to cells and brain when glucose is not available.

✔ Helps reduce inflammatory cytokines (cell-signaling molecules).

✔ Builds and regulates the production of hormones.

✔ Makes up *60 percent* of the brain and is essential for neuron communication.

Types of Fats

Fats, also referred to as *lipids*, are cellular compounds that occur naturally in food and are insoluble in water. There are four types of fatty acids:

Saturated Fat (SFA)

Polyunsaturated Fat (PUFA)

Monounsaturated Fat (MUFA)

Trans Fat (TFA)

Without getting into the chemical complexities, most foods contain combinations of these different types of fats. For example, butter contains mostly saturated fat but also contains a decent amount of monounsaturated fat and a lesser amount of polyunsaturated fat. By contrast, olive oil contains mostly monounsaturated fat and to a lesser extent saturated and polyunsaturated fats. Aside from trans fat, each of these different types of fats play a vital role in human physiology. Choosing the best types of fat in your diet can help you stay healthy, prevent disease, improve brain function, and help stabilize blood sugars (a key to good health). Here's what you need to know about the different types in order to tailor your family's diet.

Saturated Fats

Contrary to popular belief, saturated fats, SFAs, and foods that contain them are not the culprits they are made out to be. In fact, SFAs can actually *improve* inflammation and cholesterol profiles, and frankly, we need them to thrive. They are mostly found in fatty meats, lard, coconuts, coconut oil, palm oil, chocolate (cocoa butter), and full-fat dairy products like butter, ghee, whole milk, cheese, and cream. Typically, they exist in solid form at room temperature and are liquid at higher temperatures.

For the past 30 years, Mary Enig, PhD, one of the foremost research experts in dietary fats and human health, has extensively documented the critical role SFAs play in human health. There is, in fact, not one organ or cell in the body that doesn't rely on SFA for optimal function. Here are some of its key roles in the body:[174]

- **Cells:** SFAs provide energy and structural integrity (stiffness) to cell membranes and tissues. They make up 50 percent of every cell membrane, which is important for cellular communication.

- **Bones:** SFAs are required for calcium to be effectively incorporated into bone. It's most efficient when 50 percent of dietary fat is saturated.

- **Brain:** SFAs make up over half the fat in the brain needed for optimal function. This is an especially critical component for those children with attention or behavior issues and others with Alzheimer's disease, seizures, or depression.

- **Heart:** SFAs are the heart's preferred food and help lower inflammation.

- **Hormones:** SFAs are required for the synthesis of stress hormones, such as cortisol, and sex hormones, such as testosterone and estrogen.[175]

- **Immune System:** SFAs such as caprylic and lauric acids found in coconut oil and monolaurin in breast milk have antimicrobial properties that help fight viruses, bacteria, and fungi.

- **Kidneys:** SFAs help maintain blood pressure and filter toxins from the body.

- **Liver:** SFAs help clear fat from the liver and protect it from toxic insults from medications and alcohol.

- **Lungs:** SFAs, particularly palmitic acid, make up 100 percent of the fat in surfactant,

Human breast milk, the perfect diet in existence for infants, contains 54 percent saturated fat. A great example of nature demonstrating the importance of saturated fat.

the fluid that helps air exchange in your lungs.[176] Children who consume whole-milk products and butter have lower rates of asthma than those who consume skim milk and margarine.[177]

* **Metabolism:** SFAs act as a signaling messenger that influences insulin release and metabolism.

Dr. Enig has also explained the best way to evaluate fats. First, by the length of the fat molecule, and second, by how stable it is. As a general rule, the best are the shorter fat molecules and those with the least chance for oxidation (a process that causes toxic effects through the production of free radicals that damage cells). Saturated fats like butyric acid in butter and medium-chain triglycerides (MCTs) in coconut oil both make great choices because their SFAs are shorter in length and have the fewest places for oxygen to cause damage through oxidation. As a result of their unique makeup, SFAs are highly stable and are great to cook with because heat does not cause them to oxidize.

Now, all this enthusiasm about SFA does not mean you should start eating sticks of butter. At 9 calories per gram, fat is more calorie dense than carbohydrates or protein and should be consumed in moderation. Quality always matters most, and providing the necessary amounts of SFAs in the context of a healthy diet is key to performing and feeling your best. Here's what the latest evidence says about eating saturated fats:

- ✔ Most of the saturated fat and cholesterol that ends up in your blood is produced by the liver and is in response to the carbohydrates and sugar in your diet.

- ✔ Eating a lower carb, high-fiber, higher fat and saturated-fat diet improves cholesterol profiles, blood sugar, and inflammation.

- ✔ Saturated fat becomes a problem only when eaten with too many refined carbs, low levels of omega-3 fats, and low levels of fiber.

Monounsaturated Fats

One of the healthiest fat sources in the diet is monounsaturated fat (MUFA). Also known as omega-9 fatty acids, MUFAs are liquid at room temperature and are relatively stable. Healthy sources of MUFAs include olives, extra virgin olive oil, macadamia nut oil, almonds, pecans, cashews, peanuts, pistachios, nut butters, egg yolks, and avocados. They are also found in some fish, meat, and dairy foods.

Consuming foods high in MUFAs has shown great health benefits. People of Greece and

Italy, with their well-known Mediterranean diet rich in MUFAs, have remarkably low risks of heart disease as opposed to those following a typical American diet.[178] The following benefits are persuasive for consuming a diet high in monounsaturated fats:

- ✓ **Protects against heart disease:** Diets rich in olive oil and nuts have shown to protect against heart disease. Diets rich in MUFAs are also associated with improved cholesterol profiles and reduced risk of stroke.[179]

- ✓ **Rich in antioxidants:** Powerful nutrients like vitamin E help fight cell damage from free radicals all over the body.

- ✓ **Improves insulin sensitivity:** Replacing SFAs with MUFAs helps the cells respond to insulin.[180]

- ✓ **Promotes weight loss:** Studies show diets with 60 percent MUFAs can help prevent weight gain and reduce belly fat.[181]

However, there are some MUFAs that have been manufactured in ways that make them toxic to the body. Canola oil, which has been praised and promoted for many years, is a prime example. It contains around 62 percent monounsaturated, 32 percent polyunsaturated, and 6 percent saturated fat. Aside from it being one of the top seven genetically modified crops, the other egregious concern is its processing. The industrial method of extracting canola oil involves high heat and chemical solvents that turn some of its fragile polyunsaturated fatty acids into toxic compounds, including trans fat (see next two sections).[182] Avoid canola oil for cooking and use avocado oil, ghee, or coconut oil instead.

Polyunsaturated Fats

Like all natural fats, polyunsaturated fats (PUFAs), found in food (not oil) are healthy. They are found in both plant and animal foods such as fish, vegetables, nuts, seeds, and krill. PUFAs play a vital role in brain and cellular health as well as immune and hormonal functions. There are two PUFAs that are found most frequently in our foods: linolenic acid, also called *omega-3*, and linoleic acid, also called *omega-6*. They are both beneficial and considered essential, meaning the body can't make them on its own and must obtain them from food.

A proper balance of omega-6 to omega-3 is essential to maintain flexibility of cell membranes, regulate immune function, and to control inflammation.[183] Most scientists estimate that a healthy omega-6 to omega-3 ratio should be somewhere around 2:1. Today's diets are nowhere near that. The typical American diet is most likely somewhere around 25:1 and some speculate it could be as high as 40:1.

Without a doubt, omega-3 fats are one of the most important essential nutrients in our diets today, although it's estimated that 90 percent of Americans are largely deficient in this vital anti-inflammatory nutrient. The benefits of omega-3s cover many areas of health, from mental and behavioral health to cardiovascular health and cancer prevention. Of particular interest is brain health. Our brains are composed of nearly 60 percent fat, 30 percent of which are PUFAs. Of that 30 percent, half is omega-6 and the other half omega-3. It makes sense, then, in terms of brain health that an optimal omega-6 to omega-3 ratio may even be close to 1:1.

Manufacturers have caught on to the critical benefits of omega-3s, which is why we now see processed foods with artificially added omega-3s to products like peanut butter, cereals, milk, orange juice, and baby food. These products are inferior compared to whole food sources, given the changes that occur to the fatty acids in processing. The three major types of omega-3 fats are alphalinolenic acid (ALA), eicosapentaenoic acid (EPA), and docosahexaenoic acid (DHA). The omega-3s that come from food can come from plant (ALA) or animal sources (EPA and DHA), but animal sources, specifically fish, are more readily used in the body and are therefore optimal.

The two types of omega-3s linked to the most cellular benefits are EPA and DHA. You may be familiar with DHA on infant formula labels, as it's essential for a baby's brain development. Diets depleted of these essential omega-3s can affect your child's learning, behavior, and overall intellectual potential.[184] EPA and DHA keep the dopamine levels in the brain high, increase cerebral circulation, and are responsible for membrane fluidity in brain cells, which allows neurotransmitters to work efficiently. It is well known that our brains are highly susceptible to changes in body chemistry resulting from poor fat choices and nutrient deficiencies.[185]

Few nutrients have been studied as thoroughly as omega-3 fats. The benefits go far and wide and have proven beneficial with anxiety and depression, children's brain and eye health, heart disease, autoimmune disease, metabolic syndrome, and chronic inflammation, just to name a few. You should, therefore, make concerted efforts to increase omega-3 fats in your family's diet. There are no set standards for the amount of omega-3s we should consume, although the Food and Nutrition Board of the Institute of Medicine established adequate intake levels for ALA at 500 mg for infants, 700–1,200 mg for 1-to-13-year-olds, and 1,100–1,600 mg for teens and adults. It's always best to consult your integrative practitioner to obtain the proper doses for your family, as they will depend on personal health goals.

Obtaining omega-3 from food is always best, which is why I recommend both children and adults eat foods like wild-caught salmon at least two times per week. But if you prefer a

BEST OMEGA-3 SOURCES

FOOD	TOTAL OMEGA-3S	TYPE OF OMEGA-3*
Cold-pressed flaxseed oil - 1 tbsp	7,196 mg	ALA
Atlantic mackerel - 5 oz.	5,134 mg	EPA, DHA
Salmon fish oil - 1 tbsp	4,767 mg	EPA, DHA
Cod liver oil - 1 tbsp	2,664 mg	EPA, DHA
Walnuts - ¼ c	2,664 mg	ALA
Chia seeds - 1 tbsp	2,457 mg	ALA
Alaskan wild-caught salmon - 3 oz.	2,198 mg	EPA, DHA
Ground flaxseed - 1 tbsp	1,957 mg	ALA
Herring - 3 oz.	1,885 mg	EPA, DHA
Sablefish (black cod) - 3 oz.	1,806 mg	EPA, DHA
White fish - 3 oz.	1,363 mg	EPA, DHA
Sardines - 3.75 oz.	1,363 mg	EPA, DHA
Caviar (fish eggs) - 1 tbsp	1,086 mg	EPA, DHA
Rainbow trout - 3 oz.	1,051 mg	EPA, DHA
Algal oil supplement	1,000 mg	ALA
Hempseeds - 1 tbsp	1,000 mg	ALA
Anchovies - 2 oz.	951 mg	EPA, DHA
Spinach, cooked - ½ c	352 mg	ALA
Krill oil supplement	250–500 mg	EPA, DHA

* Of the 3 types of omega-3 fatty acids, DHA and EPA are the preferred sources found in cold water fish and other seafood. Plant based ALA is not the best form of omega-3s because it must be converted by a limited supply of enzymes into beneficial EPA and DHA. As a result, only a small amount of ALA—maybe 10–15 percent—gets converted to EPA and DHA. However, women are better converters of ALA (up to 21 percent), especially during childbearing years. Plant sources of ALA are still beneficial, but it's important to note that a tablespoon of flaxseed oil converts to about 700 mg of EPA and DHA. That's still better than many other foods, but far less omega-3 "strength" than what you might think you're getting from the 7,196 mg of ALA listed on a flaxseed oil label.

Sources: "Why not flaxseed oil," Harvard Medical School, last modified October 2006, https://www.health.harvard.edu/heart-health/why-not-flaxseed-oil; and Jillian Levy, "15 Omega-3 Foods Your Body Needs Now", last modified December 14, 2017, https://draxe.com/omega-3-foods/.

supplement, it's very important to do your homework in order to find a superior product because many over-the-counter fish oils are junk and potentially harmful. Here are some things to consider:

- **Source:** Fish oil must be properly sourced and processed for purity and freshness. That means making sure it doesn't contain heavy metals like mercury or other pollutants like

PCBs. It's extremely important to find a brand that is independently tested and certified.

◆ **Potency:** In order to get the most powerful anti-inflammatory product, it must contain adequate amounts of EPA and DHA. Knowing how to read a label is important. Look specifically at the amounts of EPA and DHA, they should make up the majority of the free fatty acids contained in the product.

◆ **Quality:** Natural fish oils are better absorbed than purified fish oils. It's also critical that the oil is not oxidized and rancid, which will do more harm than good.

◆ **Recommended Products:** Vital Choice Wild Salmon Oil, Nordic Naturals Ultimate Omega, and Nordic Naturals Complete Omega Jr. for kids. Appendix B provides more information in a Supplement Buying Guide.

While omega-3 fats help reduce inflammation, certain types of omega-6 fats, such as vegetable oils, promote inflammation. In fact, overconsumption of omega-6 as seen in modern America is directly associated with practically all inflammatory diseases, such as heart disease, type 2 diabetes, obesity, metabolic syndrome, IBS, arthritis, among others.[186] Since it's been well documented that inflammation is at the root of nearly all diseases, it is prudent to balance your ratio of omega-3 to omega-6 fatty acids.

But there is more to the story. Omega-6 fats have gotten a bad rap for quite some time, although it's not been entirely fair, because we weren't considering the source. Whole food sources of omega-6 like nuts, seeds, and grass-fed meats are quite different than omega-6 fats from industrialized, manufactured vegetable oils. Whole food sources are packaged with an arsenal of supportive nutrients and antioxidants that help protect unstable omega-6 fatty acids from being damaged.[187] Vegetable oils, on the other hand, easily become oxidized and damage our DNA and endothelial (the inner lining of blood vessels) function.

The Dangers of Vegetable Oils

When eaten correctly, PUFAs in their natural form can be potent regulators of health and disease. The problem is that in our attempt to modernize food and health, we've replaced natural animal- and plant-based fats with completely unnatural plant-based oils. For decades, government and food industry officials have instructed that vegetable oils were not only good for us but also essential to lower LDL cholesterol and prevent heart disease. This was clearly wrong. The dietary recommendations to increase refined corn, soybean, canola, safflower, and sunflower oils in our diets have been profoundly detrimental.

The problem lies in their highly reactive chemical structures and how we extract these oils from their seeds. The majority of vegetable oils produced today use high heat and toxic chemical solvents, like hexane, to extract the oils. Unlike MUFAs or SFAs, PUFA oils have two or more pairs of double bonds, leaving them unstable and very vulnerable to heat, light, and oxygen. In their natural seed form, such as in sunflower seed or corn, PUFAs have an arsenal of antioxidants that work together to keep their oils intact. But when these seeds are processed industrially into oil, the intense heating destroys beneficial carotenoids, tocopherols, and sterols that would normally be protective. The high heat and chemical solvents transform the once intact polyunsaturated fats into mutated, oxidized, heat-damaged oils.

To make matters worse, repeated heating of vegetable oils in your kitchen or in a deep-fat fryer at a restaurant simply amplifies oxidation, degrades the natural antioxidant vitamin E, and creates an extremely dangerous fat that is associated with cardiovascular disease risk and increased vascular inflammation.[188]

These unhealthy fats create inflammation all over the body. Consuming them contributes to poor immune function, brain dysfunction, heart disease, diabetes, dementia, and increases our risk of cancer. Oxidized PUFAs lead to the formation of free radicals in the body, which damage not only healthy PUFAs but any cell they come in contact with: cell membranes, DNA, nerve cells—the list is endless. Just remember, nature doesn't make bad fats, humans do.

The best advice I can offer is to avoid all refined polyunsaturated vegetable oils, given their unstable nature and reactivity to heat, light, and oxygen. These include soy, sunflower, safflower, cottonseed, rice bran, grapeseed, soybean, sesame, canola, and corn oils. Also pay close attention to processed and packaged goods that contain these oils. If you read labels, you will notice that soybean oil is a ubiquitous offender. Soy and corn are used by food manufacturers and restaurants ad nauseam because they are cheap, plentiful, and subsidized by the government. The only PUFA oils worth considering are unrefined, cold- and expeller-pressed flaxseed oil, walnut oil, and hempseed oil. But make sure you never heat them. The highest quality cold-pressed or expeller-pressed oils are sold unfiltered and unrefined. Look for small-batch artisanal European or California producers where the oil may appear a little cloudy, which is a good sign.

The best cooking oils are those that can tolerate heat and resist oxidation. Saturated and monounsaturated fats such as coconut oil, avocado oil, butter, lard, duck fat, and ghee are all good choices, along with macadamia nut oil at low to medium temperatures. I challenge you to inspect your pantry contents and notice how many foods contain unhealthy vegetable oils on the ingredient label. You will be shocked!

Foods with the Healthiest Fats

Animal Protein

(grass-fed, hormone, and antibiotic free):

Beef

Bison

Lamb

Elk

Venison

Poultry

(pasture-raised, GMO-free):

Chicken

Duck

Turkey

Eggs (chicken, duck and quail)

Low-Mercury Seafood:

Wild salmon (sockeye best), fresh or canned

Anchovies

Sardines, herring

Atlantic mackerel

Black cod

Sole

Squid

Trout, freshwater

Clams

Crab

Mussels

Oysters

Scallops

Shrimp

Dairy (goat or sheep preferred) and Dairy Alternatives:

Butter, grass-fed

Ghee, grass-fed

Clarified butter, grass-fed

Whole-milk kefir, organic

Cream, organic

Whole milk, organic

Artisan cheese, grass-fed, hormone-free

Almond milk (homemade)

Cashew milk (homemade)

Coconut milk (canned, bpa-free, organic)

Hemp milk (homemade)

Nuts and Seeds:

Almonds and almond butter

Brazil nuts

Cashews and cashew butter

Sunflower and sunflower seed butter

Chestnuts

Hazelnuts

Macadamias and macadamia nut butter

Pecans

Pistachios

Chia seeds

Sesame seeds

Flax seeds

Hemp seeds

Pumpkin seeds (pepitas)

Walnuts

Healthy Oils, Cold-Pressed and Unrefined:

Extra virgin olive oil (for cold applications or very low heat cooking)

Almond oil (for cold applications)

Macadamia nut oil (for low heat cooking)

Flax oil (for cold applications)

Hemp oil (for cold applications)

Walnut oil (for cold applications)

Avocado oil, organic

Mct oil (for cold applications)

Sesame seed oil (for cold applications)

Virgin coconut oil, organic

Coconut butter (for cold applications)

Krill oil, cold-pressed antarctic

Fish oil

Fermented cod liver oil

Algae oil

Other Foods:

Mayonnaise (made with 100 percent extra virgin olive oil or cold-pressed avocado oil)

Olives

Cocoa butter

Beef tallow, grass-fed, organic

Avocados

Dark chocolate, 70% or more cocoa solids

Foods with Unhealthy Fats

Polyunsaturated Vegetable Oils:

Corn oil
Soybean oil
Sunflower oil
Safflower oil
Grapeseed oil
Cottonseed oil
Rice bran oil
Palm oil
Canola oil
Peanut oil
Spray oils like pam

Trans Fats
(Read ingredient labels for these words):

Hydrogenated vegetable oil
Partially hydrogenated vegetable oil

Processed Foods with PUFAs and Trans Fats:

Cookies, breads, muffins, and other store-bought baked goods
Chips, microwave popcorn, and other snack foods
Salad dressings
Rice milk
Store-bought granola and breakfast cereals
Soy milk, soy cheese, and soy meat
Vegetable shortening (like crisco)
Margarine and non-butter spreads
Oily nuts roasted in vegetable oils
All fried foods
Fake whip cream (cool whip, miracle whip)
Coffee creamer
Fast food
Frozen meals (read labels)
Mayonnaise (made with soybean or canola oil)
Anything in a package with a shelf life, read the label

Trans Fats

Have you noticed a pattern in this book with the ill health effects of man-made food versus the positive effects of foods from nature? Here is yet another example: if there is one thing that all health experts agree on, it's that man-made trans fats are downright toxic. Trans fats were invented by scientists who converted vegetable oils into solid fat using a hydrogenation process. Once thought to be healthier than butter, we now know the opposite is true. Trans fats allow processed foods to be more shelf-stable and cheaper. Nothing good came out of this process, unless you fancy eating a donut that still appears edible five weeks after you've bought it.

Trans fats are found in snack foods, crackers, processed vegetable oils, frozen entrees, shortenings and margarines, coffee creamer, fried foods, microwave popcorn, and store-bought baked goods. In order to avoid trans fats, read ingredient labels carefully and be on the lookout for words like "hydrogenated" or "partially hydrogenated." If you want to avoid trans fats entirely, simply eliminate processed foods from your diet. According to the Center for Science in the Public Interest, the FDA has finally acknowledged that trans fats are toxic and has ordered a ban on their use. Food manufacturers have until mid-2018 to remove all trans fats from their products. Let's hope they don't replace them with a new legal toxic fat concoction!

Even though weak scientific theories and food industry products have misguided us, we can always look to historical evidence and tap into our own intuitive wisdom. Our overwhelming increase in consumption of unnatural vegetable oils, sugar, and refined carbohydrate foods has led us into the abyss of chronic disease, but we can get back to nature as soon as we choose it. Choosing healthy fats that work in unison with our body's natural lipid cycle will not only protect us from chronic disease, but also will improve our mental health and protect us from accelerated aging.

THE BEST ANTI-INFLAMMATORY FOODS: FRUITS AND VEGETABLES

Almost all food experts agree that vegetables and fruits are essential parts of a healthful diet. What makes them so special is not just their comprehensive array of vitamins, minerals, and fiber, but they also contain thousands of phytonutrients, which I like to think of as the plants' military forces. Since plants can't run from danger, they instead make an arsenal of chemical compounds that protect them from harm. Phytonutrients go to war defending the plant against protein and DNA damage caused by extreme environmental conditions like ultraviolet radiation, insects, toxins, diseases, and pollution.[189] When we eat these same phytonutrients contained in plants, we, too, reap their many benefits. Essentially, the harder a plant has to work to stay alive, the better that food is for humans.

After three decades of research, nutrition scientists have uncovered that phytonutrients play an integral part in preventing inflammatory diseases, such as cardiovascular disease, cancer, Alzheimer's disease, and diabetes.[190] Some phytonutrients also appear to help with cellular communication, others prevent mutations at the cellular level, and some act as critical antioxidants needed to help our body detoxify nasty free radicals that damage our tissues. Phytonutrients

15 Anti-Inflammatory Powerhouses

- Asian mushrooms (cooked)
- beets and beet greens
- berries
- bone broth
- broccoli and broccoli sprouts
- fermented vegetables
- flaxseed
- garlic
- ginger
- green leafy vegetables
- matcha green tea
- sardines
- turmeric
- walnuts
- wild salmon

have also been linked to improving athletic performance, boosting immunity, protecting brain health, and enhancing weight loss.[191] Substances like resveratrol in grapes, lycopene in tomatoes, luteolin in peppers, beta-carotene in orange vegetables, and sulforaphane found in cruciferous vegetables are just a few of the phytonutrients that are now under consideration as a therapeutic strategy for eradicating cancer.[192] Hippocrates is smiling at the science. These natural substances are now being considered beyond chemotherapy and radiation to get at the root cause of cancer. If that doesn't solidify the importance of our dietary decisions, I don't know what else can!

Before you run out and load up a grocery cart with fruits and vegetables, there are a few good things to know when searching for the most nutritious plants to eat. I recently came across a fabulous book written by Jo Robinson called *Eating on the Wild Side*. In it, she gives us new strategies to obtain the highest level of nutrients from the food we eat. Her sobering discoveries teach us that there are vast nutritional differences in the wild fruits and vegetables of our ancestors compared to the domesticated versions that we eat today. As we've transformed from hunters and gatherers to herders and gardeners and now to factory feedlot and monoculture farmers, our produce has ridden the wave of change not necessarily for the better.

Today we eat produce that's been manipulated by plant geneticists and breeders and assume that their goals are focused on improving the nourishment of plants. In reality, their focus lies more on improving taste, appearance, productivity, and disease resistance, rather than testing if the phytonutrient content has improved or if human metabolism is affected. Two additional unforeseen circumstances that have contributed to the nutrient loss in our food have been the depletion of soil micronutrients from conventional farming techniques and the long transportation time that food now takes to get from farm to plate.

So what is a wise, healthy shopper to do? Robinson's eye-opening research tells us, "We can choose those select varieties of fruits and vegetables that have retained much of the nutritional content of their wild ancestors."[193] It's also essential to understand how to purchase, store, and prepare your produce to get the biggest nutritional bang for your buck. For example, many people might think that heirloom vegetable varieties are always more nutritious or that pale-colored vegetables are always less nutritious, but that's not the case. Nutrients differ among varieties of a given fruit or vegetable as well as by color and preparation method. For example, Robinson states, "The old idea that a tomato is a tomato no longer holds. You'd have to eat ten of the least nutritious variety to get the same amount of lycopene as you would from one tomato of the most nutritious variety."[194] Also, some foods are more nutritious when eaten raw, but others, like carrots, provide more bioavailable beta-carotene in their cooked state with some oil or fat. Did you know that steaming artichokes increases antioxidant activity 15 times more than raw? Or that you should let raw garlic sit for 10 minutes after you chop it to let the health-promoting allicin compound develop fully before heating? I've put together a healthy produce guide to purchasing and preparing the most nutritious fruits and vegetables.

PRODUCE GUIDE TO MAXIMIZE NUTRIENT INTAKE

FOOD	HIGHEST NUTRITIONAL VALUE	PURCHASE/PREP/COOKING TIPS
Apples	• Eat the skin, more phytonutrients than flesh • Choose organic to avoid pesticides • Cloudy apple juice has 4x more phytonutrient than clear • The redder in color on all sides the more antioxidants • Granny Smith, Cortland, Discovery, and Fuji are of the most nutritious varieties of the 12 most common varieties	• Lasts 10x longer if stored in crisper drawer of refrigerator
Artichokes	• Globe artichoke most nutritious • Cooking artichokes increases antioxidant activity (steaming 15x more than raw, boiling 5x more than raw) • Inner leaves and heart more nutritious than exterior leaves • High in prebiotic inulin and fiber	• Cook artichokes as soon as purchased as they lose nutrients quickly after storing, 3 days max • Choose firm, tight leaves • Canned artichokes are very high in antioxidants; look for glass jars
Asparagus	• Steaming increases antioxidant content by 30 percent	• Loses phytonutrients rapidly; eat as soon as purchased • Look for short, dark green stems with tightly closed tips
Avocados	• Hass is most nutritious variety	• Store ripe avocados in refrigerator for 2–3 days
Beans/Lentils/Peas	• Black beans and lentils have more antioxidant activity than all other common legumes • Yellow dried peas have 6x more antioxidants than green • Dried peas and beans have more phytonutrients than fresh; fresh have more than frozen • Most nutritious legumes are dried black, navy beans, and lentils	• Pressure-cooked beans retain antioxidant values and reduce lectin content • Canned beans are higher in antioxidants than home-cooked beans • Lentils and pinto beans easiest to digest • Discard soaking liquid before cooking raw beans
Beets	• Beet greens among healthiest leaves, 7x more antioxidants than romaine, on par with kale in nutritional value • Beets without greens have more antioxidant properties than most other common vegetables (9x more than tomato and 50x more than carrot)	• Choose darkest red varieties • Purchase in bunches with leaves • Canned beets equally nutritious as fresh
Berries	• Flash-frozen berries as nutritious as fresh • Blueberries and blackberries among the most nutritious • Among the best fruits you can eat	• Cooking and canning increase phytonutrient content

FOOD	HIGHEST NUTRITIONAL VALUE	PURCHASE/PREP/COOKING TIPS
Broccoli	• All supermarket varieties are nutritious • Eating raw provides 20x more sulforaphane (anticancer property) than cooked • Broccoli sprouts have 10 to 100 times more sulforaphane by weight than mature broccoli plants • Chopping raw broccoli into small pieces and letting it sit for at least 40 minutes activates the enzyme to promote sulforaphanes • Whole head broccoli more nutritious than pre-trimmed florets due to fast decay	• Look for dark green crowns and tightly closed buds • Grow your own or purchase from farmers' market to reduce nutrient loss from transport and storage • Store chilled and eat within 1 day of purchasing; loses nutrient content fast • Steam no longer than 4 minutes until tough-tender; avoid boiling and microwaving altogether
Brussels Sprouts	• Contain powerful cancer protective phytonutrients called glucosinolates • Excellent source of vitamin K, C, and folate • Eat with healthy fat to aid absorption of fat-soluble vitamin K	• Look for bright green with tight leaves • To extract highest nutritional value, cut into quarters, let sit for 5 minutes, then steam for no longer than 5 minutes, toss with olive oil • Expire rapidly, eat within 1 day of purchasing
Cabbage	• Red cabbage has 6x more antioxidant activity than green cabbage and 3x more than savoy cabbage	• Can be stored in refrigerator for weeks without losing many nutrients • Look for heavy, firm, compact heads
Carrots	• Avoid baby carrots, they are the least nutritious. Eat whole carrots with skin, and cut into matchsticks (skin most nutritious part) • Sauté or steam makes phytonutrients more bioavailable (avoid boiling) • Deep purple carrot has 10x more antioxidants than other varieties	• Buy with green tops attached for freshness (without tops could be several months old) • Eat with fat like olive oil to allow for best absorption of fat-soluble nutrients like beta-carotene (vitamin A)
Cauliflower	• White has more cancer-fighting compounds but green and purple have more antioxidants	• Steam or sauté in olive oil, do not boil
Cherries	• Bing variety more nutritious than Rainier	• Bright green, flexible stems best indicator of freshness • Store in refrigerator in ventilated bag
Citrus fruits	• Deeper color flesh has the most phytonutrients (red and pink grapefruit vs. white)	• Store on counter or in refrigerator • Orange juice concentrate has more flavonoids than fresh
Corn	• Deep yellow varieties have up to 58x more beta-carotene than white corn • Organic has 50 percent more phytonutrients than conventionally raised • Avoid super-sweet varieties • Cornmeal made from blue, red, or purple corn has more phytonutrients than yellow	• Grilling or steaming is best to retain nutrients (the less contact with water the better)

FOOD	HIGHEST NUTRITIONAL VALUE	PURCHASE/PREP/COOKING TIPS
Garlic	• Silverskin garlic found in most grocery stores is on par with other varieties • Rich in powerful sulfur-containing compounds	• Chop and eat raw • If cooking, let garlic sit for 10 minutes after chopping, mincing, or mashing to let health-promoting allicin develop fully before heating • Store cloves in ventilated cool, dark place
Grapes	• Muscadine and Concord highest in antioxidants (Thompson seedless and pale green grapes lowest) • Buy organic • Skins contain most nutrients and polyphenols (resveratrol)	• Store chilled in refrigerator
Kale	• All supermarket varieties are high in cancer-fighting compounds and antioxidants • Most nutritious raw • Most bitter and beneficial of all crucifers	• Store in crisper and use within 2 days • Steam briefly, sauté in olive oil, or make kale chips
Leeks/ Scallions (green onion)	• Leaves and green part have more nutrients than bulb • Scallion has 140x more phytonutrients than common white onion	• Cook leeks as soon as purchased as they lose nutrients quickly, 3 days max
Lettuce	• More color = more phytonutrients • Look for red, purple, or dark green leaves • Loose-leaf lettuces have more phytonutrients • Best: red loose-leaf, bagged loose-leaf • Good: Bibb and Romaine	• Store: pull off leaves, soak in very cold water, spin dry, place in Ziploc bag removing all air, poke 15 needle holes in bag, place in crisper drawer • Tearing leaves before storing doubles antioxidant value but speeds decay
Melons	• Small seedless watermelons with deep red flesh are more nutritious than larger heirloom varieties • Melons with pale flesh have fewer nutrients than those with intense colors	• Look for watermelons without gloss with yellow ground spot and deep sound when thumped
Onions	• Skins are most nutritious (add to soups when making stock or broth) • Pungent red and yellow onions are more nutritious than sweet, all are high in antioxidant value • The smaller the onion the higher the concentration of phytonutrients • Shallots are more nutritious than most varieties of onions	• Baking, sautéing, and roasting increases quercetin content • Boiling transfers nutrients to liquid • Store in ventilated, cool, dark place
Peaches/ Nectarines	• White-fleshed peaches have 1.5x more antioxidants than yellow • Red-fleshed peaches have 9x more antioxidants than yellow • Eat the skin, it provides the most health benefits, • Buy organic	• Purchase ripe, or nearly ripe fruit

FOOD	HIGHEST NUTRITIONAL VALUE	PURCHASE/PREP/COOKING TIPS
Plums	• Darker the skin color, the more anthocyanin it contains (blue, black, and red are higher in antioxidants than yellow and green) • Dried plums (prunes) one of the most nutritious foods in grocery store	• Purchase ripe or nearly ripe fruit
Pomegranates	• Have special detox enzyme called PON-1 • POM juice has been shown to have antioxidant activity 3x higher than red wine and green tea	• Pick fruits that feel heavy and firm with no soft spots • Can be stored unopened at room temperature for 1 week or in refrigerator wrapped in plastic for 2 months
Potatoes	• Darkest flesh most nutritious (blue first, followed by red) • Skin contains 50 percent antioxidant activity • Choose organic	• Store in cool, dark place • Fresh new potatoes do not raise blood sugar as much as old • Decrease glycemic index by eating with fat, chilling for 24 hours after cooking, or flavoring with vinegar
Spinach	• Whole bunches have more health benefits than bagged leaves • Midsize leaves have more phytonutrients than small or large leaves • 1-week-old has half the antioxidants as freshly harvested	• Steam, do not boil • Store like lettuce • Extra virgin olive oil makes nutrients in greens more bioavailable
Sweet Potatoes	• Deeper the color, higher the antioxidant content • Skin more nutritious than flesh • More nutritious and lower GI than common potatoes	• Steaming, roasting, baking doubles antioxidant content; boiling reduces it
Tomatoes	• Eat whole, skin and seeds provide 50 percent vitamin C, lycopene, and overall antioxidant value • Choose deepest red color • The smaller, the more nutritious - grape, currant, or cherry tomatoes have more lycopene • Canned tomatoes have most lycopene due to heat in canning process, tomato paste 10x more lycopene than raw	• 30 minutes of cooking doubles lycopene content and becomes more absorbable form • Store fresh at room temperature, never refrigerate • Purchase in glass jars or BPA-free cans

Sources: George Mateljan Foundation, The World's Healthiest Foods, www.whfoods.com; Jo Robinson, Eating on the Wild Side; and *J. W. Fahey, Y. Zhang, and P. Talalay, "Broccoli Sprouts: An Exceptionally Rich Source of Inducers of Enzymes that Protect against Chemical Carcinogens," Proceedings of the National Academy of Sciences of the United States of America 94 (September 1997): 10367–10372. https://doi.org/10.1073/pnas.94.19.10367

SUMMING UP: THE FOOD TRIBE MEAL PLAN

The eating philosophy that I prescribe to my patients, as well as the one we practice at home, focuses on nutrient density, microbial balance, and hormonal response. It includes healthy fiber, rich carbohydrates, protein, and fats, along with healing herbs and spices, prebiotic and probiotic foods, and supplements as needed. The Food Tribe approach is not a diet, it's a lifestyle. It's not about being perfect, it's about educating ourselves and doing the best we can for our families. The table below breaks down the types of food that can be readily included in this eating philosophy.

WHOLE FOOD EATING PLAN

PROTEIN 4–6 OZ.		HEALTHY FATS		NON-STARCHY VEGGIES	
• Wild salmon†	• Hormone-/ antibiotic-free turkey	• Cold-pressed extra virgin olive oil †	• Organic coconut milk	• Asparagus	• Celery
• Hormone-/ antibiotic-free chicken	• Wild halibut or flounder	• Grass-fed butter/ ghee	• Avocado†	• Spinach†	• Tomatoes†
• Grass-fed bison or elk	• Wild shrimp/ Scallops	• Seeds (hemp, chia, flax)†	• Dark chocolate	• Cucumbers	• Sea vegetables
• Tofu (fermented organic soy)	• Rainbow trout†	• Nuts & nut butters (walnut, almond, cashew)†	• MCT Oil	• Bell peppers	• Artichokes
• Grass-fed beef	• Lamb	• Virgin coconut oil†	• Cold-pressed avocado oil	• Kale and leafy greens†	• Broccoli†
• Pasture-Raised Eggs	• Venison	• Grass -fed cheese	• Cold-pressed macadamia nut oil	• Cauliflower†	• Green beans
• Sardines/ anchovies†	• Spirulina	• Olives	• Omega-3 fish‡ †	• Brussels sprouts†	• Carrots
	• Nutritional yeast		• Whole Greek yogurt	• Asian mushrooms†	• Bok choy
				• Onions	• Bean sprouts
				• Microgreens	• Cabbage
					• Fennel

STARCHY VEGGIES, LEGUMES		SPROUTED WHOLE GRAINS*		FRUIT	
• Beets†	• Turnips	• Amaranth	• Groats	• All Berries†	• Cantaloupe
• Green peas	• Yams	• Buckwheat	• Wild Rice	• Peach	• Watermelon
• Potatoes	• Pumpkin	• Oats	• Non-GMO corn	• Apple	• Lime
• Rutabaga	• Plantains	• Quinoa	• Black rice	• Kiwi	• Pear
• Sweet potatoes	• Butternut squash	• Brown rice	• Red rice	• Grapefruit	• Pineapple†
• Acorn squash	• Lentils	• Sorghum	• Non-GMO polenta	• Oranges†	• Plum
• Parsnips	• Beans	• Teff	• Einkorn	• Cherries†	• Pomegranate†
	• Yucca	• Millet	• Kamut	• Papaya	• Lemon

BEVERAGES		ANT-INFLAMMATORY SPICES†		PRE- AND PROBIOTIC FOODS	
• Filtered water	• Green vegetable juice	• Turmeric	• Thyme	• Kefir	• Miso†
• Soda water with fresh citrus	• Bone broth†	• Ginger	• Garlic	• Kimchi†	• Gherkin pickles
• Filtered lemon water	• Kombucha†	• Cloves	• Nutmeg	• Kombucha or jun†	• Jerusalem artichoke
• Herbal tea	• Fruit-infused water	• Rosemary	• Mustard	• Sauerkraut†	• Tigernuts
• Green, red, white, black tea†	• Unsweet ice tea	• Cinnamon	• Curry	• Acacia gum (or gum arabic)	• Leeks
• Coconut water	• Club soda with lime	• Oregano	• Cumin	• Unpasteurized pickled veggies	• Raw Jicama
• Green matcha tea†	• Turmeric milk	• Cayenne pepper	• Black pepper	• Raw goat's and sheep's milk cheese	• Green bananas
	• Lemon ginger tea	• Sage	• Basil		• Garlic and onions

† Strong anti-inflammatory foods

‡ Omega-3 Fish = sardines, mackerel, wild salmon, black cod, herring, anchovies. arctic char

Optimum calorie levels differ for everyone based on age, gender, size, activity level, genetics, and microbiome composition. As we become better skilled at choosing the right kinds of foods in the right balance, calorie levels become less important and the food quality becomes paramount. Once you adopt this whole foods eating approach, your natural appetite control kicks in, along with sustained energy and steady blood sugar levels. Our bodies speak to us on a daily basis. We need to carefully listen to their cues to ascertain which foods make us feel the best. Perfect proportions of fats, carbohydrates, and proteins don't exist. But there are essential principles that your family can learn to maximize digestion and optimize microbial balance, and in turn achieve peak health.

Food Tribe Principles

1. **Balance Your Meals.** Balance each meal with lean protein, healthy fats, and fiber-rich vegetables to help keep digestion slow and blood sugar levels steady throughout the day. And balanced blood sugar is the secret ingredient to great energy levels, positive moods, restful sleep, crystal clear focus, healthy weight, and fewer sugar cravings.

2. **Eat mostly plants.** Strive to eat mostly vegetables, preferably the non-starchy kind, at mealtimes—leafy greens are the superstars. Try to eat a rainbow of colors, the deeper the color the better. Fresh or frozen veggies are great choices. Most are best consumed raw or lightly cooked. Eat starchy vegetables such as sweet and white potatoes and whole grains like quinoa in smaller quantities. Serving size is about ½ cup cooked.

3. **Choose well-sourced protein.** Think of meat and animal foods as condiments or a small side instead of the main player at a meal; proteins should make up about a quarter of your plate. Serving size is about the palm of your hand or 4–6 oz. for most lean, grass-fed meats, pasture-raised poultry, and wild-caught, low-mercury fish. Beans and lentils with the right cooking preparation can be a great source of plant-based protein and fiber and are best paired with healthy fat and non-starchy vegetables. Eat in moderate amounts (up to 1 cup a day).

4. **Eat healthy fats every day.** Choose two to four servings of healthy fats per meal. The best sources come from whole foods like avocados, nuts, seeds, olives, eggs, grass-fed butter, ghee, organic virgin coconut oil, fatty fish, and organic coconut milk. A typical serving of fat is 1 tbsp of oil or grass-fed butter, half an avocado, 4 oz. of cold-water fatty fish like salmon,

a handful of nuts or seeds, 1 tbsp nut butter, ¼ cup coconut milk, or 6 olives. Make an effort to include omega-3 fats in your family's diet every day from sources like wild salmon, ground flax, walnuts, and trout.

5. **Eat whole, intact, preferably gluten-free grains.** Buckwheat, quinoa, and wild rice are all good choices, but remember that all grains can raise your blood sugar and insulin levels, so eat them in smaller quantities. I'm partial to gluten-free grains simply because so many people feel better without gluten. (See Appendix A where I thoroughly discuss my concerns with grains and gluten.) Grains are best paired with healthy fat, non-starchy vegetables, and protein. Serving size is about ½ cup. Proper preparation methods like soaking and sprouting are important to lower anti-nutrient load. See chapter 10 for cooking methods.

6. **Enjoy fruit every day.** Choose one to two servings of fresh or frozen whole fruit a day. The average serving size is ½ cup or one piece of fruit. Berries are the best choice. Higher sugar dried fruits, such as dates, raisins, cranberries, and prunes, should be kept to a minimum. Avoid all canned fruit in syrup and fruit juice.

7. **Feed and support your microbiome every day.** As described in chapters 5 and 6, prebiotic and probiotic foods are essential for optimal health. Think about fiber every time you eat. Adults and children should aim for 40–50 g of fiber per day (at least 10 g per meal and 5 g per snack) from foods like peas, lentils, beans, artichokes, leeks, berries, quinoa, chia seeds, Brussels sprouts, and pears. Other resistant starches like unmodified potato starch, chicory, tigernuts, and green banana flour are also excellent choices. Fermented foods also help balance gut bacteria by inoculating and feeding the gut. My family's favorites are kombucha, kimchi, pickles, miso, and kefir made with cashew milk.

8. **Eat foods and spices that fight inflammation.** Chronic inflammation is the source of many, if not most, diseases, and your diet is key to reducing it. Ounce for ounce, herbs and spices are the most potent anti-inflammatory ingredients in your kitchen. Some of the big hitters are cloves, ginger, rosemary, turmeric, cinnamon, and oregano. Other powerful foods include omega-3-rich fats like those found in wild salmon, dark leafy greens such as kale or Swiss

chard, matcha green tea, deeply pigmented fruits like blueberries and pomegranate, Asian mushrooms like shiitake, and garlic. And since most inflammatory diseases start in your gut, it's wise to nourish your microbiome by eating fermented foods like sauerkraut, kombucha, and kimchi or by taking a probiotic supplement.

9. **Drink water.** People underestimate the power of hydration. It's vitally important for keeping your body functioning at its best. If you are not well hydrated, your detoxification pathways become inefficient, your stress hormones increase, fatigue develops, and cravings ensue. Clean, filtered water is optimal, but other decaffeinated beverages like bone broths, kombucha, herbal teas, lemon water, and green vegetable juices are also good choices. A general rule of thumb is to shoot for at least 8 c of fluid a day from both food and water sources. Aim for your urine to be colorless or light yellow.

10. **Avoid foods with pesticides, hormones, antibiotics, GMOs, and artificial food additives.** One of the best ways to avoid toxic ingredients is to buy organic. I realize that organic foods can be expensive, which is why I created my Healthy Eating on a Budget Guide located on my website, www.nicolemagryta.com. As far as food additives go, we need to stop letting the food industry decide what is safe for us to eat. We must read labels and vote with our pocketbooks. Do you really want your kids drinking Mountain Dew with synthetic food dyes (made from petroleum—yes, the same ingredient in gasoline!), high fructose corn syrup, and brominated vegetable oil (flame retardant used in rocket fuel)? More on food additives in chapter 8.

11. **Avoid sugar in all its forms.** It's really important to take inventory of your family's diet and assess the areas where sugar sneaks in. Sugar, refined flour, and processed carbohydrate foods all contribute to rapid spikes in blood sugar and insulin levels. One of the biggest offenders in kids' diets is sugar-sweetened beverages (and cereals are in second place). I always tell parents, if you don't buy it, they won't consume it (at least at home). With a little creativity, we can make healthier sugar swaps for our kids. And when they do want a sugary treat, it's best we teach them to eat sweets sparingly, not every day.

TIPS FOR PANTRY AND KITCHEN MAKEOVER

If you are serious about changing your family's food habits, a pantry and kitchen makeover are essential for success. We know that if kids meander into the pantry after school with a grumble in their tummy, and find cream-filled cookies, cheesy snack foods, multicolor candies, and flavored juice drinks, they will be sure to grab it and gobble it. As discussed, this processed junk food offers your kids zero nutrition. Alternatively, if the selection in the pantry consists of nuts, granola bars, canned fish, beans, fruit, trail mix, organic popcorn, almond butter, oatmeal, and herbal tea, their bellies will be filled with a whole different nutrient profile. The fruit basket on the counter will all of a sudden look more appealing. Removing tempting unhealthy food options from your house is really a game changer. In today's world, snacking accounts for almost 25 percent of your child's daily opportunity to obtain good nourishment. I promise you, that if the pantry is filled with whole foods instead of processed junk, your kids will reach for the good stuff, and they will have a much better chance at meeting their growing bodies' high demand for nutrients.

The makeover starts with taking inventory of everything on your shelves and in your refrigerator and freezer. Read ingredient labels and get rid of any toxic inflammatory foods. Remove food items with chemical additives, preservatives, food dyes, added sugars, and anything made with soybean oil, vegetable oils, or hydrogenated fats. Toss artificial sweeteners, prepackaged baked goods, breakfast cereals, low-fat dairy products, and anything with more than five ingredients on the label. Get rid of sugar-sweetened yogurts, fake butter replacements, and all sweetened beverages like soda, sweet tea, juice, and sports drinks. Imagine creating a food environment that sets up your whole family for success. Then, when cravings strike, nourishment will be exponentially better. Instead of grabbing ice cream, you might make fresh fruit with coconut whipped cream, or instead of grabbing cheese puffs, your kids might satisfy their salt craving with a couple of handfuls of nuts, a pickle spear, olives, or homemade organic popcorn. Here is a look at some of the healthy food items that make up a well-stocked pantry, kitchen, and freezer.

PANTRY AND KITCHEN ESSENTIALS

DRINKS

- Almond, coconut, hemp, or cashew milk, unsweetened (homemade or without carrageenan)
- Raw coconut water
- Coconut milk
- Vegetable juices
- Kombucha/jun
- Unsweet teas
- Herbal, green, white, red or black teas
- Coffee
- Water/sparkling water

WHOLE GRAINS AND PASTA

- Rice (wild, black, brown, red)
- Steel-cut or rolled oats
- Oat groats
- Buckwheat
- Amaranth
- Teff
- Millet
- Sorghum
- Quinoa
- Granola (homemade, low-sugar or bought without PUFAs)
- Sprouted grain cereal (Ezekiel)
- Sprouted grain breads (Ezekiel)
- Quinoa, lentil, or buckwheat pasta
- Sprouted whole-grain, brown rice, GMO-free corn, or gluten-free tortillas

DAIRY AND EGGS

- Organic plain whole-milk yogurt
- Organic whole-milk kefir
- Hormone-free raw cheese
- Eggs (local, pasture-raised or organic)

COUNTER STAPLES

- Fresh fruit
- Assorted nuts

SWEETENERS

- Local raw honey
- Maple syrup (grade B)
- Coconut palm sugar
- Date sugar
- Chicory root syrup
- Stevia
- Monk fruit

SNACKS

- Mary's Gone Crackers and Pretzels
- Bean chips
- Snack bars (Kind Bars, look for less than 6g sugar and >3g fiber)
- Organic popcorn (homemade)
- Trail mix (homemade)
- Seaweed snacks
- 70%+ Dark chocolate
- Dill pickles
- Beef or turkey jerky (grass-fed)
- Salmon jerky (wild)
- Olives

FREEZER FOODS

- Frozen berries and fruit
- Frozen veggies
- Frozen bone broth
- Guacamole
- Pesto
- Grass-fed beef (ground or burgers)
- Veggie burgers (no soy or GMO)
- Acai frozen packets
- Hormone-free chicken tenders
- Frozen turkey meatballs
- Frozen wild shrimp
- Wild-caught salmon
- Sprouted whole grain breads (Ezekiel)
- Gluten-free bread (Three Bakers)
- Sprouted grain tortillas

BEANS AND NUTS

- Beans (adzuki, black, chickpeas, pinto, white northern, cannellini) (BPA-free cans)
- Lentils (red, green, yellow, brown)
- Nuts and seeds, raw (almonds, walnuts, cashews, pistachios, hazelnuts, Brazil nuts, sunflower seeds, sesame seeds, pumpkin seeds, hempseeds, chia seeds, flaxseeds)
- Almond flour
- Coconut flour

OTHER STAPLES

- Smoked wild salmon
- Wild-caught salmon (canned or packet)
- Hummus
- Tahini
- Salsa
- Bone broth
- Low-sodium chicken/veggie broth
- Garlic
- Onions
- Canned coconut milk/cream (BPA-free can)
- Cultured sauerkraut
- Himalayan or Celtic sea salt

SPREADS, DRESSINGS & CONDIMENTS

- Nut or seed butter (almond, cashew, sunflower)
- Marinara sauce
- Mustard
- Balsamic vinegar
- Salsa
- Pesto
- Mayonnaise (made without GMO soybean or canola oils)
- Apple cider vinegar
- Tamari
- Unsweetened coconut flakes
- Raw cacao powder

COLD-PRESSED OILS AND FATS

- Extra virgin olive oil (very low or no heat)
- Grass-fed butter (low heat)
- Grass-fed ghee (high heat)
- Avocado oil (high heat)
- Extra virgin coconut oil (high heat)
- Macadamia oil (low heat)
- Fish oil (as supplement)
- Almond oil (med heat)
- Peanut oil (high heat)
- Walnut oil (no heat)
- Flax oil (no heat)
- Sesame oil (no heat)
- MCT oil (as supplement to food)

DESSERTS AND SWEETS

- Dark chocolate (70%+ cocoa solids)
- Chia pudding
- Smoothie popsicles
- Banana ice cream
- Homemade treats

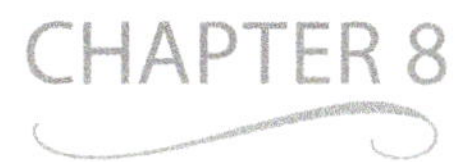

CHAPTER 8

REDUCING YOUR FAMILY'S TOXIC BODY BURDEN

Our grandparents undoubtedly faced their own unique stressors, but they were nothing like the barrage of chemicals, heavy metals, radiation, electromagnetic frequencies, and pollution that batter people today. Although the human body has an innate capacity to detoxify itself, people now are exposed to a level of consumer, agricultural, and industrial toxins that the human organism never evolved to handle.

—Dr. Joseph Pizzorno

*N*ourish Your Tribe is a blueprint for human health and longevity; however, over the last half-century we have learned that nourishing your tribe can also be sabotaged by toxins that have invaded our environment. The research is very clear that excessive toxin exposure plays a significant role in today's chronic disease crisis. The volume of agricultural, industrial, and household toxins introduced in the twentieth century has tipped the balance sheet on our toxic load, and these toxins affect us through all stages of our life cycle. Children are particularly vulnerable because their cells are rapidly developing, and they are exposed to more chemicals per kilogram of body weight. In this chapter, you will learn how toxins damage our bones, our organs, our DNA, our hormones, and modify our gene expression. I will show you that among the fastest and easiest ways to reduce your family's toxic load is to eat whole organic fruits and vegetables, filter water, replace plastic food containers with glass or stainless steel, and avoid large game fish high in mercury, thus altering your children's health trajectory.

Have you ever heard the term chemical body burden? It refers to the total amount of chemicals and pollutants that accumulate in the body and can be detected at any time in blood, urine, and breast milk. Think heavy metals like lead or mercury, synthetic ingredients like food dyes, industrial pollutants like PCBs, or known carcinogens like Monsanto's deadly Roundup. Toxic chemicals are everywhere—in our food, our cooking utensils, and in our plastic drinking containers—and most of us are unaware that we carry toxic compounds in our bodies. It's been estimated that 24 percent of all worldwide diseases are caused by exposure to environmental chemicals.[195] Many experts, such as Dr. Joseph Pizzorno, agree that our toxic body burden is a key factor in many health problems, ranging from asthma and cancer to infertility and endocrine dysfunction.

TOXIN OVERLOAD

It's important to first get a sense of just how many chemicals are now produced and used in society. Five hundred years ago, chemicals where quite limited and for the most part were extracted directly from the natural world through wood, metals, and natural resources. The Industrial Revolution brought many new chemical discoveries, but it wasn't until the twentieth century that rapid development occurred. Over the last 75 years, expansion of pharmaceuticals, synthetics, plastics, solvents, and petrochemicals have exploded into the marketplace. Between 1970 and 1995, the volume of synthetic organic chemicals produced tripled, from about 50 million tons to around 150 million tons. Today we have nearly 84,000 chemicals in commerce in the United States. The volume of chemicals used worldwide is expected to dramatically outpace the increase in population by 2050.[196]

The Majority of Chemicals Are Unregulated

The United States—unlike the European Union—does not have sound laws that protect us from exposure to a multitude of industrial chemicals. In fact, the majority of the 84,000 chemicals that have been allowed on the market have not been tested for safety and are, for the most part, unregulated. For instance, most Americans assume that the chemicals in their shampoos, cosmetics, and household cleaners have been thoroughly tested and proven safe. Unfortunately, they are mistaken. No premarket safety testing is required for the 10,500 industrial chemicals that go into our personal care products.[197]

Testing for industrial chemicals on our food is no better. The USDA does not require any heavy metal testing of our food, regardless of whether the food is organic. Persistent organic pollutants like pesticides, insecticides, and herbicides are also a concern given the volume of use in our food supply. Think for example, of glyphosate, the active ingredient in Monsanto's toxic herbicide Roundup that is used extensively on non-organic crops and is now also being used just prior to harvest to speed plant drying time. Sadly, in the United States, not only do we widely use it on GMO crops, but the EPA's relaxed rules allow 50 times more glyphosate on corn grain now than in 1996.[198]

Another point to consider is that the research we do have on environmental toxins does not paint an accurate picture of our true risk. Most of the research done to date examines only one toxic compound in isolation (and not usually in people). The reality is, we are exposed to endless combinations of chemicals and it's the combined effect that has yet to be assessed.

The Uncontrolled Chemical Experiment in our Bodies

The problem of toxic overload is real. And children and teens are at the greatest risk because their cells are rapidly developing and their bodies are less able to detoxify.[199] Developing babies and infants are particularly vulnerable because they lack a fully developed blood-brain barrier, the structure of the central nervous system that prevents the passage of chemicals between the bloodstream and the neural tissue. Scientific organizations such as the Environmental Working Group were the first in 2004 to test the presence of chemicals in umbilical cord blood from 10 random babies across the country. They made the shocking discovery of 287 industrial chemicals and pollutants in the baby's blood, 180 of which we know cause cancer in humans or animals and 217 that are known to be toxic to the brain and nervous system.[200] For a deeper look into the findings, I strongly encourage you to watch the "10 Americans" presentation given by Ken Cook found at www.ewg.org.

Another study conducted by Mount Sinai School of Medicine found a total of 167 different chemicals in the blood and urine samples of nine volunteers, with each person averaging 91 toxins. The toxins included lead, dioxins, PCBs, phthalates, DEHP, as well as compounds that have been banned for more than a quarter century.[201] Another study done by the US Centers for Disease Control found 148 different chemicals in 2,400 Americans. The report documented bigger doses in children than in adults, the most common being a mixture of pesticides, an automobile toxin called benzoapryene, and oxybenzone (a common toxin in sunscreen).[202]

How Toxins Damage Your Body

When a toxic chemical enters your body, it does not necessarily mean that it will cause harm, because your body has a built-in metabolic detoxification system to eliminate harmful compounds. The liver, intestine, kidneys, lungs, and brain all play important roles in transforming, conjugating, and transporting toxins out of the body. We know that a healthy body can handle a certain number of chemicals, but we don't know what that number is—and it's most likely different for everyone. Today's world exposes us to hundreds of toxins on a daily basis. In fact, we all have some load of toxic chemicals stored in or passing through our bodies.

But it appears that the rate at which new chemicals are introduced is faster than our bodies can adapt. Even the healthiest of bodies may have trouble filtering out the tremendous volume of present-day toxins. In the past, toxin concern was reserved for those we knew had occupational exposure, such as coal miners. Today is a completely different environment. We are the canaries in the coal mine because of our exposure to toxins in modern society. We store them in our bones, in our brain, in our blood, and in our fat. They have the ability to alter our genes, leaving us vulnerable to a variety of diseases and disorders.

Here are three significant ways toxins impair the body's functions:

1. **Toxins damage our organs.** Of particular concern are our own detoxification organs: gastrointestinal tract, liver, and kidneys. If they are impaired, we cannot heal and recover from environmental insults.

2. **Toxins damage DNA and modify gene expression.** Epigenetics has taught us that our genes are switched on and off by environmental influences. Many toxins activate or suppress our genes that result in unwanted conditions.

3. **Toxins interfere with hormones and undermine countless bodily functions.** Toxins can imitate hormones, increase or decrease production of certain hormones, and interfere with hormone signaling. Your endocrine system is an elegantly interconnected network of chemical messengers. Even tiny amounts of hormone disturbance can have huge effects in the body. Endocrine-disrupting chemicals have been linked to reproductive disorders, endometriosis, adrenal imbalances, thyroid issues, insulin resistance, diabetes, obesity, and a variety of cancers.

TIPS TO REDUCE TOXIC BODY BURDEN

Toxins exist everywhere. They are in our air, food, water, furniture, household cleaners, children's toys, plastic containers, building materials, and the list goes on. There is a push-pull between nutrients and toxins in the body. We need to do everything we can to minimize the toxin influence so that the scale is not unfairly weighted. I feel compelled to go beyond the scope of food in this chapter as this topic is critical to the development of human disease. So the question is, what can we do, personally and as a society, to reduce our burden of exposure? The laws that are in place to ensure our safety against exposure to commercial chemicals are pathetically ineffective, to say the least. The long-term solution involves a collective effort among citizens to rise up and demand better regulation of chemicals in our environment. In the meantime, there are tangible steps we can all take to help reduce our exposure. While we cannot control industrial smokestacks pumping out volatile organic compounds or BPA on grocery store receipts, we can control the items we purchase, the products we ingest and put on our skin, and the chemicals we allow in our homes. Although it can all seem daunting, this information is meant to empower you with knowledge rather than overwhelm you. What follows are suggested ways you can begin to reduce your family's toxic body burden.

> *Why should you care about pesticides? According to the Environmental Working Group (EWG), there is a growing consensus in the scientific community that small doses of pesticides and other chemicals can have adverse effects on health, especially during vulnerable periods such as fetal development and childhood.*
>
> —Dr. Andrew Weil at drweil.com

- **Eat organic.** From a toxic exposure standpoint, there's no doubt that organic foods are healthier. They protect us from consuming herbicides, pesticides, antibiotics, and hormones. Each year, the EWG produces its *Shoppers' Guide to Pesticides in Produce*, which reports fruits and vegetables with the highest pesticide load. Here you will find a single strawberry sample can harbor up to 22 different pesticide residues and spinach can harbor relatively high concentrations of permethrin, a neurotoxic insecticide banned in Europe. You can lower your pesticide intake substantially by buying organic versions of fruits and vegetables on their list. Or better yet, grow them organically yourself. Included here is EWG's 2018 results of their "Dirty Dozen" and "Clean 15" lists. Conventional meat and dairy foods are also high in environmental contaminants like synthetic growth hormones, antibiotics, and pesticides. Choose pasture-raised, organic, grass-fed varieties. Or better yet, get to know your local farmers who practice humane chemical-free farming, and buy directly from them.

Top 12 Produce with Highest Pesticides*	Top 15 Produce with Fewest Pesticides*
1. Strawberries	1. Avocados
2. Spinach	2. Sweet corn
3. Nectarines	3. Pineapples
4. Apples	4. Cabbages
5. Grapes	5. Onions
6. Peaches	6. Frozen sweet peas
7. Cherries	7. Papayas
8. Pears	8. Asparagus
9. Tomatoes	9. Mangos
10. Celery	10. Eggplants
11. Potatoes	11. Honeydew melons
12. Sweet bell peppers	12. Kiwi
	13. Cantaloupes
	14. Cauliflower
	15. Broccoli

Visit the EWG's web page to get updated lists each year at www.ewg.org.

◆ **Eat foods high in antioxidants and plant polyphenols.** Consume bright-colored fruits and vegetables (try to eat a rainbow of colors), green and white teas, and herbs and spices like ginger, turmeric, garlic, cinnamon, oregano, and rosemary. Cruciferous vegetables like broccoli, bok choy, cauliflower, Brussels sprouts, and broccoli sprouts are enormously detoxifying. Their sulfur-containing chemicals produce glutathione, a powerhouse antioxidant.

◆ **Eat iodine-rich foods.** Iodine deficiency increases our vulnerability to the effects of certain environmental pollutants, such as nitrate (found in contaminated well-water), thiocyanate (in cigarette smoke), and perchlorate (in drinking water).[203] Adequate iodine intake is necessary to produce thyroid hormone, which is particularly important for pregnant or lactating moms because thyroid hormone is required for healthy brain development in children. Check with your healthcare provider to see if you are deficient. Good dietary sources of iodine include sea vegetables such as kelp, cranberries, wild-caught cod, Greek yogurt, navy beans, pastured eggs, and organic strawberries.

◆ **Limit your intake of rice.** The levels of arsenic found in certain foods, such as rice, are alarming and carry a risk for adults, and even more so for children and pregnant moms. Between 2012 and 2014, Consumer Reports tested 128 samples of basmati, jasmine, and sushi rice as well as reviewed FDA data on various rice products and found that one 2-oz. serving of rice pasta or 2 c of rice milk puts a child over the weekly limit of arsenic. And only two ¼-cup servings of most types of rice puts an adult at their weekly limit.[204] Regular exposure to low doses of inorganic arsenic over time has been shown to cause a variety of cancers, diabetes, cardiovascular disease, reproductive problems, impaired brain development, and a compromised immune system.

To minimize your exposure choose alternative grains with lower arsenic risk like quinoa, millet, or amaranth. Do not feed infants or children under five years of age (or pregnant moms) rice products, including infant rice cereals, rice milk, rice crackers, rice pasta, rice cakes, or whole grain rice. Brown rice generally has 80 percent more arsenic than white because arsenic accumulates in the grain's outer layers, which are removed when processed into white. Brown rice, however, has more nutrients, so if you do choose to eat rice products occasionally, eat no more than twice per week and choose brown basmati or white rice products from regions known to have lower arsenic levels such as California, India, or Pakistan. Organic rice does not offer protection from arsenic. You can reduce 50–80 percent of the arsenic in rice by using a traditional Asian cooking method: soak rice overnight and rinse. Then cook 1 cup of rice in 5 c of water, and drain the excess water afterward.

◆ **Invest in a high-quality water filter.** Water quality issues are very real in the United States. Under the 1976 Safe Drinking Water Act, only 91 contaminants are mandated to be regulated. The problem is, there are now over 85,000 approved chemicals on the market. This translates into 84,909 unregulated chemicals potentially in our water. Contaminants like fluoride, chlorine, lead, mercury, PCBs, arsenic, perchlorate, dioxins, nitrates, micro-plastics, and MTBE (a gasoline additive) are a few of the nastier contaminants that still manage to make it into our glasses. If you want safe, clean water for your family, regardless of whether your water comes from an in-ground well or from the city, invest in a water filtration system. Carbon filters are a good choice, but an even better option is a reverse osmosis filter or an under-the-counter multi-stage filter. A great guide to help you choose the best filter can be found at www.ewg.org. Also carry your filtered water in a glass or stainless steel container.

- **Drink plenty of water.** Once you've filtered your water, drink a lot of it! Not only does water keep your body and your cells hydrated, but it helps move waste products and toxins out of the body.

- **Sweat!** It's the best all-natural method for detoxification. Exercise, steam room, infrared saunas, or relax in a hot Epsom-salt bath.

- **Place plants in your home.** Indoor air pollution is most commonly caused by adhesives, carpets, paper products, furniture, household cleaners, paint, and pressed-wood products. NASA studied houseplants in an effort to find the most effective common indoor plants for filtering harmful toxins and pollutants from the air. They found that certain plants were better at filtering the air and removing volatile organic compounds (VOCs) than others. Plants can reduce many air pollutants such as formaldehyde, microbial pathogens, ammonia, and benzene.[205] NASA research suggests having at least 1 plant per 100 square feet of home. Some of the most beneficial plants include aloe, spider plants, English ivy, peace lily, snake plant, rubber plant, golden pothos, Boston fern, and palms (bamboo, date, and lady varieties).

- **Switch to eco-friendly cleaning products.** Children and pets have been shown to have the highest levels of many harmful chemicals in their bodies. It's not surprising given that they are constantly close to the ground and have a lot of hand-to-mouth behaviors, which make them more vulnerable to exposure. The EWG has an excellent "Guide to Healthy Cleaning" on their website at https://www.ewg.org/guides/cleaners. Brands like Aspen, Attitude, BuggyLove, Fit Organic, and Green Shield routinely get high marks. As eco-friendly products tend to be more costly, a more economical solution is to make your own cleaning products with essential oils. A good resource for recipes is www.motherearthliving.com.

- **Reevaluate your personal care products.** About 60 percent of what we put on our skin is absorbed into our bloodstream. From lead in lipstick and mascara to phthalates in creams and deodorants to oxybenzone in sunscreens, we have enormous toxic exposure. Teenagers in fact use more personal care products than any other market. I highly advise women and teen girls to switch to tampons made with organic cotton. Ninety percent of the non-organic cotton in the United States has been genetically modified, which means it's been sprayed with glyphosate. Tampons also contain dioxins—chemical by-products of the bleaching process that are categorized as a "known human carcinogen" by the WHO. Fragrances in tampons are also a concern because their formulas are considered "trade secrets" and have been known to contain dozens of chemicals linked to hormone disruption. The vagina is a highly permeable space which allows toxins to be readily absorbed into the bloodstream. Cumulative monthly exposures to a cocktail of chemicals (placed directly in our bodies) over time presents many health risks. Go to EWG's Skin Deep website at https://www.ewg.org/skindeep to explore safe personal care products and harmful ingredients.

- **Avoid canned foods with BPA.** Bisphenol A is a synthetic estrogen found in the lining of food cans and is a known endocrine disruptor, which has the potential to affect virtually all aspects of the body's metabolism and function. When you eat canned soup from a BPA-coated container, you increase BPA levels more than tenfold.[206] The EWG website reports which companies use BPA in their packaging. Some popular BPA-free brands include Amy's, Earth's Best, Health Valley, Native Forest, and Imagine.

- **Get rid of plastics.** Plastic containers leach endocrine-disrupting chemicals like BPA into the food and liquids we store them in, especially when heated. Recycle plastic water bottles and plastic storage containers and replace with glass or stainless steel. If you need to reheat foods do not use plastic steam bags or plastic containers often found in packaged frozen foods. Transfer food to glass or stainless steel and reheat.

- **Avoid large game fish high in mercury.** This is the number one cause of mercury exposure in America due to air and water pollution settling in our oceans. Avoid big species of fish like king mackerel, marlin, orange roughy, shark, swordfish, tilefish, and tuna. Eating smaller fish lower on the food chain is best, such as wild salmon, wild flounder, anchovies, or sardines.

- **Avoid GMO foods.** By design, GMO foods are coated with chemical herbicides and pesticides. The top GMO foods are corn, soy, canola, alfalfa, sugar beets, cotton, papaya, summer squash/zucchini, and meat from animals fed GMOs. Apples and potatoes are the newest members to the list, with even more worrisome genetic modification risks using double-stranded RNA technology.

- **Throw out non-stick pans.** Toxic fumes from non-stick pans like Teflon occur when pans are used on high heat, particularly over 350°F. The non-stick chemicals, called perfluoroalkyls, used on these pans break down and absorb into the foods we cook and eat. They are made using fluorine, an element that takes decades to break down in our bodies and has been shown to cause cancer in laboratory animals.[207] Instead, choose 18/8 food-grade stainless steel or cast-iron for stove-top cooking or glass, ceramic, or stainless steel for oven baking.

- **Use safe cooking methods.** Cooking meat and fish (as in grilling, broiling, or pan frying) at very high temperatures, particularly above 300°F, can lead to the creation of dangerous carcinogenic compounds called heterocyclic amines (HCAs), polycyclic aromatic hydrocarbons (PAHs), and advanced glycation end products (AGEs). Essentially, the hotter and longer a meat is cooked, the more HCAs, PAHs and AGEs.[208] The best ways to reduce these DNA-damaging compounds include; adopt slower, indirect-heat cooking methods such as stewing, braising, boiling, steaming or poaching; turn meat often over a high-heat source to reduce HCA exposure; avoid burning, charring or cooking meat to well done; marinate your meat before you cook it in an acidic mixture such as lemon juice or vinegar; and add spices to your meat prior to cooking at high temperatures. Rosemary, in particular, has been found to significantly reduce the production of HCAs in beef cooked at high temperatures.[209]

- **Eat probiotic-rich foods or consider supplementation.** Probiotic bacteria are capable of helping your body detoxify some of the most highly toxic chemicals in our environment. For example, two common probiotic strains, *Bifidobacterium breve* and *Lactobacillus casei*, have been shown to reduce absorption of BPA and enhance its excretion.[210] It's also well known that probiotic bacteria, such as Lactobacilli, bind heavy metals, preventing their entry into the body. Research has shown many other examples of bacteria strains that are capable of reducing our toxin exposure. Make an effort to eat probiotic-rich foods like kimchi, sauerkraut, kefir, and kombucha so they can go to work for you. If you choose a daily probiotic supplement instead, make sure you consume it with nourishing prebiotic foods.

◆ **Make sure you and your kids poop every day.** One or two well-formed bowel movements a day is essential to remove toxins from the body. Take this seriously! Address constipation with dietary changes like increasing fiber and water intake and reducing dairy consumption. If you are unsure what a healthy stool should look like, look up Bristol Stool Scale to view pictures of a well-formed poop.

AVOID FOOD ADDITIVES: READ FOOD LABELS

Since the average American spends the majority of their food budget on processed foods, it's safe to say that exposure to artificial food additives is quite high. Food additives are used to extend shelf life, improve appearance, and ease processing. There are so many foreign substances on food labels that it's hard to know which ones are safe. Here are my top 10 food additives to avoid.

Food Dyes

All the FDA-approved food dyes are chemicals derived from petroleum (crude oil), which as you likely know, is also the source of gasoline. Artificial food colors (AFCs)—Red 40 and Yellow 5 and 6 are the most widely used—are found in a wide assortment of foods like sports drinks, sodas, fruit-flavored drinks, energy drinks, candy, ready-to-eat cereals, desserts, snack foods, salad dressings, butter, skins of fruit, casings of hot dogs, any packaged food, and even toothpaste and pediatric medications. Once you start to read labels more carefully, you will be alarmed at the variety of products that contain food dyes. Children's Motrin and bouillon cubes are two that surprised me.

Food dyes add zero nutritional value to the foods we eat, trigger behavior and learning problems in some children, and potentially carry a cancer risk. American processed foods contain much greater concentrations today than they did 50 years ago. Remove them from your family's diet. Investigate food labels, eat whole foods, cook food at home, and spread the word about the potential impact of food dyes on children's ability to learn.

Another contributing factor to higher consumption of AFCs is the significant increase in processed junk food available on our grocery store shelves. In 1970 supermarkets carried an average of 7,800 items compared with 43,844 items in 2013, according to a report by the Food Marketing Institute. The increase reflects the enormous expansion of processed junk food, much of which contains food dyes.

I grew up eating processed food with food coloring and I turned out just fine. What's changed?

My favorite frozen treat as a kid was the Bomb Pop, with stripes of red cherry, white lime, and blue raspberry. The excitement came at the end, when my tongue turned a solid dark blue. I'm sure you recall similar childhood favorites. Perhaps what is most concerning about such treats is that an FDA report shows the total amount of dyes certified by the FDA has increased *five-fold* in the last 60 years—from 12 mg/per capita/per day in 1950 to 68 mg/per capita/per day in 2012.

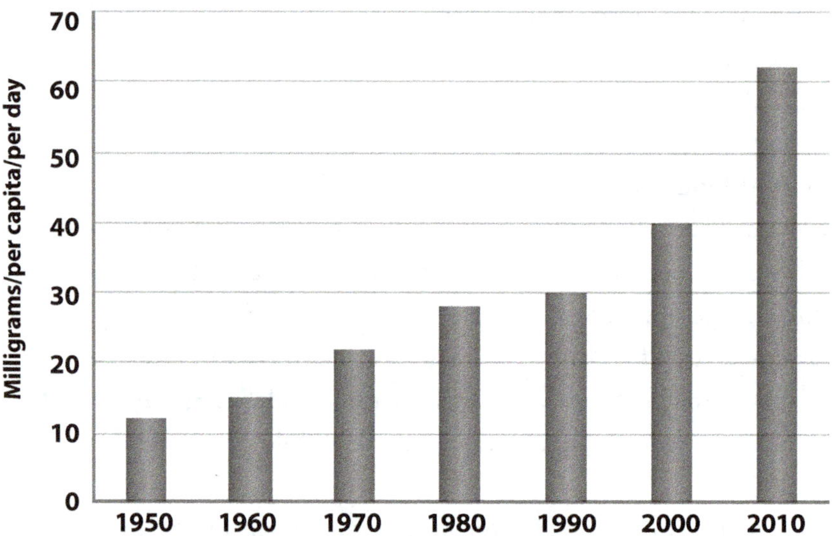

Trends in the amount of artificial food colors manufactured for the US market since 1950 as certified by the FDA for three common food colors and the total of all colors

Source: Laura J. Stevens et al., "Amounts of Artificial Food Colors in Commonly Consumed Beverages and Potential Behavioral Implications for Consumption in Children," Clinical Pediatrics 53, no. 2 (Feb 2014): 133-40, https://doi.org/10.1177%2F0009922813502849.

Lastly, concentrations of AFCs per serving have increased in individual products in the United States, specifically in candy, cereals, and baked goods—much of which is marketed specifically to our children. For example, Generals Mills decided Trix cereal, introduced in 1955, needed a newer, brighter look in 1995, so the company increased Yellow 6, Blue 1, and Red 40, which now account for a whopping 36 mg of AFCs per serving. And what growing kid eats just a

1-cup serving of this stuff? None that I know. Cap'n Crunch Oops! All Berries cereal, introduced in 1997, contains four times the amount of AFCs as the Original Cap'n Crunch version, which I unfortunately ate as a kid in the late 1970s.

Behavioral studies show that a greater proportion of children react to doses greater than 50 mg and that younger children are more reactive than older children.[211] A real-life scenario makes it easy to comprehend how an average American child can consume a considerable amount of food dye each day: Fruity Cheerios (31.8 mg) for breakfast; Yoplait Strawberry Kiwi Yogurt (4.5 mg) and Kraft Macaroni and Cheese (17.6 mg) for lunch; Keebler Cheese & Peanut Butter Crackers (14.4 mg) and Fruit Roll Ups (3 mg) for snacks; Hamburger Helper for Dinner (7.7 mg), Orange Powerade (55 mg) and 2 Little Hug Grape Juices (30.8 mg) to drink; and a couple handfuls of M&Ms (29.5 mg), and their daily AFC total could be over 200 mg (and more than 115 g of sugar)!

Interestingly, in 2009, Britain's Food Standards Agency (our FDA counterpart) asked food companies to voluntarily ban the use of six common synthetic food dyes (which included the three dyes most widely used in the United States). A year later the European Parliament also enforced a labeling requirement on all products containing dyes to carry a warning label that reads: "May have adverse effect on activity and attention in children." Since then, many American-based companies now make two different versions of their products so that they can be sold in Europe and the United States. Companies like Kellogg's use Red 40, Yellow 6, and Blue 1 to color their Pop Tarts in the United States, but in the UK you will find only natural colorings of beet juice, annatto, and paprika. This sort of comparison goes on and on with sodas, packaged goods, candies, and more.

Artificial Sweeteners

Whether you are using artificial sweeteners to prevent sugar spikes or to avoid calories, they are doing far more harm than good. They are found everywhere from candy and breakfast cereals to processed foods and beverages. They also surprisingly show up in children's vitamins and liquid medicines. It's essential to read labels in order to avoid them. Some of the most common artificial sweeteners are aspartame (NutraSweet, Equal), neotame, saccharin (Sweet 'N Low, Sweet Twin), sucralose (Splenda), erythritol, sorbitol, xylitol, maltitol, and acesulfame potassium (Sunette, Ace K).

New research has confirmed three significant reasons to avoid these ingredients: 1) they confuse the body's hormone signaling, causing increased insulin production, storing more fat, and slowing metabolism; 2) they can become addictive and actually cause us to crave more sweets; and 3) they disrupt our microbiome [212](by far the most important reason to avoid them). Artificial sweeteners shift the balance toward harmful bacteria that increase our risk for diabetes and obesity. If that information doesn't seal the deal to avoid them, I don't know what else can.

For a safer alternative, choose all-natural sweeteners including stevia, monk fruit, raw local honey, or maple syrup in moderation. Make sure to look for pure organic stevia leaf in powder or liquid form. Avoid highly refined varieties (like Truvia) that have been chemically processed and contain added bulking agents like maltodextrin (corn) and "natural flavors."

High Fructose Corn Syrup (HFCS)

As described in chapter 2, HFCS is a chemically processed, refined-sugar product that's been pumped into a plethora of processed foods: sodas, baked goods, jams, candies, crackers, and dairy products. This artificial syrup is derived from genetically modified corn and is made up of both fructose and glucose. For most of human history, we consumed no more than 15 g (3 tsp) of fructose a day from natural fruit.[213] Today that number is up to 82 g (19.5 tsp) a day due to our overindulgent consumption of HFCS products.[214] Unlike glucose, excessive fructose is solely and rapidly metabolized in the liver and stored as fat, leading to chronic health problems such as obesity, insulin resistance, pancreatic cancer, and heart disease.[215] This ingredient should be avoided at all costs. The best alternatives to HFCS are natural sweeteners like dates, bananas, raw local honey, maple syrup, blackstrap molasses, pure whole-leaf stevia, and coconut sugar.

MSG

Commonly known for its presence in Chinese food, monosodium glutamate—commonly known as MSG—is an amino acid used as a flavor enhancer in a number of processed foods like soy sauce, soups, chips, bouillon cubes, stock, canned foods, prepared meals, and fast food. The real bonus for companies that use this ingredient is the substance not only makes the food irresistible, but it also allows them to reduce the amount of real ingredients in their food. MSG is a known excitotoxin, which means it excites neurons in the brain and has shown in studies to cause neuron death. There is no doubt that some people are sensitive to MSG, causing instant headache, nausea, vomiting, dizziness, pain in the back of the neck, and heart palpitations.

Although glutamates occur naturally in some foods like dried mushrooms and soy, when they're consumed as free unbound MSG, the body may handle them differently. As with all nutrients, when glutamates are packaged with fiber and other food components, the body is naturally inclined to manage its digestion. It is also thought that only small amounts of MSG can cross the blood-brain barrier, but now that we know "leaky brains" exist, it's very possible that this substance is causing much more harm than once believed. MSG is hidden under many different ingredient names on food labels. Here are a few common ones: autolyzed yeast, hydrolyzed protein, yeast extract, natural flavoring, and glutamic acid.

BHA and BHT

It's always shocking to hear of preservatives that are banned around the world, yet the United States drags its *regulatory* feet with the attitude, "It's only a *probable* carcinogen." Why not adopt a precautionary principle to protect consumers until we know for certain that these chemicals are safe? Why not demand that companies actually use known safer alternatives that work just as well? The European Union classifies BHA (or butylated hydroxyanisole) as an endocrine disrupter, but it's also been shown to lower testosterone, thyroid hormones, and alter sperm quality.[216] BHT (or butylated hydroxytoluene) is also to be avoided for the same reasons. There are much safer options for companies to use, such as vitamin E as a natural replacement. Avoid these two processed food preservatives along with TBHQ and propyl gallate. They are found in the cereal aisle, but are also found in chips, preserved meats, and chewing gum.

Potassium Bromate

This food additive by itself is a known carcinogen. Countries all over the world, including Canada, those in the European Union, and the UK have banned its use, but Japan and the United States are still not budging. The state of California has even listed potassium bromate as a known carcinogen. Potassium bromate has long been used to improve the structure of baked goods like bread and rolls. Some proponents say that once bread is baked, potassium bromate is converted to non-carcinogenic potassium bromide. A 1994 UK study disproved this claim by showing significant detectable amounts in commercial baked bread products.[217] Look for this ingredient in all bread and flour products, including frozen pizza crusts and processed baked goods.

Artificial and Natural Flavors

These two terms on a nutrition label tell us absolutely nothing about what's actually in a product. It's simply a sneaky way for food manufacturers to add in cheap toxic ingredients such as synthetic chemicals (like propylene glycol), preservatives (like BHA), and glutamine by-products (like MSG). Legally, food companies can use these vague terms to keep from disclosing almost any ingredient they want. In fact, the term "natural flavors" could represent over 100 substances on a single package, many of which are designed to hijack your taste buds and manipulate your appetite. Stay away from foods with these terms on their labels, unless you want to play chemical roulette with your body. Certified "organic natural flavors" labels will provide protection from synthetic and GMO ingredients.

Carrageenan

This red seaweed derivative is used in thousands of products as a thickening, gelling, and stabilizing agent. The food industry uses carrageenan in a wide array of products, such as dairy, dairy alternatives, jelly, infant formula, salad dressing, deli meat, frozen dinners, and toothpaste. Although the ingredient is a controversial topic, independent researchers like Joanne K. Tobacman, MD, have shown that exposure to carrageenan causes inflammation and that the amounts in food products are enough to cause harm.[218] The Cornucopia Institute also agrees: "Animal studies have repeatedly shown that food-grade carrageenan causes gastrointestinal inflammation and higher rates of intestinal lesions, ulcerations, and even malignant tumors."[219] It's also hard to ignore the numerous people that have reported improvement in gastrointestinal symptoms once they eliminated this substance. I suggest erring on the safe side and avoiding this ingredient altogether.

This chapter on toxins and how to minimize exposure to them is weighty, I know. But it's because of their pervasiveness that we need to arm ourselves with the sort of information I've presented here so that we can better protect our families. Obtaining optimum health for your family is not so complicated, it just takes educating yourself about our modern-day environment. If we give our bodies what they need, fill in our nutritional deficiencies, and remove from our bodies what harms them, meaning toxins, the body will heal itself and thrive.

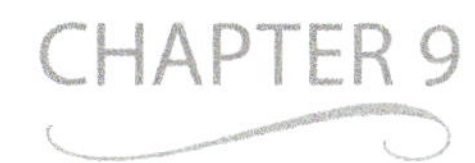

"JUST ONE MORE BITE":
Eating Behaviors and Strategies to Encourage Healthy Choices

It is not what you do for your children, but what you have taught them to do for themselves that will make them successful human beings.

—Ann Landers

One of the curses of modern parenting is the picky eater. The kid's meal and kid-friendly foods have stacked the deck against the parent and home cooking. We know that it's our job as parents to model and teach our kids healthy habits as they grow. In this chapter you will learn that an authoritative parenting style produces the most positive outcome when feeding kids. This type of parenting reads kids' cues, has a high degree of control, but is also responsive and nurturing. It's important that two-parent households work as a team and that all parents model good behaviors, but also that they learn how to deliver a positive message without showing anger and frustration at every meal. A healthy, nourished family requires parents to learn basic cooking skills and adopt some tricks of the trade. By the end of this chapter, you will be empowered to succeed and sleep well at night knowing that you have set your tribe up for optimal health and wellness.

Nutrition is one of the most important modifiable factors that can significantly affect a child's brain development, immune function, gut health, and behavior. As parents today, we need reminding of this. Nurturing nutritional well-being and health is a lifelong process, with each phase influencing the next. Food and health connect children to life, and we need to prepare them for the world that lies before them. Teaching children good nutrition also teaches them how to respect their most precious gifts: their minds and their bodies so that they can survive the world's diverse stressors. A well-nourished body is fundamental to peak performance, no matter where you live or what line of work you choose. Imagine if you had been taught healthy self-loving behaviors as a child and were taught to listen to your body and respond wisely to its messages. Might you have a different relationship with food today? One of my goals for my children is to empower them with the wisdom to nourish themselves with healing foods and to be consciously aware of their bodies' messages. What a gift these would be to our next generation of children!

SHIFTING PERCEPTION

In my line of work, I hear many reasons, roadblocks, and justifications from parents as to why they feed their children poor-quality food. Here are a few of the more common statements:

"My kids are so picky, all they will eat is pizza, cheese, bread, and crackers. There is really nothing else I can do."

"My kids are 'fine.' They eat broccoli and carrots at dinnertime."

"They don't like what my husband and I eat each night, so I prepare them a 'kid-friendly' meal."

"Frankly, at the end of the day, I'm just too tired to argue with my kids about what they eat."

"My husband has a horrible diet and my kids eat just like he does."

"I cannot afford healthy food."

"I give them a good multivitamin every day, so they are covered."

"I have four kids, and there's just no way I can manage all their eating habits."

"I ate crap when I was young, but look at me now, I turned out okay."

I realized that after hearing responses like this over and over, parents' perspectives on nourishment can be skewed. Now that you've read about how necessary healthy nourishment is, how can we give it as much attention and reinforcement as we give good manners and good study habits? I'll be the first to tell you it's not easy. Frankly it's difficult. But what part of *good* parenting is easy? Parents first need to understand that changes, though challenging, are worth it. I trust that by now you have a better understanding of our broken modern food environment and how it negatively affects our children's built-in impulses and shapes our culture-wide acceptance of suboptimal nourishment.

Even if your child is plotting a steady curve on their growth chart, it does not mean they are nutritionally sound. In other words, growth is not a good measure for a healthy immune system, a well-functioning mind, or a healthy digestive tract that resists disease. When I think of my family's nourishment, I ask questions such as, "What harm are unhealthy chemical fillers doing to my children's lifelong gut health and metabolic processes? What effect does chronic exposure to inflammatory foods like refined sugar, white flour, processed chemicals, and HFCS have on my family's overall health? How can food defend against the damage of increased environmental toxins? Does the food my children eat significantly alter their behavior or attention capacity, cause headaches or stomachaches? How are my kid's food choices affecting their academic performance? Are they optimally nourished during the most critical periods of rapid growth? What lifelong nourishment lessons am I teaching my kids by modeling poor food choices? Do I model disease avoidance or promotion?" These types of questions help us look at the bigger picture of nourishment and the significance it plays in the growth and development of a modern-day child.

Here is my best advice: Don't follow the masses! Don't conform to what Americans are choosing to eat just because that's our norm. It's killing us and crippling our kids' health. What are we teaching the soccer team when we give them cupcakes and Capri Sun after a game? Does your dentist give out lollipops to kids after their appointments? Mine does. (And I don't feel better knowing they are sugar-free.) It's simply modeling a sugar prize after a potentially stressful event, not to mention the contradictory message it sends from a dental health professional.

Be brave. Set an example for your fellow soccer moms, your colleagues at work, your siblings, or your child's school teachers. Don't let other people's actions determine how you feed your children. The fractured food world outside your home is largely uninformed, wildly hectic, manipulative for profit, and suffering. Thankfully, there is a growing chorus of health experts, parents, scientists, and policy makers that is starting to create positive change. Pay attention to their messages, because the health of our next generation depends on it.

So by now you may be thinking, "Okay lady, I screwed up the younger years: I gave in to my kids' tantrums, I asked the wrong questions, and I fed my kids junk. Now what do I do?" First, don't beat yourself up. I made many mistakes too. Parenting is a learning journey for all of us. The most important thing is your attitude moving forward. No matter what your child's age, there are always opportunities to improve your food culture at home. I promise it's not an impossible feat. It just takes the same persistence and effort that you put towards all the rest of your parenting goals. You are your children's greatest teacher. It's not your job to please them all the time and make their life easy. It's your job to love them and teach them the skills to become independent adults who will know how to nourish themselves well, and eventually, perhaps their own children also.

The next three sections in this chapter outline the key factors to create a healthy food tribe at home. First is understanding a little more about the physical and psychological nature of kids when it comes to food and eating. Second is the importance of bringing awareness and consistency to your and your spouse's feeding styles. And third is empowering you, as parents, with solutions to help end mealtime struggles and navigate our crazy modern food culture.

KIDS' EATING BEHAVIORS

I will never forget feeding my son's first taste of solid food. His face lit up like a Christmas tree as he gobbled the pureed sweet potatoes off the spoon. It's not uncommon to hear stories about one-and-a-half-year-old babies who gobble up any kind of food that's placed on their trays. It's somewhere between two and four years old when this happy food frenzy stops in its tracks. It's not a coincidence that feeding struggles begin at the same time toddlers are introduced to processed foods, sweeteners, and salt. When it comes to taste, whole food from nature can never compete with processed food that's been engineered to encourage addiction. This is an important fact to remember when you are introducing new foods.

Eating is a developmental process for toddlers. They reach an age where having control in their world is important. They have little understanding of how other people feel and are motivated almost entirely by their own desires. So when young Johnny's mother asks him to give up his diapers or eat his broccoli, Johnny robustly refuses. Elimination and eating are probably the two activities that toddlers have the most control over. Although this is normal in development, parents often worry as frustration, anxiety, and power struggles become more prevalent. It's important to remember that, if you haven't already passed the toddler years with your children, this phase will pass as your child develops cognitively. But how you as a parent handle this stage of eating will be critical in shaping your child's food habits later on in childhood.

Developing Taste Buds

At the tender age of four, Johnny, and probably most of his posse at preschool, have an innate preference for sweet foods and an intolerance for bitter foods. This taste preference was actually quite useful in the days when our ancestors foraged for food: bitter meant poisonous and sweet meant safe. While there are good evolutionary reasons for this preference because some bitter plants contain alkaloid toxins, there are many plants that don't, particularly vegetables. In fact, compounds such as glucosinolates and phenolics found in vegetables like broccoli and kale, contribute to the taste of bitterness but are actually the same compounds that act as antioxidants, protecting against cell damage. So we still need to teach Johnny that vegetables are important and are vital to growing well and strong. As Johnny's parent, it's your responsibility to teach him which foods are safe and important, just as you would have done foraging for food a century ago.

Food Neophobia

Let's face it, when it comes to food, many kids are neophobic (experience a fear of new things). Studies have found that food neophobia actually reaches its peak between the ages of two and six years, when rejection of vegetables and new flavors peak. Neophobia might be another evolutionary survival tactic. My son, at age 10, still had this character trait going strong. I made a bean dish in the crockpot with healthy local chicken sausage and spinach that I thought he'd be sure to love. It had ingredients he likes with seasonings he was used to. He took one look at the new entree and literally jumped out of his seat. After a half-hour of discussion, pouting and antics, and a rumble of his tummy, he decided to try it. He couldn't hide his smile. He was actually slightly embarrassed to admit how much he liked it. The next morning, he asked for it in his lunchbox. New food acceptance does not always follow this pattern; in fact, as you probably know, it can often lead to much more arguing from a child. Sometimes it ends with flat-out refusal of the food.

Here's what you may not know: research tells us that children may have to be introduced to a new food as many as 12–15 times before they develop a taste for it. As frustrating as that might sound, food refusal is a natural part of a child's growth and development. It's our job as parents to teach and model new food acceptance, just as we would teach our children to say thank you, which also requires time and a lot of repetition.

Picky Eaters

If words could exhaust their usefulness, the term "picky eater" would be removed from our vocabulary. This overused term describes an era of children who are being raised in a toxic food environment by parents who have unwittingly conformed to our cultural food norms. The term has become an excuse—a "get-out-of-jail-free card"—for parents and pediatricians to allow unhealthy eating to progress throughout childhood. Let me be clear: children are picky by nature. Food preferences are developed by trial and error. Children will learn to eat and accept new foods because we guide them to.

But there is more to the story. As mentioned, kids' taste buds and brains are wired to hunt down sweet and avoid bitter. So when food companies defy nature by making products with enormously high levels of fat and sugar, a child's biology responds by telling them to "eat more." We can't blame kids for craving food that's been specifically designed to target their evolutionary impulses. Blame can be placed on the makers of such products. Better yet, we can resist their manipulative tactics by refusing to purchase their unhealthy products.

Kids don't "outgrow" picky eating: parents must teach children how to accept new foods via repetition and modeling healthy habits. Letting children choose everything they eat does not work, especially if the choices are processed foods with high volumes of sugar and salt. When we try to please our kids all the time by giving them unhealthy foods they might be craving, we end up undermining our leadership, which means we enable unhealthy food choices. Parents must sit in the driver's seat and take a more directed approach to feeding. Never has there been a more critical time to teach children where food comes from, how it's made, and how it affects their metabolism.

Some parents fear that directing a child's food choices will create an eating disorder. This is not the case. There is a big difference between constantly speaking about weight loss, diets, and/or "being thin" and sending messages of self-love through healthy eating and the notion of honoring one's body. The energy behind the two stances looks and feels very different. Certainly, kids need to feel they have some control in their world. Give them choices, but control the options, for example, offer a choice between an apple with peanut butter or carrots with hummus. It's okay for children to be hungry between meals. A little rumble in their tummies will set up a greater acceptance of healthy offerings and more willingness to try new foods. When it comes to eating, we need to raise our expectations for what our kids can handle, just as we do with all other social behaviors. They will surprise you with how adaptable they are. Perhaps most

Super-Tasting Tongues

You may have noticed that some people—both kids and adults—are supersensitive to bitter tastes like broccoli, while others are not bothered by them at all. As it turns out, about 25 percent of the population are considered super-tasters, in other words, they are highly sensitive to bitter flavors because they have an unusually high number of taste buds.[220] There are a few different ways to test who in your family might be a super-taster. There is a Sweet-N-Low test, a blue tongue test, a PTC paper test, and a tonic water taste test, which all can be found with an internet search. (I tried the PTC taste test with my family. Turns out, we are all average tasters.) Studies suggest that there may be correlations between the ability to taste PTC and preferences for certain types of foods. Aside from a genetic test, I'm not convinced entirely of their accuracy; nonetheless, they could be a fun home experiment to entertain curiosity. The point is to be aware that some children are genetically more sensitive to bitter foods than others. They will require a more compassionate approach to feeding but still the discipline to keep it based on whole foods and healthy.

importantly, don't give in when your child says no. Stay calm and try not to show frustration. Getting upset only fuels an argument.

Lack of Oral Motor Skills and Sensory Dysfunction

Sometimes children are selective about the food they eat because they lack the oral motor skills needed to sustain resistive chewing or the ability to move a mouthful of food in their mouth. The term *oral motor* refers to the use and function of the muscles of the face (lips, jaw, tongue, palate, and/or pharynx). Mealtime can often be stressful and exhausting when a child has limited movement, coordination, and/or strength in his mouth. Here are some symptoms of a child that might have this type of eating difficulty:

- Very selective about foods, particularly meats and raw vegetables
- Problems with ability to take food into the mouth
- Poor coordination and timing of the suck-swallow-breathe sequence
- Overstuffs mouth with food

- Frequently bites on cups or straws to stabilize jaw for drinking (cups are chewed up)

- Tongue protrusion, spoon biting, and head retraction to remove food from a spoon

- Frequent gagging, choking, and/or vomiting

- Failure to gain weight

- Holds food in mouth for long periods of time

- Swallows food before it has been adequately chewed, often leading to a hard swallow

- Suckles instead of chews food to assist with oral transport of food

If you feel your child may have oral motor deficits, visit with your pediatrician who can refer you to a licensed speech-language pathologist or occupational therapist. For more information on oral motor skills and treatments visit the American Speech-Language Hearing Association at www.asha.org.

It's also important to differentiate between a picky eater and a child with a true sensory dysfunction. Children with a sensory processing disorder (SPD) can present with specific tactile or oral sensitivities, which can greatly affect their eating habits. They often have difficulty with texture, temperature, taste, and/or smell. Review this list of SPD characteristics:

- Limited diet of less than 20 foods

- Gags or chokes when eating or frequently vomits with introduction of new foods

- Inability to transition to new foods at milestones (i.e., difficulty going from pureed food to whole food)

- Difficulty with breast or bottle feeding

- Mealtimes create constant stress, possibly to the point of avoiding eating

- Meals and snacks need to be predictable and without surprises

- Sensitivities to sound, light, touch, or taste

- Gets anxious when messy or if certain fabrics rub a certain way

- Irritability when one food touches another on a plate

- Foods that are sometimes dropped are not reacquired or replaced by alternatives

If more than a few of these symptoms fit your child, you may want to speak to your pediatrician and visit with an occupational therapist trained in Sensory Integration Theory. Additional resources to learn more about food sensory dysfunctions include SPD Foundation www.spd-foundation.net; Kay A. Toomey, PhD, www.sosapproach-conferences.com; and Feeding Matters www.feedingmatters.org.

FEEDING STYLES

Have you ever thought about your feeding style and how similar or different it is to your spouse's or partner's? Every household is unique. For those with two parents, they may come from two totally opposite ends of the world. Many have different perspectives, values, and childhood belief systems. You need to be aware of how you developed your specific feeding style so that you can objectively evaluate whether or not it's serving your children. In Deborah Kennedy's fabulous book *The Picky Eating Solution*, she teaches parents how to overcome their current problematic eating environments and create healthy eaters. Here are some factors to consider that Dr. Kennedy points out:

Childhood Patterns: Every parent has at least one feeding perspective: the one they were raised with. Did your parents force you to sit at the table and clean your plate, or did you sit in front of the TV and eat with your siblings during mealtimes? Did your mother bake a lot and prepare elaborate meals, or did she despise the kitchen and celebrate the convenience food gods? Good or bad, our food upbringing is what's familiar to us. The key is to be aware of your childhood feeding patterns. Often, there is room for improvement.

Ethnicity: Appreciate and acknowledge the significant impact ethnicity has on food choices, eating styles, food traditions, and feeding expectations. Consider how your ethnic background may influence your child's food choices.

Health Concerns: Food allergies, obesity, and mood disorders are just a few examples of conditions that demand more of a parent's energy, and likely more control and emotion over a child's choice of foods. Stress is also a health concern where food comes into play. Some parents use food as a reward when their children are emotionally distressed, anxious, or depressed. Be aware of how these behaviors feature in your feeding routine and whether it's setting up healthy or unhealthy eating habits.

Parent's Disposition: Your personality plays a central role in your feeding style. Are you laid-back, patient, strict, bossy, controlling, or indifferent? How about the rest of your family? Interactions among family members elicit varied responses that can create happy or unhappy food tribes.

Every parent, at some point, questions whether they are being too demanding or too lenient. We question if we are showing enough love and affection while still creating reasonable boundaries and teaching self-regulation. Every child is different and every family's dynamics is unique. As I'm sure you've discovered, there's no one size fits all when it comes to parenting practices. As a parent of two children with opposite personalities, my parenting approach looks a bit different with each child.

What's Your Feeding Temperament?

Mainstream psychologists generally recognize four main parenting styles that are based upon the landmark discoveries of clinical and developmental psychologist Dr. Diana Baumrind. The four parenting styles are *authoritarian*, *indulgent*, *uninvolved*, and *authoritative*. As you might expect, the parenting style that produces the most positive outcomes overall is the *authoritative* approach.

Deborah Kennedy explains in *The Picky Eating Solution* how each of these parenting styles pertains to addressing kids' eating. Below is an outline of each parenting style based on how Dr. Kennedy relates them to eating and mealtimes.

Authoritarian ("Mr./Mrs. Strict")

- regarded as "old school" approach
- big on control and override of a child's preference

A Mother's Diet Affects Her Child's Food Preferences

Research has shown that a mother's food intake while pregnant and breastfeeding may have a significant effect on a child's acceptance of new foods during childhood.[221] There is evidence that amniotic fluid and breast milk are "flavored" by a mother's food intake and result in preferences for these foods later in life. As a pregnant or lactating mother, if you eat garlic, your child will taste garlic. If you eat curry, your child will taste curry. It's nature's way of introducing baby to a family's food culture before they are born. It tells us that early exposure to healthy flavors before and after birth will positively influence food recognition as a child transitions to solid foods.

- often force a child to clean his plate

- often scare children by using force, yelling, and screaming, creating a lot of anxiety during mealtimes

- style is strict and sometimes inconsistent

Indulgent ("The Spoiler")

- the most common approach

- warm and nurturing, but primary concern is an enjoyable experience which translates into giving children whatever foods or treats they want

- let kids make all the food decisions to facilitate a positive, fun experience

- little attention to encourage nutritious options because fun trumps nutrition

- fear that if they push too hard at the table, they will create an eating disorder in kids

- style works for special occasions like birthdays but will deprive children of essential nutrients if used daily

Uninvolved ("Hands-Off")

- parents are checked out and don't monitor food intake at all

- unresponsive to children's needs and let them choose their own meals

- children tend to eat large quantities of junk food in excess

- style is not recommended and will set children up to be deficient in micronutrients

Authoritative ("The Teacher/Coach")

- the best approach

- in full control but responsive and nurturing with children

- able to read children's behaviors at mealtimes and provide reasoning and structure to encourage eating

- constantly balancing between parental control and children's autonomy, depends greatly on child's individual eating personality, parent's intuition, and behaviors parent displays around food

◆ sets rules and consequences that are non-threatening and child-focused

Perhaps you recognize your parenting style in the above descriptions. Wherever your approach falls in these standard categories, the next section recommends feeding practices essential for developing healthy eating behaviors. You will learn how to become an effective teacher and coach so that your children can flourish in our current food environment.

EMPOWERING STRATEGIES TO CREATE A HEALTHY FOOD CULTURE FOR YOUR TRIBE

After counseling many patients over the years, I've come to realize educating families is the easy part. The hardest part of my job is motivating people to make enduring changes. Most people make changes after they have developed an ailment or their child has a chronic problem. Maybe my perspective is different because both my husband and I work on the front line of defense: we witness the effects of our toxic food environment and see firsthand the undeniable power of good nourishment. It truly is profound, and frankly, it's what has motivated me to write this book. The previous chapters have concentrated on *why* healthy nourishment is vital for families and growing children. The upcoming section focuses on *how* to create a culture among your tribe that supports this goal.

First, get in touch with your motivation for change. Ask yourself, "How will this or that suggestion fit and serve my family?" There's no single solution that works for everyone. You know your children better than any doctor, teacher, or nutritionist. Don't overwhelm yourself by trying to implement everything you read to start the evolution of change in your home.

The information below is based on science, my experience as a nutrition consultant over the past twenty years, and my experience as a wife and mother raising two energetic, strong-willed children. There is no magic here, just hard work, dedication, and a lot of love. I'd be lying if I told you this process is easy. Parenting is always a work in progress, isn't it? It took me a while to find confidence in my approach. After reading volumes of scientific articles and attending lectures for decades, I knew exactly *what* to feed my family, *how* was the difficult part. Parents hear and read far more about *why* vegetables are important rather than what to do when their kids throw them back. Our goal is for our kids to be nourished but also balanced emotionally around food. It requires daily effort and patience, but with the right approach, the result is empowered, intuitive, healthy kids.

I now realize, much to my relief and surprise that kids will eat healthy and will actually enjoy their meals given the right environment! My ongoing mission is to help children become intelligent eaters who listen to their bodies' cues, choose foods that propel them to peak health, and understand the manipulative marketing environment that surrounds them. Let's get started.

Be a Calm Gladiator

At mealtimes, parents tend to talk too much. The minute we start bribing, coaxing, or making a big deal out of eating a particular food, it tells kids the food must not be that good. When is the last time you said, "Oh, you just have to try a little bite of this super yummy chocolate chip

Food Arguments and Conversations

There are moments when kids need to understand the reasons for your food choices. Here is a healthy dialogue with a seven-year-old who asks on the way home from school, "Why are you always so mean and make us eat healthy food all the time? I don't want split pea soup for dinner!"

A mom might respond, "I am your mother and I love you. One of my many *jobs* as your mom is to *protect* you and to help you to stay healthy. To do that I make sure your body and brain are getting the best foods possible. It's my job to introduce you to new foods and teach you how to take care of your body. Mommy is wise. It's because I love you so much that I prepare healthy meals for you."

It's very possible that your child might tightly cross her arms and say something like, "Lucky me," or "I love you too, but I really want pizza," or even "I don't care, it's not fair!" If so, repeat the message but use slightly different words. If you have strained conversations about food with your kids, be firm, but not harsh. Firm parents set secure boundaries with thoughtful consequences that are set up to help their kids grow. Harsh parents use angry words to try to force their intentions, which usually backfires with more resistance. You know the best way to connect with your child. The important thing is that you remain cool, calm, and collected. In other words, be very conscious of your body language and the language you use during and after your conversation. Children watch every single twitch and sound you make and if they suspect anger, control, or frustration, they end up absorbing a whole different experience rather than the one intended, which came from a place of love.

cookie, it melts in your mouth and will give you tons of energy!" Never. So when a mealtime comes around, serve your prepared meal, tell them what they are eating, and move on. If questions come up, explain why it's healthy for them, that there will be no alternatives, and that they are expected to eat what is served.

Don't give up if the first few days are difficult introducing this new approach. It's completely *normal* to have pushback. If a tantrum or argument arises from your child, stay calm! When we behave as if their tantrums don't bother us, we starve our kids of their argument fuel. Respond with loving, simple, one-line answers like, "I love you and it's my job to feed you good food." Kids want to get a reaction out of you. It's their way of testing the waters and learning (a) how to get more attention and (b) if they can argue you into submission. They are experts at figuring out the weakest links in the family. Give them time to learn new expectations and food rules.

Okay, bear with me, as I am about to compare parenting your kids to training your dog. I promise there's a point in the end. When we first brought home our ridiculously cute 10-week-old golden retriever, Nala, 14 years ago, we really failed miserably at her training. She'd cry in the middle of the night and instead of letting her cry through it, we'd take her out of her crate and put her in bed with us (a big no-no). When Nala was six months old, we hired a fancy trainer to come and teach her how to walk on a leash without pulling our arms out of their sockets. You guessed it, we failed. We soon came to the conclusion that Nala was an untrainable dog with a mind of her own. *Wrong!*

One day, after reading a book by world-famous dog trainer Cesar Millan, I realized that the problem wasn't my dog, it was *me*! Training your dog to become an admired family member is all about respect, tone of voice, repetition, and consistency. Dog trainers train *people*, not dogs. Can you guess where I'm going with this? If we want our kids to respond positively to a new healthy food culture, we as parents need to change *our* behaviors and responses when feeding our kids. We need to learn how to deliver a positive message without showing anger and frustration at every meal. It's a shift in emotion and patience. Be a calm gladiator.

Be a Good Role Model

I wake up every day hoping to put my best foot forward for my children. As their role model, I know that I am a driving force in creating their map of the world. My daily interactions with my husband, neighbors, strangers, and even animals are constantly being downloaded into their brains' hard drives. I know that nonverbal behavior is the most crucial aspect of communication.

As most of us learned in communication class, your nonverbal behavior represents 55 percent of what actually influences people. Kids learn far more from what they observe than from what they are told. In other words, the more your children see you eating and choosing healthy foods, the more they will do the same. This is one of the most important tools to creating a healthy food culture at home, and often the hardest. As many of us remain selective eaters as adults, it doesn't mean that we can't model healthy efforts and bravery in trying new things.

Let's pick on dads for a moment. Surely, this is not true in all households, but I find that there are many more mothers reporting their efforts being sabotaged by their husbands than vice versa. If Mom takes the time to cook a healthy meal for the family and Dad complains about eating his vegetables or picks apart all the healthy foods and pushes them aside on his plate, who do you think children will choose to model? Or, if Mom is away and dad decides to pack candy and donuts in lunch boxes and visit fast-food drive-thrus at dinnertime, what model is Dad portraying for his behavior sponges in the back seat? It is not necessary for parents to enjoy every

Ways to Model Healthy Eating Habits

- Drink water or unsweetened tea instead of soda or juice.
- Eat fruit for dessert.
- Eat healthy balanced meals that include protein, healthy fat, and whole, intact carbohydrates.
- Avoid labeling food as "good" or "bad," instead teach kids the importance of quality, nourishing food.
- Choose restaurants that offer healthy selections.
- Eat consciously, sitting together rather than in front of the TV, computer screen, or mobile devices.
- Limit snacking, especially late at night.
- Reward with non-food items when celebrating.
- Engage kids with meal planning and food preparation.
- Try new foods with your kids and fill your plate with the same type of foods.
- Limit processed junk food and sweetened beverages in the house.
- Prepare visually appealing colorful vegetables and eat them together.
- Both parents speak pro-health language.
- Avoid packaged foods with more than five ingredients, especially if you can't pronounce them.

fruit or vegetable on their plates, but they should model trying and tasting new flavors each time they are presented with a new food. If dads have limited palates, they can model a powerful message that says, "It's hard for me too, but I like trying new healthy things, and I will keep trying because I know it's the best thing to do for my body and mind."

Aim to ensure both parents in the same household are a united front. If Mom and Dad speak the same pro-health language, enforce the same food rules, and model nourishing behaviors, then the rate of success for kids following suit goes up exponentially. Even if your children don't follow your lead initially, they will emulate it over time. As kids grow to become teenagers and young adults, they will most likely continue to adopt your healthy habits, and will practice the skills you teach them throughout their lives. Consistent modeling reaps long-term rewards!

Adopt a Healthy Home Environment: Cook, Eat, Teach

Someone asked me as I was writing this book, what would be the most important thing he could do to make positive, healthy changes for his family. My answer was simply, "Learn to cook." I'm not saying become Julia Child; I'm saying take the time to get out your cookware and learn to cook some basic healthy dishes that are quick, easy, and tasty. According to Dr. Mark Hyman, a four-time *New York Times* bestselling author, "In 1900, 2 percent of all meals were eaten outside the home. In 2010, 50 percent were eaten away from home and one in five breakfasts is from McDonald's. Family meals happen about three times a week, last less than 20 minutes, and are spent watching television or texting while each family member eats a different microwaved 'food.'"[222]

Let's face it, how many fruits and vegetables do your kids get when you eat food on the run? The reality is very little—and ketchup doesn't count! Cooking at home is cheaper, allows you to offer a variety of foods, empowers you to have complete control over the ingredients, and brings families together. If you want to have healthy eaters, this is a critical piece of the puzzle.

Raising my kids over the past 14 years, I have also realized there's an art to introducing new foods, flavors, and textures to kids. Below are some helpful hints to make your food journey a little easier if your kids are resistant.

Cooking and Feeding Tips for Parents

- ◆ **Hold off on introducing processed food to infants and toddlers.** Real whole foods cannot compete with processed food in taste. Nature simply doesn't produce food with five times the salt and sugar content that addicts the human taste bud. The longer you expose young children to whole food, the more likely they will accept the textures and flavors as they grow.

- **Do not give your kids juice.** In terms of glycemic load, offering juice is like giving kids a soda. It also fills their bellies up with empty calories. If you let your toddler or adolescent get nice and hungry prior to a meal, the likelihood of healthy eating rises greatly. Water is the best beverage for kids.

- **Enroll in a healthy cooking class.** The more skilled you are, the easier and quicker mealtime preparation becomes, and you will feel more comfortable trying new foods. Online cooking classes are a great option for busy parents; you can learn and cook in your own kitchen!

- **Ease into new foods.** For example, if your goal is for your kids to drink unsweet tea instead of sweetened, initially mix the sweet tea with half unsweet tea, and gradually reduce the sweetened portion. If your kids love rice but your goal is for them to eat quinoa, start serving half rice and half quinoa gradually transitioning to all quinoa. This strategy works for weaning off foods high in salt and sugar too.

- **Use familiar flavors and textures to introduce new foods.** My kids love pesto. I make it fresh from my garden each summer. I also prepare and freeze about 20 extra Mason jars of pesto that feed us through the winter. Given the choice, my son would probably eat pesto pasta for dinner each night for the rest of his life. Knowing this, I used this flavor to introduce him to new foods. At first he wasn't a fan of grilled zucchini, but as soon as I added a little pesto to it, he gobbled it off his plate. Other kids prefer flavors like salsa, tomato sauce, or guacamole. Don't be afraid to combine these flavors with new foods. It not only makes the food more familiar but appeals to kids' taste buds and adds nutrients.

- **Don't stress if it's not nutritionally perfect.** It's okay to add small amounts of less healthy foods to broaden acceptance. For example, sometimes I roast butternut squash with a little maple syrup. If necessary, you can slowly decrease the amount of the less desirable ingredient as your children get used to the new flavors.

- **Cook soup.** This is one of the best ways I know to get kids to accept and eat vegetables, not to mention the great taste and benefits of bone broths. Chicken, lentil, minestrone, and beet soup are our family favorites. Pureed soup chock-full of vegetables is also a good alternative. Soup makes an easy lunch box meal, too.

- **Add little extras.** Try adding little portions of new vegetables to dishes that your children already enjoy eating. My kids love eating sautéed lentils, for instance. To boost nutrition, I started chopping up small pieces of greens (kale, spinach, or chard) and added them at the end. The key was chopping the greens small so they were not pronounced when the dish was complete. (I wanted them to know it was in there; I just didn't want them to think it was the main player in the dish.) Another tactic would be if your child likes pasta or brown rice, add little extras like peas or small pieces of broccoli when you prepare it. Start with just a little, then add more. (This works great with soup, too.)

- **Learn what a healthy serving size is.** Too often, parents put adult-sized portions of food in front of kids, which creates instant panic. At mealtimes, especially at dinner when I serve more unfamiliar foods, I give my kids very small portions to start, usually about two to three bites, which exposes them to the smell, texture, and taste. We expect them to finish it before they get anything else. Sometimes they decide they like it, sometimes they decide to go hungry, and sometimes they plug their noses while chewing and then move on to something they enjoy. Although it takes time, they undoubtedly expand their palates and get braver and more accepting.

- **Serve healthy foods first.** One of the best tricks in my arsenal is knowing how to leverage hunger. Most days, my kids sit down to dinner quite hungry. As I'm preparing our food for supper, I will cook their vegetables just ahead of the rest of the food. Often, I will serve up a bowl of broccoli and butter, a fresh green salad, or a plate of sliced raw veggies with hummus as a pre-meal appetizer. Knowing their tummies are rumbling means their food acceptance scale is much higher. I use this technique when we eat in restaurants, too. My husband and I will order veggies or big salads as appetizers to share so that we can be assured the best nutrition enters their bodies first.

- **Implement an "ask before you snack" rule.** Too often parents let their kids pull out whatever they want to eat at whatever time of day. With younger children, it helps to have them communicate when they are hungry so that you can steer their food choices in a healthy direction. Since snacks make up such a large part of your child's nutrient profile, it's wise to have them ask before they snack.

- **Avoid manipulating eating habits.** Although sneaking healthy ingredients into entrees is great for increasing nutrition content, it fails to teach fundamental goals of establishing good eating patterns. It's not that I don't ever use the "sneak tactic," but I also know that

Finger Food Snacking Tips for Babies and Toddlers

On-the-go parents often reach for processed, refined-grain snack foods like teething crackers, biscuits, cookies, and cereal (like Cheerios). Unfortunately, these foods offer very little nourishment and in addition to being addictive, they are also inflammatory.

Snacks that provide better nourishment include foods like jiggly gelatin (pure and unprocessed, not instant), avocado chunks, ripe bananas or other soft fruit, well-cooked veggies, hard-boiled egg yolks, dehydrated fruits, and sweet potato pancakes (see recipe below).

SWEET POTATO PANCAKES

1 egg yolk

⅛ tsp of pumpkin pie spice or ground cinnamon

¼ cup previously baked sweet potato

⅛ tsp Celtic sea salt

¼ ripe banana (1.8oz)

2 tbsp butter, ghee, or coconut oil (melted)

¼ cup coconut flour

¼ tsp vanilla

2 tbsp butter, ghee, or coconut oil (for the skillet)

1. Combine first 8 ingredients in a small mixing bowl. Form into 1-inch balls by working batter between your hands. Flatten into mini round circles.

2. Melt butter in a cast-iron skillet on medium-low heat. Cook mini pancakes rounds for about 4-5 minutes on each side or until golden brown.

3. Serve hot or store in a sealed container in refrigerator for one week. This is a great grab-and-go snack that can be eaten as small rounds or broken into bite-sized "pincher grasp" pieces.

I don't want my 14-year-old son to scream at the sight of spinach because I haven't taught him the look, feel, and taste of this green leafy food. I sometimes sneak a few extra superfoods into my kids' smoothies in the morning, but after they slurp it down with a smile, I tell them exactly what's in it. (My son now makes his smoothies with spinach.) Once a child is able to distinguish taste, they need to see food in its original state, so that they learn where it comes from and that it's safe to eat.

◆ **Published studies' tips for improving fruit and vegetable acceptance with children:** Small children prefer having their veggies cut into slices and sticks or fun shapes and figures (the star shape usually gets the highest rating).[223] Serve vegetables with dips like salad dressing and even peanut butter. Using fun names for vegetables like "X-ray vision" carrots or "tiny tasty tree tops" for broccoli increases consumption.[224] Research concurs that the most important predictor of children's fruit and vegetable consumption is the model the parents set up for their kids.[225]

Involve Children with All Aspects of Food

It's human nature to be wary of things that are unfamiliar. The more we are acquainted with and educated about the things that scare us, the more open-minded and fearless we become. When it comes to food and eating, kids only know what you expose them to. If you want your kids to be more accepting of the food you serve, involve them in the process of cooking, teach them where the food comes from, and expose them to community events that provide new ways to view food. Here are four ways to expand your child's curiosity about the foods they eat.

- **Cook with them.** Not only does this provide a wonderful bonding experience with your child, but it also exposes them to the sight, smell, and texture of different foods. Encourage kids to open, stir, cut, strain, measure, mix, and *taste* as they go along. Get messy. Talk about the physical properties of the food and allow them to squash it, smell it, play with it, and pour it in different containers if desired. These activities influence their perception of food, and the repeated exposure will broaden their acceptance, dissolving fears.

- **Food shop with them.** As children get older and begin to read, there is great opportunity to teach them how to identify healthy food products and how to navigate grocery stores. Simple lessons like shopping the perimeter of the store or looking for labels with less than five ingredients are good places to start. Invite them to help you pick out new fruits and vegetables each week. Teach them how food makers try to manipulate their taste buds and how manufacturers' food claims and packaging are misleading. Point out the list of ingredients on a food label and educate as to how it helps your family make healthy choices, maximize nutritional value, and avoid potential harmful ingredients.

- **Garden with them.** There are few things children and adolescents enjoy more than digging in the dirt and exploring Mother Nature. A vegetable garden inspires wide-eyed wonderment by allowing kids to cultivate their curiosity and explore and eat foods that they would otherwise avoid. Kids love to choose seed packets, inspect worms and bugs, and water newly seeded plants. If you really want to watch their excitement come alive, get them their own gloves and spade and assign them their own plot in the garden. Fun veggies to plant are tomatoes, peppers, radishes, broccoli, snap peas, carrots, beets, lettuce, and rainbow chard. Herbs are also fun like basil, cilantro, parsley, dill, mint, and stevia. Not only will kids feel a sense of accomplishment, they will be more likely to enjoy growing healthier foods on their own.

◆ **Teach them where food comes from.** As unstructured outdoor play has declined in today's technological world, so has our kids' awareness of where food comes from. It's not uncommon for kids to think that strawberries grow on trees or that chicken comes from the supermarket. In his book *Last Child in the Woods*, journalist and child advocate Richard Louv directly links our children's "denatured childhood" to some of our greatest childhood health epidemics such as obesity, attention disorders, and depression. He reminds us of the large role nature plays in child development. Here are some creative ways to teach your children about where food comes from:

- Farmers' markets are a perfect venue for teaching children about the food they eat. Many markets have interactive programs that engage and teach kids how to make food source connections.

- Visit a pick-it-yourself farm. Even adults can find excitement in picking their own strawberries, pumpkins, apples, and peaches.

- Go clamming at the beach, fishing at a lake, or crabbing off a dock.

- Join or visit a community farm. Observe a chicken coop, see what the pigs eat, and watch the labor involved in picking a whole row of vegetables. Many communities also have farm tours that are offered in the fall and spring.

- Volunteer gleaning for a day or weekend. You will help a team pick fruits and vegetables that would otherwise be left to rot in the field at the end of the growing season. Gleaning combines charity, agriculture, and firsthand contact with the process of feeding the less fortunate. Check out www.endhunger.org/gleaning_network.htm.

- Sign your kids up for a summer farm camp.

Setting Food Rules and Independence

For many parents, food represents love, which ironically perhaps, is one of the reasons parents fail at sticking with their best intentions. Setting food rules can be uncomfortable, especially if tantrums ensue or a child refuses to eat. When we fall into the "food is love" belief by letting kids eat anything they want, we let guilt and pleasing steer us, instead of leadership and nurturing. Some parents mistakenly believe that food rules and consequences may even lead to an eating disorder. In fact, eating disorders are complex medical and psychiatric illnesses; they are not caused by parents.[226]

Think of all the behaviors that we parents have rules for. With rules come consequences. What consequences have you set if your child doesn't go to bed on time, behaves poorly at school, speaks disrespectfully, mistreats a sibling, or refuses to do chores? There is no difference when it comes to eating behaviors. Remember that the "food represents love" message does not come from the food itself. Rather, your love is expressed through the effort, time, and nurturing involved in preparing or offering the food to your child, your ability to stay calm during any pushback, and the verbal messages your child hears during mealtimes. My kids routinely hear, "this food is perfect nourishment for your growing body, and it's my *job* as your mom to teach you how to take care of it."

So at what age should your children start choosing foods on their own? The answer involves many variables. Age, motivation, understanding of healthy foods, sibling influence, food access and acceptance, and a child's personality all play a role. Children do not have the cognitive ability or maturity to fully understand how food affects their brains and bodies. The same holds true for teens.

World-renowned neuroscientist, psychiatrist, and brain imaging expert Dr. Daniel Amen speaks passionately about the need for parents to protect adolescent brains by supervising what they eat. He notes that part of our brain, particularly the prefrontal cortex (PFC), does not finish developing until we are in our mid-twenties. The PFC is responsible for cause and effect, judgment, forethought, impulse control, and learning from our mistakes. In his book *Making a Good Brain Great*, Dr. Amen remarks,

> *One group of people who need to have the best diets are teenagers and young adults, as their brains are still developing. Unfortunately, they are famous for having the worst diets. Many teens and adults have little education in nutrition and give in to their desires for "bottomless fries" or "supersized meals" without thinking about the consequences. Because of their underdeveloped prefrontal lobes, teens succumb to their impulses and eat whatever they want, whatever tastes good, whatever is on the table. Yet teenage obesity and adult-onset diabetes in teens are reaching epidemic proportions. The teenage and young adult brain is going through vast changes, and*

Family Table Rules

Here are simple and effective food rules to create a healthy food tribe.

- Only one nourishing dinner will be served. No extra "kid's meals."
- Everyone helps prepare the food and clear the table afterwards.
- Mealtimes equal family time.
- No food rewards will be offered, meaning no sweet treats for eating vegetables.
- Use respectful language about the food that's served.
- No electronics (phones, computers, TV, etc.) at the table.
- Everyone must at least try everything on their plate (be sensitive to serving sizes).
- No snacking before dinner.
- Be thankful.

giving it proper nutrition helps to build better adults. Parents and schools need to take an active role in teaching kids how to eat, not just abdicate our role because we think our teenagers won't listen to us.[227]

Before you establish your family's food rules, you must be certain that you are ready to uphold them. Consistency is key for success. If you waver in your leadership, then your kids will pick up on it and use their finely tuned manipulation skills (whining, negotiating, and begging) to satisfy their whimsical desires. I can guarantee your patience and decisions will be tested. You must use your own intuition to decide what's best for your child without sabotaging all your efforts, and at the same time honoring their needs.

Food on the Run: Restaurant Eating

The American Restaurant Association projected industry sales of $799 billion in 2017 and equal to 4 percent of the US gross domestic product. This is an enormous change from 1970, when total restaurant sales were only $42.8 billion.[228] Since eating out is now fulfilling such a large part of our so-called nourishment, it is wise to be a savvy consumer and capitalize on the many advantages of eating out instead of falling prey to the traps that can send your family's nutrition down the drain. Below are some on-the-go tips for the whole family when eating outside the home.

- **Set clear parameters.** Before entering the door to any restaurant, kids should have clear expectations on what they are allowed to order. This will save you hours' worth of arguing at the table. For example, allow only water to be ordered with meals and/or expect a vegetable of choice to be ordered with every entree. Imagine the reduction in sugar intake, let alone the money saved by ordering water.

- **Avoid ordering from the kids' menu.** It is challenging today to find a restaurant without a kids' menu, and they all pretty much offer the same thing: cheeseburgers, french fries, pizza, chicken fingers, macaroni and cheese, and ice cream. Not only do kids' menus offer our children the least nutritious choices, they have also set the American cultural food bar for families who now think that it's typical for kids to eat this way at a restaurant. In truth, there's nothing normal about it.

  Order from the main menu and ask to have an adult entree split in half if the portion is too big. Most restaurants will accommodate this request or even provide a smaller portion at a reduced cost.

- **Don't be afraid to make special requests.** You hold the cards when it comes to choosing food that nourishes and supports you. It's called taking care of yourself and your family. So go ahead and ask for vegetable substitutions or if your meal can be grilled or sautéed in healthy fat instead of fried, or ask the waiter to check if certain food items contain gluten or dairy if you are avoiding specific foods for sensitivities.

- **Hold the bread and corn chips.** Be sure to decline the basket of bread or the GMO corn chips that come before the meal so that your kids stay hungry right before the good nourishment arrives.

- **Let hunger be your helper.** When kids are hungry, they are most likely to eat healthier foods that they typically would turn their nose up to. Order your kids a healthy side vegetable or salad as an appetizer. Restaurants often prepare tastier vegetables than you typically do at home. This is a great way for kids (and parents) to learn new flavors and gain respect for a few more green things on their plates. If they come with heavy sauces, ask for the sauce on the side. If your kids typically refuse a salad at home but will eat salad at one of their favorite restaurants, ask to purchase a container of the restaurant's salad dressing, and take it home to duplicate the salad. My kids actually prefer a mixed greens salad at home over any other vegetable.

- **Choose balanced meals and vary choices.** Many kids want to repeatedly choose only pasta and butter, pizza, or a burger and french fries. Try to include lean protein, healthy fats, fruits, and vegetables at mealtimes. Avoid fried foods altogether. Penne pasta with butter is not a nutritionally sound selection for anyone. However, a mixed green salad with veggies and nuts paired with a plate of penne pasta with olive oil and broccoli is a great choice for kids.

◆ **Avoid fast-food restaurants!** I can proudly say that my kids have never eaten at a fast-food restaurant. I know, unheard of, right? But very doable with a little planning and a shift in how you think about mealtimes. I am an on-the-go mom, driving between 8 and 18 hours a week just for after-school activities. Review restaurant menus online and plan ahead. Look for restaurants that have a lot of variety as well as those that are proud of the quality of their food. They might use words like "fresh," "local," "seasonal," "organic," or "grass-fed." Call ahead orders to your favorite restaurants. Visit grocery stores that have nutritious hot/cold food buffets like Whole Foods, Wegmans, and Earth Fare.

◆ **Travel with a small cooler with emergency food.** This is great not just for on-the-go snacking but also for those times when you get to a restaurant and your kids are so hungry that they just can't wait for their meals to be served, or if by chance the restaurant doesn't have the healthiest options. Some cooler ideas include:

- snack bags of mixed nuts

- snack bags of veggies (carrots, red peppers, cucumbers, etc.) with a container of hummus

- hard-boiled eggs

- canned or sealed packets of salmon or trout

- small containers of apples (lemon juice to prevent browning) with almond butter packs

- individual kefir or yogurt containers with small bags of chia seeds and nuts

- avocados (and a knife for cutting fresh and a spoon for eating whole)

- pickles with sliced turkey roll-ups

- container of chickpeas with olive oil and seasoning

- individual baggies of protein powder (made yourself), coconut milk (some milks even come in individual easy-open containers) and shaker cup

YOUR FAMILY'S PATH TO NOURISHMENT

Once you've finished this book, I hope that you will see food for what it truly is: *information.* The amino acids and carbon chains at the end of your fork speak loudly to each and every one of your 10 trillion cells. Food is language, and your body is its translator. We've been lulled into a health-threatening sense of complacency about our diets that's killing us and crippling our kids' health. I have seen thousands of patients, family members, and friends with many ailments—acne, arthritis, migraines, constipation, eczema, irritable bowel, poor lipid panels, ADHD, diabetes, low thyroid function, poor concentration, and the list goes on—that can be alleviated, if not cured, from evolving their diets. Of course, change is not easy; sometimes it takes months or years to really take hold, but when we consider what's at stake and that results are life-changing, there's no turning back.

I frequently use the term "evolution of eating" to describe each person's journey with food as it relates to his personal health. It seems we all eventually take steps to improve our baseline behaviors that were formed when we were children. The difference is the timing of our awareness that change is needed, and our readiness to shift our core values. As Charles Darwin once said, "It is not the strongest of the species that survive, nor the most intelligent, but the one most responsive to change." I hope you're inspired to raise the level of nourishment in your home. I hope you're feeling empowered with the knowledge of why it's necessary and how to get there. At this very moment in time, we have ample wisdom to not just heal our loved ones' ailments but also to teach a generation of children a new way of thriving. It begins with food, the nourishment we put on their plates.

Peace, love, and good nourishment to all.

CHAPTER 10

NOURISHED TRIBE RECIPES AND MEAL PLANS

Well, you have reached the fun part: eating! I really wanted to call this chapter "Nicole's Food Lab" because sometimes I feel more like a mad scientist than a chef in my kitchen. That's probably because I am not only trying my best to create healthy food that tastes good, but also I'm always looking for ways to enhance the nutritional value. My kids, of course, are my biggest critics. If they don't give it their stamps of approval, then the recipe finds its way to the trash can. But I never give up. (My daughter tells me I'm like Disney's Moana in the kitchen.) A snarl or an eye roll from the peanut gallery just motivates me to keep developing and creating new, tasty dishes for their ever-changing palates.

SEVEN DAYS OF FOOD TRIBE SAMPLE MEALS

The following meal plan is designed to help give you an idea of how simple it is to incorporate healthy food into your lifestyle. Based largely on the upcoming recipes, these plans are designed for all types of families: those who need help transitioning from processed foods to whole, clean options; those who are looking to maximize their children's nourishment; and those who just want a few new ideas to add to their already stellar dietary plan. When choosing your family's meals and snacks, focus on a basic template of lean protein, high-fiber carbs, healthy fats, and non-starchy vegetables (especially leafy greens). What you will find below are fresh, whole, nourishing foods that balance blood sugar, slow digestion, and feed good bacteria. What you won't find are refined sugars, processed foods, or artificial ingredients. Remember, it's equally important to keep harmful foods out of your diet as it is to put the good stuff in. We need to know what exactly is in our food because, frankly, some of the foods in our homes are toxic.

We have an enormous opportunity to rethink food and learn what our kids need in order to truly maintain optimal health. Start with one or two things that are easiest for your family to implement or modify. You become an instrument of change even with the smallest effort, and a lot of small efforts eventually become big changes.

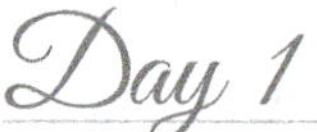

Day 1

Breakfast: Power Porridge (page 192)

Lunch: Roasted Garlic Hummus (page 232) & Veggie Wrap (hummus, mixed greens, broccoli sprouts, tomato, mint, cucumber, green onion, salt, and pepper) wrapped in a sprouted grain tortilla, with side of dill pickles (traditionally fermented), and a small piece of seasonal fruit

Dinner: Chimichurri Shrimp Skewers (page 220) with Cucumber Dill Salad and Italian Pesto (page 189) zucchini noodles (or chickpea pasta like Banza)

Snack: Banana Chia Pudding (page 244)

Day 2

Breakfast: Green Monkey Smoothie (page 190)

Lunch: Grandma's Chicken Soup (page 200) with side of Guacamole (page 233) and cucumbers (or black bean chips), and ½ cup pomegranate seeds

Dinner: One-Pan Baked Fish with Asparagus (page 217) with Quinoa Pilaf (page 225)

Snack: Miso Tahini Dip with Veggie Crudités (page 231)

Day 3

Breakfast: Sweet Potato Turkey Hash (page 197)

Lunch: Finger Food Box of raw red peppers and Roasted Garlic Hummus (page 232); Anjou pear; hard-boiled egg; raw milk, hormone-free cheddar-cheese cubes; 1-oz. piece of dark chocolate (70% or more cocoa solids)

Dinner: Wild-Caught Salmon Lollipops (page 221) over Pesto Pasta Primavera (mixture of zucchini, peas, and broccoli) and Red Cabbage Roast (page 211)

Snack: Piña Colada Smoothie (page 191)

Day 4

Breakfast: On-the-Go Grub of 1 apple sliced, 2 tbsp almond butter, 1 tbsp hempseeds, and 4 oz. kefir (made from cashew milk, coconut milk, or goat milk)

Lunch: Potato Leek Soup (page 201), with side of sliced kiwi

Dinner: Chicken Curry with Green Peas (page 219), with cauliflower rice

Snack: Fresh Berries with Coconut Whipped Cream (page 230), topped with chopped Brazil nuts

Day 5

Breakfast: Mixed Berry Smoothie (recipe at nicolemagryta.com)

Lunch: Working Mom's Black Beans (page 223), with brown basmati rice, and a side baby greens salad with pistachios, goat cheese, and Balsamic Vinaigrette (page 207)

Dinner: Lentil Meatballs (page 226), with Guacamole (page 233) and a side Green Kale Salad with Tahini Dressing (page 203)

Snack: Hard-boiled egg, with a handful of Roasted Almonds (page 227)

Day 6

Breakfast: Quinoa egg spinach scramble, with ½ grapefruit

Lunch: Meeska's Minestrone Soup (page 199), with a side mixed greens salad (butter lettuce, shaved carrots, chopped cucumbers, cherry tomatoes, broccoli sprouts, sliced avocado, and chickpeas drizzled with Creamy Yogurt Dill Dressing or Basic Vinaigrette Dressing (page 206-208)

Dinner: Nic's Black Bean Burger (page 222), with sweet potato fries and steamed broccoli and butter

Snack: Avocado Toast (page 228)

Day 7

Breakfast: Weekend Waffles (page 196), with fresh berries

Lunch: Curry Fish Salad (page 218), stuffed in a half raw red pepper, with half an avocado with a squeeze of fresh lemon and a pinch of garlic seasoned salt, and a small piece of seasonal fruit

Dinner: Thomas's Bison Meat Loaf (page 216), with Cauliflower Mashed Potatoes (page 212), and Roasted Brussels Sprouts (page 209)

Snack: Cashew butter sprinkled with chia seeds on celery

Drinks: Filtered water, Bone Broth (page 198), Fruit Water (page 238), herbal tea, fresh-squeezed Green Juice (page 241), kombucha, fermented pickle juice shots

RECIPES

n the following section, I share over 65 of my favorite quick and easy recipes that my family enjoys. I am happy to report that every single recipe in this section has been approved by both the little and big people in my family. While all the recipes contained within this book are gluten-free, they may be further modified if you have food allergies or sensitivities. A note on the mention of canned foods: every mention of a canned product should be understood as recommending BPA-free cans. I hope you enjoy nourishing meals together with your family, in good spirits and with happy, healthy tummies. *Buon Appetito!*

BUILDING BLOCKS

BREAKFAST

SOUPS AND SALADS

VEGGIES

Roasted Brussels Sprouts........... 209
Prosciutto Wrapped Asparagus......210
Red Cabbage Roast 211
Cauliflower Mashed Potatoes.......212

Roasted Butternut Squash...........213
Italian Stuffed Artichokes............214
Sautéed Spinach with Garlic.........215

MEAT AND SEAFOOD

Thomas's Bison Meat Loaf..........216
One-Pan Baked Fish
   and Asparagus 217
Curry Fish Salad...................218

Chicken Curry with Green Peas 219
Chimichurri Shrimp Skewers........ 220
Wild Salmon Lollipops
   with Italian Pesto 221

BEANS, LEGUMES AND GRAINS

Nic's Black Bean Burgers........... 222
Working Mom's Black Beans........ 223
Creamy Herbed White Beans 224

Quinoa Pilaf....................... 225
Lentil Meatballs....................226

SNACKS

Roasted Almonds 227
Avocado Toast 228
Baked Cinnamon Apple Chips 229
Fresh Berries with Coconut
   Whipped Cream 230
Miso Tahini Dip
   with Veggie Crudités..............231

Roasted Garlic Hummus.............232
Guacamole 233
Homemade Popcorn............... 234
Kale Chips 235

BEVERAGES

Homemade Cashew Milk........... 236
Homemade Lemon Ginger Tea 237
Fruit Water........................ 238

Sensible Soda......................239
Upgraded Hot Chocolate........... 240
Green Juice 241

DESSERTS

Dark Chocolate Bark
   with Super Seeds and Sea Salt 242
Frozen Chocolate Banana Bites 243

Peach Yogurt Ice Pops..............243
Banana Chia Pudding 244

Building Blocks

Homemade Ghee

MAKES 1 16-OZ JAR

Ghee is similar to clarified butter, except it's simmered a bit longer to bring out butter's inherent rich nutty flavor. As an ancient healing food of India, ghee is a staple in my kitchen for numerous reasons. This traditional food is made by boiling butter and removing its milk solids, making it suitable for those unable to tolerate milk protein or casein. It's also free of lactose. Because of its high smoke point at 485°F, ghee makes a perfect cooking oil for baking, sautéing, and roasting. Ghee is made up of about two-thirds saturated fats and one-third mono and polyunsaturated fats. Its saturated fat is mostly made up of butyric acid, which is an all-star nutrient for gut health and reducing inflammation. Ghee also contains antioxidants, CLA, and fat-soluble vitamins. I use ghee for just about everything: on veggies, eggs, sweet potatoes, popcorn, the list is endless! Give it a try, it's easy to make and tastes delicious.

1 **lb. unsalted organic butter from grass-fed cows (I like Kerrygold Pure Irish Butter)**

DIRECTIONS:

1. In a 2-qt saucepan, bring butter over medium heat to boiling. Adjust heat to maintain slight rolling boil. The butter will sound like its crackling as it boils. White foam collecting at the top will condense and thicken. Skim off the white foam with a spoon or a mash skimmer and discard.

2. After about 20–25 minutes, the loud boiling will stop, and the ghee will be transparent and slightly golden brown. Just make sure it's not burnt. The dark brown sediment that has adhered to the bottom of the pan is what gives the ghee its distinctive flavor. Remove from heat. Pour ghee through strainer lined with cheesecloth into a glass Mason jar. Cool and cover. Ghee can be stored for 12 months in the refrigerator or in a cabinet for up to 3 months away from direct light.

Homemade Avocado Mayonnaise

MAKES 1 16-OZ JAR

I'm not one for creating extra work for myself in the kitchen unless it makes a big impact nutritionally, and this one fits the bill. Almost all commercial mayonnaise is made with inflammatory oils, such as soybean or canola oils, which are also genetically modified. Even those mayos made with olive oil still have unhealthy soy or canola mixed in with it. My mayo recipe below is made with real, whole foods without GMOs, pesticides, or additives. The oils are also anti-inflammatory and it's truly a snap to make. Highest quality oils are imperative for this recipe, since that's the main reason for making it in the first place.

- 1 pasteurized egg yolk (room temperature, organic)
- 1 pasteurized whole egg (room temperature, organic)
- 1 tbsp apple cider vinegar
- 1 tbsp lemon juice, freshly squeezed
- 1 tbsp water
- 1 tsp honey Dijon mustard
- 1 tsp sea salt, or pink Himalayan salt
- 2 tsp raw local honey
- ¼ tsp garlic powder
- 1¼ c organic, expeller cold-pressed avocado oil
- 2 tbsp organic, expeller cold-pressed extra virgin sesame oil

DIRECTIONS:

1. Add egg yolk, whole egg, vinegar, lemon juice, water, mustard, salt, honey, and garlic powder to immersion blender cup. Pulse for 10–15 seconds.

2. Add the avocado and sesame oils to the blender cup. Place the head of the immersion blender at the bottom of the cup and pulse for 10 seconds as the emulsion begins to form. Begin to carefully and slowly lift the head of the immersion blender away from the bottom of the cup until emulsion is entirely formed and mayonnaise is thick and creamy.

3. Adjust seasonings to taste. Transfer to a covered Mason jar and store in refrigerator for up to 1 week.

MAYONNAISE-BASED SAUCES:

Tartar Sauce

- ½ c homemade mayo
- 3 tbsp finely chopped onion
- 2 tbsp chopped dill pickles
- 1 tsp lemon juice
- 1 tbsp chopped fresh parsley
- ½ tsp Dijon mustard
- dash pepper

Smoky Mayo

- ¼ c homemade mayo
- 1 tbsp BBQ spice (I like Savory Spice Shop's BBQ blends)

Curry Mayo

- ¼ c homemade mayo
- ½ tsp curry powder
- ½ tsp fresh lemon juice
- salt to taste

Chipotle Mayo

- ½ c homemade mayo
- ¼ tsp chipotle powder
- ¼ tsp garlic powder
- 1 tsp lime juice
- ⅛ tsp paprika
- ¼ tsp salt

Umami Mushroom Powder

MAKES A LITTLE LESS THAN ½ CUP

This powder is unbelievably versatile and adds a magical depth of flavor to almost any dish. We add it to soups, meats, burgers, veggies, or anything that we think could use a kick of umami.

½ oz. dried porcini mushrooms

¼ c sea salt, or pink Himalayan salt

1 tsp red pepper flakes

1 tsp dried thyme

1 tsp dried chives

1 tsp dried parsley

DIRECTIONS:

1. Grind dried mushrooms in clean coffee grinder until they resemble fine powder. Transfer to small bowl.

2. Grind the herbs into fine powder. Mix together with mushroom powder and store in a spice jar or airtight container.

Italian Pesto

MAKES ABOUT 20 OZ.

Pesto is a very versatile food. You can use it to flavor chicken or fish, add it to roasted vegetables, use it as a dressing for salads, mix it with zucchini noodles, or use it as a spread for burgers or sandwiches. I grow basil in my garden every summer and then make pesto during the fall, which I freeze to last us the winter months.

½ c (rounded) walnuts

8 cloves garlic

5 c basil leaves, firmly packed (or 4 c basil and 1 c baby spinach)

1 tsp salt

1 tsp pepper

1¼ c extra virgin olive oil

¾ c Pecorino Romano cheese (optional)

DIRECTIONS:

1. In a large food processor, blend nuts and garlic until combined. Add basil leaves (and spinach, if using), salt, and pepper. Pour in oil with food processor running, to desired pesto consistency. Add more oil if you prefer a thinner pesto.

2. Add cheese and blend for 30 seconds.

3. Store in a covered Mason jar in the refrigerator for 4 weeks or in the freezer for 6 months.*

**I store pesto in small Mason jars with plastic wrap directly on its surface which prevents it from oxidizing and turning brown. You can also pour a layer of olive oil on the top of the pesto before sealing the jar to get the same benefit. Another good option is to freeze fresh pesto in ice cube trays for 2-3 hours, then transfer to airtight container in freezer.*

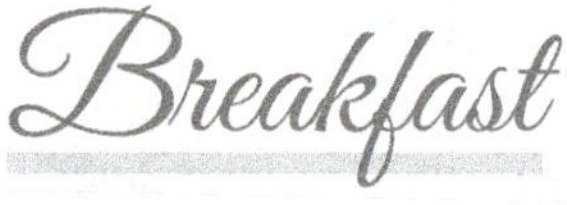

Green Monkey Smoothie

SERVES 1

This is my son's favorite smoothie. I had to give it a fun name because initially the green color gives some kids pause. Not to worry though, once it passes their lips, they suddenly realize it tastes similar to a peanut butter cup. The only sugar found in this recipe comes from the natural sweetness of the banana, which you can adjust with its ripeness. The greener or less ripe the banana, the more resistant starch it contains. I buy a couple of bunches and then break them into 3-in. pieces and freeze them in plastic bags for quick access. I buy fresh bags of organic greens and spinach, store them in the freezer, and pull out handfuls as I need them.

- ½ c unsweetened almond milk (or any non-dairy milk)
- 1 frozen banana
- 2 tsp raw cacao powder, or cocoa powder
- 1–2 c spinach, kale, or mixed baby greens
- 2 tbsp almond butter
- 2 tbsp hempseeds, or 1–2 scoops vanilla protein powder
- 1 tbsp unmodified potato starch (GMO-free) (optional prebiotic to feed good bacteria)*
- 1–2 tsp chia seeds (optional)
- ½ c ice, (optional)

DIRECTIONS:

1. Add ingredients to high-speed blender in order listed. Add more milk if you like your smoothie thinner, and less if you like it thick.

2. Cover and blend until smooth. Enjoy!

**If you are new to potato starch, start out with 1 tsp and work your way up to 1 tbsp to avoid stomach discomfort or gas. It's a great flavorless healthy addition.*

Piña Colada Smoothie

SERVES 2

After a recent trip to Mexico, both my kids came home with a new favorite drink: "virgin" piña coladas. It's not surprising, since they are loaded with sugar when made at a resort bar. At home, I wanted to make a healthier version without any added sugar, so I created a more balanced version with whole fruit, protein, healthy fat, and fiber. After a few attempts at pleasing their palates, this is what I came up with. My kids enjoy this as an after-school snack or sometimes on fast-paced school mornings.

- ½ c frozen pineapple pieces
- 1 frozen banana
- 1 c organic canned coconut milk
- ¾ c ice cubes
- 2 scoops of protein powder (I like Pure Planet Plant Protein, Vanilla Coconut flavor)
- 1–2 tbsp chia seeds (optional)
- 1–3 tsp unmodified potato starch (GMO-free) (resistant starch to feed good bacteria)

DIRECTIONS:

1. Add all ingredients to high-speed blender in order listed. Adjust thickness with more or less coconut milk. My kids like it thick and sometimes eat it with a spoon.

2. Cover and blend. Enjoy!

Power Porridge

SERVES 2

When my kids ask for oatmeal in the morning, I want to give them something that will fuel them until lunchtime. My Power Porridge has only 1 tsp of added sugar but also contains brain-boosting healthy fat along with protein, fiber, and essential nutrients.

1 tsp coconut oil or ghee	¼ tsp cinnamon
½ c old-fashioned oats	¼ c pepitas, ground (raw pumpkin seeds) or 2 tbsp chia seeds
1 c water	
⅛ tsp sea salt	2 tbsp almond milk
1 egg	1 tsp maple syrup, stevia, or monk fruit (optional)

DIRECTIONS:

1. In a 2-qt saucepan over medium heat, add coconut oil, oats, and salt. Cook covered for about 5 minutes or until oats have absorbed all the water and mixture looks creamy.

2. Turn the heat to low and crack the egg into the pan. Vigorously stir until the egg incorporates with the oat mixture and starts to cook, about 1 minute. If you don't stir quickly, the egg will cook on top of the oats. Add cinnamon, ground pepitas, and almond milk. Let mixture heat all the way through for another 2–3 minutes.

3. Serve in breakfast bowls and drizzle with a little maple syrup to taste.

Variations: My dear friend Beth adds 1 tbsp peanut butter and ¼ c fresh or frozen berries instead of adding the pepitas and syrup.

Oat & Pumpkin Pancakes *(Gluten-, Dairy-, and Egg-Free)*   **SERVES 8–10**

(Adapted from "The Detox Challenge Dietary Guidebook" by Deanna Minich, PhD, in collaboration with the Institute for Functional Medicine)

These delicious little morsels are exploding with flavor and make busy mornings carefree and healthy. The warm comforting flavors of fall come shining through with each bite. I double the recipe and freeze a bunch because they go quickly in my house.

- 2 c gluten-free, old-fashioned rolled oats (I buy mine at Trader Joe's)
- 1/4 c sesame seeds
- 4 tsp cinnamon
- 1/2 tsp nutmeg
- 1/2 tsp ginger powder
- 1 tsp salt
- 1 tsp baking soda

- 1 1/3 c pumpkin puree
- 2/3 c applesauce (substitute more pumpkin or sweet potato for FODMAP diet)
- 2/3 c unsweetened coconut beverage, or almond milk
- 4 tbsp coconut oil, melted
- 2 tbsp maple syrup
- 2 tsp vanilla extract

EGG REPLACER:

- 1/4 c freshly ground flaxseed
- 3/4 c water

DIRECTIONS:

1. Heat oven to 350°F, convection preferred.

2. Prepare the egg replacer by mixing the freshly ground flaxseed and water. Allow to sit for 5–6 minutes to thicken.

3. Grind oats in blender until finely ground. Pour into large mixing bowl. Add spices, salt, and baking soda, and blend until incorporated.

4. In another medium bowl whisk together wet ingredients.

5. Add egg replacer to wet mixture and blend.

6. Add wet mixture to dry ingredients and combine.

7. Spray cookie sheet with coconut oil spray and place dollops of batter onto the cookie sheet and form into pancakes (about 4–5 in. diameter and 1/2 in. thick).

8. Bake for approximately 25–35 minutes, flipping halfway through cooking. (Pancakes are ready when you can get a spatula under them to flip with ease. All ovens are different and you may need to cook these more to firm them up.) Pancakes will firm up a little as they cool.

9. Eat hot out of the oven with a little coconut oil, ghee, or nut butter spread.

Tips: *These pancakes freeze very well. Freeze in an airtight container or plastic bag, separating layers with parchment paper. When ready to eat, grab from the freezer and pop in the toaster. You may need to toast them twice to ensure the center is thawed.*

Creamy Apple Breakfast Bowl

SERVES 1

This dish tastes like a creamy apple peanut butter pie, but offers a lot more nutrition. It can be eaten for breakfast or as a snack. It's balanced with healthy fat, protein, carbs, and a large dose of healthy fiber. It also has 8 g of resistant starch, which is a prebiotic fiber that feeds your good bacteria along with probiotics in the yogurt. If you're dairy-free, substitute with non-dairy, low-sugar yogurt and add some hempseeds for protein. Try this recipe first without the honey. If you think it needs a little sweetness, add a little to taste.

- ½ c organic plain Greek yogurt (from grass-fed cows) (I like Maple Hill Creamery), or Goat Milk Yogurt (I like Redwood Hill Farm)
- 1 tbsp almond butter
- 1 tbsp unmodified organic (non-GMO) potato starch (I like Anthony's or Bob's Red Mill)
- 1 tsp local raw honey, or monk fruit powder (optional)
- ¼ tsp Ceylon cinnamon
- 1 small apple, with skin, sliced into bite-sized cubes
- 1 tbsp chia seeds, or hempseeds (optional)

DIRECTIONS

1. Stir to combine first five ingredients in a bowl.

2. Fold in apple pieces and sprinkle with chia or hempseeds.

Spaghetti Squash Hash Browns   SERVES 4–6

*If you are in the mood for comfort food but also want to eat something that loves you back, these hash browns will do the trick. They require a little extra prep, but you can roast the squash ahead of time and store the squash in the refrigerator until you are ready to use it. They are an anytime food, eaten for breakfast, lunch, or dinner. These make simply flavored patties that kids will enjoy.**

1 spaghetti squash

2 tsp ghee

1–2 eggs, pasture-raised

1/2 tsp garlic powder

1/2 tsp onion powder

1/2 tsp sea salt

1/4 tsp black pepper

3–4 tbsp arrowroot starch

1–2 tbsp ghee

DIRECTIONS

1. Preheat oven to 375° F, convection preferred.

2. Slice the spaghetti squash in half and scoop out the seeds to discard. Rub 2 tsp of ghee on flesh of each half. Place cut side down on a rimmed sheet pan. Roast for 45 minutes, or until flesh is tender. Let cool.

3. Scoop out flesh of spaghetti squash with fork and place in medium-sized bowl. With a clean kitchen towel, wrap squash in towel and squeeze out as much water as possible. Discard water and place spaghetti squash back in bowl.

4. Stir in egg, garlic powder, onion powder, sea salt, pepper, and starch until combined.

5. Heat 1 tbsp ghee in cast-iron skillet over medium-high heat.

6. Place 4–5 small patties on skillet and pan fry 4–5 minutes on each side. They should be rather thin in order to crisp up. Patties are ready to flip when they are golden brown on each side.

7. Serve by themselves, with eggs, or simply with grass-fed butter.

** For more adventurous eaters, I like to add more texture and color with scallions, fresh herbs, fresh garlic, or minced onion.*

Weekend Waffles

Every now and then my kids request waffles. Of course, I want to feed them a dish with a pumped-up nutrition profile yet also give them something that will please their taste buds. My weekend waffles are made with gut health in mind and are packed with nutrients and fiber—insoluble, soluble, and resistant starch. I use a Belgian waffle maker to prepare these, which makes 10 waffle squares. Each 4.5-in. waffle square has roughly 9 g of fiber.

1 c old-fashioned oats, ground in mini food processor (I like Trader Joe's gluten-free)

½ c almond meal

½ c freshly ground flaxseed

¼ c chia seeds

½ c teff flour * (I like Bob's Red Mill Teff Flour)

1 tsp salt

1 tsp baking powder

½ tsp baking soda

1 c plain, grass-fed Greek yogurt (goat milk preferred), or dairy-free yogurt or kefir

1¼ c unsweetened almond milk (or other milk alternative, cashew, coconut, etc.)

4 eggs

3 tbsp ghee (warmed to liquid form)

coconut oil spray

DIRECTIONS

1. Preheat waffle iron.

2. Combine oat flour, almond meal, flaxseed, chia seeds, teff flour, salt, baking powder, and baking soda in a medium bowl. Stir to combine.

3. In a separate bowl mix yogurt, milk, and eggs. Add to flour mixture and stir to combine. Stir in ghee. Let sit for 5 minutes.

4. Spray waffle iron inside on top and bottom with coconut oil cooking spray. Pour waffle batter into waffle iron and cook waffles until brown and crisp. (Cook less if you prefer tender waffles.)

5. Top waffles with grass-fed butter, and fresh berries. Enjoy! (If more sweetness is preferred, sprinkle a pinch of monk fruit extract or a ½ tsp of maple syrup on top of waffles.)

** I occasionally use tigernut flour in this recipe and replace the almond or teff flour with it. Tigernut flour is gluten- and grain-free and has a high level of resistant starch.*

Sweet Potato Turkey Hash

SERVES 6-8

This dish can truly be for breakfast, lunch, or dinner. Turkey can sometimes be dry when you cook it, but not in this dish. That's because of my secret ingredient—mushrooms! They blend right into the meat mixture, and your kids won't even know they are there. In fact, my son rated this dish a 9 out of 10. I hope your family enjoys it as much as we do. My kids like this dish as is or with avocado. My husband enjoys 2 flipped eggs over the top with all the fixings.

- 9 cremini mushrooms (about 5 oz.)
- 2 garlic cloves
- 1 lb. ground turkey (look for breast and dark meat, this is important to producing moist meat)
- 3 tbsp plus 2 tsp taco seasoning (see homemade recipe below)
- 1 tbsp ghee

- ¾–1 c chicken broth or bone broth
- 1 medium yellow onion, diced
- 1 large sweet potato, skin on, cut into small ½-in. cubes
- 2 c spinach, roughly chopped
- 1 tsp sea salt

Optional Toppings: Flipped eggs, avocado, jalapeños, green onions

DIRECTIONS:

1. Place mushrooms and garlic in mini food processor and pulse until the mixture resembles ground turkey consistency.

2. In a medium bowl, combine the ground mushroom and garlic mixture, raw ground turkey, and 3 tbsp of taco seasoning. Blend together with hands until all ingredients are fully incorporated.

3. Place a 5-quart, stainless-steel sauté pan over medium-high heat. Once the pan is hot, add 1 tsp ghee, the raw turkey mixture, and ¼ cup chicken broth to the hot oiled skillet. Using a wooden spoon, break up the mixture into smaller pieces as the meat cooks, stirring constantly. Remove turkey from pan and set aside on separate plate with juices. Don't overcook the turkey or it will get tough. Turkey is cooked once it reaches 165°F.

4. In the same sauté pan, add 2 tsp ghee, onion, ½ tsp salt, and dash of pepper over medium heat. Sauté until onion becomes translucent and slightly brown, about 4–5 minutes. Add sweet potatoes, 2 tsp taco seasoning, ½ tsp salt, and ½ cup chicken broth. Cover and cook for about 20–25 minutes, or until sweet potatoes are tender. You may need to add a little more chicken broth if the mixture appears too dry as it cooks. Add chopped spinach and cover again until spinach wilts, about 1 minute.

5. Fold in turkey meat to sweet potato mixture and heat through.

Homemade Taco Seasoning

- 2 tbsp chili powder
- 2 tsp cumin
- ½ tsp coriander

- 1 tsp oregano
- 2 tsp onion powder
- 1½ tsp garlic powder

- ⅛ tsp cayenne
- 1 tsp salt

DIRECTIONS:

Combine all the above spices in a small bowl. Store in sealed container for 6–8 months.

Soups and Salads

Delicious Chicken Bone Broth

MAKES ABOUT 1 GALLON OF BROTH

If you are wondering if all the hype about bone broth is true, it certainly is. Our ancestors were definitely on to something, and now we have the science to prove it. The components of bone broth influence almost every aspect of our health: bones, joints, skin, heart, brain, gut, and digestion. Rich in the amino acids glycine, proline, and glutamine, bone broth helps heal the gut, strengthen the immune system, and reduce inflammation. It's also packed with minerals and collagen, which is the jiggly gelatin that forms when your broth is cooled. It helps break down proteins and increases the digestibility of beans, legumes, and meat.

10 lb. of bones from pasture-raised organic chickens, or local hormone-free chickens (use 1–2 necks, 7 backbones, 1–2 feet) (If you can't find feet you can use wings or more backs.)*

4 qt cold filtered water (or enough to cover bones)

2 tbsp apple cider vinegar (important: helps extract minerals from bones)

3 large onions with skin, roughly chopped

3 large carrots with skin, chopped into 1-in. pieces

4 celery stalks, roughly chopped in 1-in. pieces

4 garlic cloves with skin, roughly chopped

1 tbsp peppercorns

3 bay leaves

1 bunch fresh parsley, about 2–3 oz. (or 2 tbsp dried)

2 tsp thyme, dried

1 tsp rosemary, dried

1 tsp sage, dried

1 tsp ground turmeric, dried

sea salt, or pink Himalayan salt to taste

**Using bones with some meat attached will give your broth more flavor. Bones can be obtained from local butchers, farmers' markets, saved from organic rotisserie chickens, or last night's chicken dinner. Quality is important when making bone broth. Always use bones from organic or pasture-raised, hormone-free animals.*

DIRECTIONS:

1. Preheat oven to 425°F, convection if possible.

2. Optional Step. Place bones (except feet) on a rimmed baking sheet and roast in oven for 1 hour. Turn after the first 30 minutes. (You can skip this step if you want to save time. Roasting the bones simply adds another layer of flavor.)

3. Place all the bones in a 16-qt stockpot along with enough water to cover the bones by at least 2 in. If the bones are floating around you've added too much water. Add the vinegar along with the rest of the ingredients, except the salt. Turn the burner to high heat and bring covered pot to a boil. As soon as the liquid boils, reduce heat to low and let simmer uncovered (very gentle bubbles will rise

to the surface) for 6–12 hours. Stir every 45 minutes to make sure all bones are submerged under water and breaking down. Skim off any scum that rises to the surface as needed throughout the cooking process.

4. Remove bones and strain the stock through a fine mesh strainer (add cheesecloth to bottom of strainer for clearer broth) into large empty stock pot.

5. Season broth with sea salt to taste while broth is still hot. Transfer to a shallow, wide container to encourage quicker cooling. (In the winter, I place my pot outside in the cold temperatures to let cool.) Once cooled, transfer container to refrigerator and let cool overnight.

6. The next day, if desired, skim off fat from top and transfer broth into freezer-safe Mason jars or other glass containers. When chilled, broth should look like jiggly semi-solid gelatin. That's the good stuff! (Be sure to leave 1 inch of space at top of Mason jar for ice expansion.) Store in refrigerator for 1 week or in freezer for up to 6 months. Broth can be used as stock in soup, as a warm beverage, or as a cooking liquid in recipes.

Meeska's Minestrone Soup

SERVES 8-10

This is a fabulous fall or winter soup recipe that I make regularly for my family. Change up the vegetables as your taste prefers. Peppers, mushrooms, green beans, or any other beans work well in this recipe too. This soup is nutritious, filling, and a great way to introduce vegetables to your family's palate.

2 large onions, diced

3 cloves garlic, minced

2 tbsp olive oil

3 carrots, diced (leave skins on)

1 zucchini squash

1 yellow squash

1 tsp dried thyme

1 tsp dried basil

½ tsp dried savory

½ tsp dried oregano

2 qt bone broth, or low-sodium chicken or vegetable broth

1 15-oz. can pureed tomatoes, or canned diced petite tomatoes

1 15-oz. can cannellini beans, or any of your favorite beans

1 c frozen peas

Sea salt and pepper to taste

DIRECTIONS:

1. In soup pot, sauté onion and garlic in oil to soften.

2. Add carrots and squash; sauté 5–8 minutes, or until softened.

3. Stir in thyme, basil, savory, and oregano. Add stock, tomatoes, beans, peas, salt, and pepper.

4. Bring to boil; simmer 20 minutes. Adjust seasoning as needed.

Grandma's Chicken Soup

If you are looking for a classic chicken soup recipe that will be a home run with your kids, this is it. It's a staple in my house all winter long.

1 tbsp expeller-pressed avocado oil

2 chicken breasts, bone-in, skin on (about 2–2½ pounds)

1 large onion, diced

5 garlic cloves, minced

6 large carrots, chopped into ½-in. thick half-rounds

6 celery stalks, chopped into ¼-in. thick slices

1 large leek, diced

1 tsp salt

1 tsp pepper

8 c chicken bone broth (homemade, p. 196, or low-sodium boxed chicken broth or stock)

2 bay leaves

1 tsp dried thyme

1 tsp dried dill

1 tsp dried parsley

DIRECTIONS:

1. Heat avocado oil in 8-qt soup pot on medium heat. Sear the chicken breasts skin side down until nice and brown (about 4 minutes). Turn chicken over and quickly sear boney side for another 1–2 minutes. Remove chicken from pan and set aside.

2. Add onion, garlic, carrots, celery, leek, salt, and pepper into the soup pot with the oil left over from searing the chicken. Sauté for about 5 minutes to soften vegetables.

3. Add bone broth, along with bay leaves, dill, thyme, and parsley. Add chicken breasts back in pot. Bring pot to a boil then reduce to a low simmer. Cook on a low simmer for 2–3 hours. Turn off heat.

4. Remove chicken breasts from soup. Discard skin and bones and chop breast meat into bite-size pieces. Add breast meat back to soup pot and stir. Remove bay leaves. Ladle into soup bowls and devour.

Potato Leek Soup

SERVES 6–8

This soup can fit almost any kind of eater. It can be easily adjusted for the omnivore or vegetarian with just a few quick substitutions. It pleases mature taste buds with its flavor combinations but also suits baby as a nutritious puree.

- 1 tbsp coconut oil or ghee (if you don't like strong coconut flavor, use ghee)
- 1 yellow onion, chopped
- 2 large leeks, chopped
- 2 medium carrots, diced
- 2 celery stalks, diced
- 3 Yukon gold potatoes, chopped into 1-in. cubes
- 1 qt chicken stock (or veggie stock if vegetarian or vegan)
- 4–5 garlic cloves, chopped
- ¼–½ c coconut milk (can substitute any milk if you don't like coconut flavor)
- 1–2 oz. fresh dill, chopped
- 1¼ tsp sea salt
- ¼ tsp freshly cracked pepper
- crispy bacon and scallions (optional toppings)

DIRECTIONS:

1. Add 1 tbsp coconut oil or ghee into a 4-qt Dutch oven. Add onion, leeks, carrots, celery, 1 tsp salt, and ¼ tsp pepper. Sauté until veggies begin to soften, about 10 minutes. Add garlic and sauté another 1–2 minutes.

2. Add potatoes and stock to vegetable mixture and cook covered until potatoes are soft, about 20–25 minutes. Puree with a hand immersion blender until smooth. Stir in coconut milk and dill. Season with salt and pepper to taste. Enjoy!

Cabbage Soup

Although it looks like iceberg lettuce, cabbage is actually from the cruciferous vegetable family along with kale, broccoli, and Brussels sprouts. I consider them all "super-veggies" because they contain powerful disease-fighting phytochemicals such as sulforaphane that have been shown to stop the growth of cancer cells. This is a quick and easy soup to prepare. It's best eaten with a little bite left to the cabbage.

- 1 tbsp unrefined cold-pressed avocado oil
- 1 large onion, diced
- 3 celery ribs, diced
- 3–4 carrots, diced
- 1/4 tsp salt
- 1/4 tsp pepper
- 4 garlic cloves, minced
- 1/2 tsp dried basil
- 1/4 tsp dried dill
- 1/2 tsp dried parsley
- 1/2 tsp dried thyme
- 1 head green cabbage, chopped into small pieces in a food processor or grated by hand
- 8 c of bone broth or chicken broth (see Delicious Chicken Bone Broth, page 198)
- salt and pepper to taste

DIRECTIONS:

1. Heat oil in a Dutch oven or medium soup pot and add onion, carrots, celery, 1/4 tsp salt, and 1/4 tsp pepper. Cook for 5–6 minutes until softened. Add garlic, basil, dill, parsley, and thyme to soup pot, and sauté for another minute. Add cabbage and bone broth and cook until cabbage is tender, about 10 minutes. Season with salt and pepper to taste.

Green Kale Salad with Tahini Dressing   SERVES 4–6

What I love most about this salad is the nutritional punch you get from all its different ingredients. The kale is loaded with vitamins like K, A, and C and is a powerful anti-inflammatory agent. Tahini, which is simply ground sesame seeds, is rich in minerals like phosphorus, magnesium, copper, iron, and zinc. Fermented organic miso is filled with beneficial, live probiotic cultures that work to balance gut bacteria. And last but not least is the garlic. Its sulfur compounds work their anti-inflammatory and immune-boosting effects all over the body. But the best part about this salad is probably the surprising taste. My kids were pleasantly surprised that it went down as a yummy creamy salad with a slightly nutty taste.

1 large bunch of curly kale, washed, stems removed

Tahini Dressing

2 garlic cloves

1/2 c raw sesame tahini

1 1/2 tbsp organic traditional red miso (I like Miso Master)

3/4 c water

1 tbsp lemon juice

1/4 c olive oil

2 tsp local raw honey

sea salt and freshly ground pepper to taste

OPTIONAL TOPPINGS:

roasted sunflower seeds, handful to taste

raisins, to taste

slivered almonds, pine nuts, or any favorite nut

pumpkin seeds

dried cranberries

grated carrots

crispy prosciutto or pastured bacon

DIRECTIONS:

1. Carefully stack kale leaves and use kitchen knife to slice into bite-size pieces. Place in serving bowl and set aside.

2. Blend garlic, tahini, miso, water, lemon juice, and olive oil in a small food processor until smooth. Add more water if dressing is too thick.

3. Start with about 1/2 cup of dressing and pour over kale greens. With clean hands, massage dressing into kale leaves, making sure to coat all the pieces. Adjust amount of dressing to taste. You will have extra dressing left over for another salad later or to use as a dip.

4. Add preferred toppings. My family enjoys shaved almonds, carrots, raisins, crispy turkey bacon, and salt and pepper.

Note: *You can make this salad ahead of time. As the dressing sits on the kale leaves it makes them a little more tender. I also love this salad the next day out of the refrigerator.*

Cucumber Dill Salad

Light and refreshing, this salad pairs great with just about any dish or it can be enjoyed as a cool after-noon snack. It takes about 10 minutes to prepare and tastes amazing.

2 cucumbers, cut lengthwise, seeded, then thinly sliced (1 peeled, 1 left with skin on)

DRESSING

- ¼ cup plain full-fat goat yogurt
- 1 tbsp rice vinegar (white wine vinegar or fresh lemon juice will also work)
- 1 medium garlic clove, minced
- 2 tbsp fresh dill, finely chopped
- ½ tsp raw local honey
- ½ tsp salt
- ½ tsp freshly ground pepper
- 2 tsp chia seeds (sesame or poppy seeds will work too)

DIRECTIONS:

1. Combine and stir all dressing ingredients in a small bowl. Dressing can be used immediately or refrigerated for a hour to let the flavors meld even further.

2. Right before serving, stir to combine sliced cucumber and yogurt dill dressing in medium bowl.

Mix and Match Leafy Green Salads

Not all salads are created equal. To get the biggest nutritional bang for your body, you need to pay attention to each of the components that make up a salad and follow a few easy steps.

1. Choose a good foundation. Throw out the iceberg lettuce, and look for lettuce with dark green or red leaves like mesclun, spring mix, or baby spinach.

2. Pile on as many colorful veggies as you can—cucumber, tomato, broccoli, carrots, etc.

3. If the salad is your main meal, add some protein like beans, lentils, eggs, chicken, or fish.

4. Add some healthy fat like avocado, nuts, seeds, or cheese.

5. Choose a dressing that's not full of sugar or unhealthy polyunsaturated vegetable oils (like canola or soybean).

   The goal, of course, is to find which flavor combinations suit your family's palate the best. Here are a few ideas you may want to try (recipes for dressings follow):

- **Butter lettuce + Chickpeas + Cucumber + Avocado + Shaved carrots + Cherry Tomato + Creamy Yogurt Dill Dressing**

- **Mixed baby lettuces + Pistachios + Goat cheese + Red bell pepper + Balsamic dressing**

- **Romaine lettuce + Black beans + Cherry tomatoes + Green onion + Avocado + Bell pepper + GMO-free corn + Avocado Lime Dressing**

- **Mixed baby lettuces + Beets + Green onion + Goat cheese + Walnuts + Maple Dijon Vinaigrette**

- **Mesclun greens + Avocado + Tomato + Olives + Cucumber + Orange pepper + Red onion + Olive + Wild salmon + Pinch of sea salt + Basic Vinaigrette**

- **Romaine lettuce + Red bell pepper + Red onion + Cucumber + Olives + Cannellini beans + Feta cheese + Tomato + Greek Dressing**

Basic Vinaigrette*

The foundation to any classic vinaigrette is the combination of an oil and an acid; traditionally, two to three parts oil to one part vinegar. If you want a less acidic dressing, use less vinegar and replace it with water instead. What really brings a dressing to life further are the spices and the emulsifiers. As you know, oil and water (and vinegar for that matter) don't mix, so if you don't use an ingredient that will force them to blend, then you often end up with oil-soaked lettuce leaves and vinegar at the bottom of the salad bowl. Good emulsifiers are foods like mustard, mayonnaise, tomato paste, avocado, honey, and egg.

- 2/3 c extra virgin olive oil
- 3 tbsp white wine vinegar, or lemon juice (I like champagne vinegar)
- 1 tbsp water

- 1 tbsp Dijon mustard, more or less to taste
- 1/2 tsp salt
- 1/4 tsp freshly ground black pepper

OPTIONAL ADDITIONS:

- 1–2 garlic cloves, minced
- 1–2 tbsp fresh herbs (basil, thyme, dill, parsley, oregano, or chives)

- 1 tbsp onion or scallion, minced

DIRECTIONS:

1. Combine in a Mason jar, cover and shake vigorously until ingredients are emulsified. You can also blend in a small food processor if you like a smooth dressing. Add a little more water for a thinner consistency.

**Once you find a flavor combination you like, you can add it to leafy salads, bean salads, fish salads, or use as a dressing over vegetables.*

Maple Dijon Vinaigrette

SERVES 4

Recipe shared from Bruce Bradley at www.brucebradley.com

3 tbsp extra virgin olive oil

1 tbsp apple cider vinegar

1 tbsp pure maple syrup

1/2 tbsp Dijon mustard

1 tsp garlic, minced

freshly ground black pepper to taste

DIRECTIONS:

1. Mix together all the ingredients. Make sure the dressing is well-blended before pouring on your salad. If you don't like garlic pieces, you can place in a mini blender and make it into a smooth dressing. This dressing can be made ahead of time. (It gets more flavorful the longer it sits in the fridge.) If you make it ahead of time, just pull it out 30 minutes prior to serving so that it can come back to room temperature before serving.

Balsamic Vinaigrette

MAKES ABOUT 3/4 CUP

1 shallot, skin on

1/2 c extra virgin olive oil

3 tbsp balsamic vinegar, good quality

2–4 tbsp water (adjust based on desired consistency of dressing)

1–2 tsp Dijon mustard

1 garlic clove

1/4 tsp sea salt

1/4 tsp freshly ground pepper

Note: *A good-quality balsamic is thick and sweeter tasting. If you are using a lesser quality balsamic the dressing will taste less sweet and slightly more acidic, which can always be balanced with a 1/2 tsp of honey if desired.*

DIRECTIONS:

1. Preheat oven to 425°F. Place shallot on aluminum foil and rub skin with olive oil. Roast for 45 minutes. Remove from oven and let cool slightly on stove. You can skip this step and use 1 tbsp raw shallot instead if desired.

2. Combine olive oil, vinegar, water, roasted shallot with skin removed, mustard, garlic clove, salt, and pepper in a mini food processor. Blend until smooth. Taste and season with salt and pepper as desired.

Avocado Lime Dressing

Adapted from www.thegardengrazer.com

¼ c extra virgin olive oil

1½ tsp apple cider vinegar

1 c cilantro, stems removed

½ large avocado

2 tbsp fresh lime juice

2 garlic cloves

½ tsp cumin

1 tsp maple syrup

¼ tsp salt, or more to taste

DIRECTIONS:

1. Place all ingredients in a food processor and blend until smooth. Adjust salt, cumin, maple syrup, or lime to taste.

Creamy Yogurt Dill Dressing

¾ c full-fat goat yogurt

2 tbsp avocado oil mayonnaise (See recipe, page 188)

1 tbsp dried parsley

1 tsp dried chives

1 tsp onion powder

1 tsp garlic powder

½ tsp dried dill

¼ tsp sea salt

¼ tsp freshly ground black pepper

DIRECTIONS:

1. Place all ingredients in a small food processor and blend until smooth.

2. Use immediately or store in the refrigerator for 1–2 weeks.

Greek Dressing

¼ c extra virgin olive oil

2 tbsp lemon juice

1 tsp dried oregano

¼ tsp dried dill

¼ tsp black pepper

1 tsp garlic, minced (about 1 large clove)

sea salt to taste

DIRECTIONS:

1. Place all ingredients in a small bowl and whisk until combined. There is no emulsifier in this recipe, so it's important to whisk just prior to pouring on salad to get even distribution of ingredients.

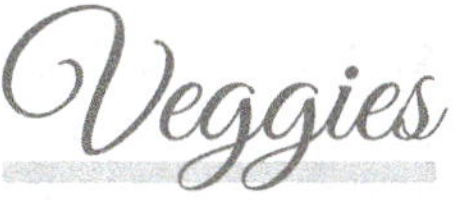

Roasted Brussels Sprouts

SERVES 4

Brussels sprouts are loaded with nutrients and are particularly high in vitamins K and C. They have been largely studied for their cancer prevention properties because of their special nutrient support they provide to the body's detoxification, antioxidant, and anti-inflammatory systems. They have one of the highest concentrations of glucosinolate, which is an important cancer-protective phytonutrient. To avoid overcooking Brussels sprouts, cut them into smaller pieces to reduce cooking time.

- 1 lb. Brussels sprouts, washed, trimmed, and cut in half, or in quarters if sprouts are large
- 2 tbsp ghee
- 1 tsp dried parsley
- 1 tsp dried basil
- 1 tbsp Pecorino Romano or Parmesan cheese
- ½ tsp garlic salt
- ¼ tsp black pepper

DIRECTIONS:

1. Preheat oven to 425°F.

2. In a medium roasting pan, combine all ingredients. Mix with hands to ensure ghee and spices and cheese are covering each Brussels sprout. Place in hot oven and roast for 25–30 minutes, stirring halfway through cooking. They should be slightly browned and tender.

Prosciutto Wrapped Asparagus

SERVES 6–8

Prosciutto is an uncooked Italian ham, made by rubbing salt, spices, and lard on the outside of meat and then slowly air drying for one to two years. Unlike American ham or bacon that's been cured or smoked, traditionally made good-quality prosciutto has no added preservatives such as nitrites or nitrates. Prosciutto is an important aspect of Italian cuisine and is part of a typical Mediterranean diet. It is enjoyed in small quantities as an accompaniment to fruits and vegetables. This simple dish is fun to make with your kids and can be eaten with your fingers.

16 asparagus spears

8 prosciutto slices (thin)

ghee

DIRECTIONS:

1. Wash asparagus spears and cut 1 in. off bottom of tough stem.

2. Slice each piece of prosciutto in half lengthwise. Wrap each asparagus spear with a half slice of prosciutto. This works easiest by wrapping on an angle so that most of the stem gets covered. The end product will have a little bit of green asparagus sticking out of each end.

3. Heat cast-iron pan with 1 tbsp of ghee. Place wrapped spears in pan and cook, turning until each side gets brown and crispy, about 2–3 minutes on each side.

Red Cabbage Roast

This delicious dish is a quick vegetable dish that can be paired with any meal. I like to roast the cabbage until it's slightly browned on the edges, giving it some texture.

- 1 red cabbage, small head chopped into 1-in. pieces (about a pound chopped)
- 1 onion, sliced thin
- 5 garlic cloves, minced
- 1 tbsp avocado oil
- 1 tbsp ghee
- salt and pepper

Directions:

1. Preheat oven to 425°F, convection preferred.

2. Heat a medium sauté pan on medium heat and add ghee to pan. Add onion and ¼ tsp salt and ¼ tsp pepper to pan. Cook until onion softens, about 5 minutes. Add garlic and sauté another minute and remove from heat.

3. Place chopped cabbage in roasting pan and pour onion mixture on top along with avocado oil and ½ tsp salt and ¼ tsp pepper. Mix with hands so that all the cabbage pieces are coated with oil and onion mixture.

4. Roast for 30 minutes, stirring halfway through roasting.

Variations: *For those days that I don't have time to sauté onions, I simply combine 1 head of chopped red cabbage with dried shallots, extra virgin olive oil, and Herbamare seasoning in a large roasting pan. I convection bake at 425° F for about 25 minutes, stirring once or twice to ensure even cooking.*

Cauliflower Mashed Potatoes*

SERVES 6–8

I can confidently say that this recipe was kid tested and mother approved. Both of my kids gobbled up this cauliflower puree and demanded more. Ahh, music to any mother's ears! I highly recommend purchasing a hand-held immersion blender, for those who haven't been introduced to this fabulous piece of machinery. It's by far the most valuable tool in my kitchen (aside from my kitchen knife). While extremely versatile, a hand mixer saves time and dirties fewer dishes. What a treat for a busy mom!

1 cauliflower, large head

¼ c bone broth, or low-sodium chicken broth

1 tbsp extra virgin olive oil, or ghee

dried herbs like thyme, rosemary, chives, or parsley

garlic salt and ground pepper to taste

DIRECTIONS:

1. Cut and stem cauliflower into florets. Place in steamer basket fitted to saucepan and steam until cauliflower is fork tender.

2. Drain water from saucepan and leave tender cauliflower in warm saucepan. Add chicken bone broth, olive oil, ½ tsp thyme, ½ tsp chives and ½ tsp parsley. Puree cauliflower with hand mixer until cauliflower has a smooth consistency.

3. Season to taste with garlic salt (about ½ tsp) and pepper (about ⅛ tsp). Serve hot with a spoon and enjoy!

   ***Variation:** Try this puree mixed with zucchini noodles or your favorite lentil pasta (cooked al dente) or serve as a dip with cut raw or roasted veggies.*

Roasted Butternut Squash

This recipe is easy and delicious. Let the squash brown and caramelize before taking it out of the oven. There won't be any leftovers.

1½ lb. butternut squash, peeled and ¾-in. diced

2 tbsp expeller-pressed avocado oil

1 tbsp grade B maple syrup (optional)

Himalayan salt and freshly ground black pepper

DIRECTIONS:

1. Preheat the oven to 400°F. (Convection oven works great when roasting vegetables.)

2. Place the butternut squash on a roasting pan. Pour avocado oil over diced squash, with 1 tsp salt and ½ tsp pepper and toss by hand. I only use maple syrup if the squash is out of season and might need a little hint of sweetness.

3. Roast for about 20–25 minutes until it's nicely browned and tender. Stir with a large spoon about halfway through cooking so that squash roasts evenly and doesn't burn.

Italian Stuffed Artichokes

This recipe was passed down from my paternal grandmother. I think it was one of my favorite veggies to eat as a kid. Don't forget to eat the "heart" of the artichoke after you have finished with the leaves. Simply scoop the inedible fuzzy hair layer that sits right inside the middle of the choke above the heart base. The bottom layer is the heart and is absolutely delicious!

2 large artichokes (look for fresh chokes with tight leaves)

10 large garlic cloves, finely chopped

4 tbsp extra virgin olive oil

5 tbsp Italian-style breadcrumbs, (gluten-free work great)

1 tsp Celtic sea salt

¼ tsp pepper

DIRECTIONS:

1. Trim artichoke by cutting 1 in. off the top of each choke and trim pointy end off each leaf. Next cut bottom with stem so that each artichoke can sit up on its own. Then trim stems so that you are left with 2–3 in. cylinder with outer skin removed. Set aside.

2. With your fingers, gently fan out artichoke leaves so that space is formed between leaves. Evenly stuff chopped garlic cloves (about 5 cloves per artichoke) inside each of the leaves and on top of artichoke. Repeat with breadcrumbs (about 2–3 tbsp per choke). Pour 2 tbsp olive oil over each artichoke and sprinkle with salt and pepper.

3. Fill a large pot with about 2 in. of water. Place artichokes and stems in the pot and cover. Bring to a boil and let simmer for about 45 minutes. Be sure to check the water level periodically to make sure it has not all evaporated. If so, add more hot water to the pot as needed. The artichokes are done when the leaves remove from the choke with ease and are tender.

4. Place artichokes and stems in a bowl and pour the remaining artichoke juice from the pan over the center of the choke. The juice is wonderful as a dip eaten with the heart.

Sautéed Spinach with Garlic

SERVES 4–5

Oxalic acid is a natural compound found in high concentrations in certain plant foods like spinach, rhubarb, chard, and beet greens. It imparts a sharp, bitter taste in these foods and also interferes with the absorption of many nutrients like iron, vitamins A and E, fiber, zinc, and calcium. However, by lightly cooking these foods the oxalic acid starts to break down and doesn't interfere with the absorption of these nutrients. This sautéed spinach recipe is the same recipe that my mom made for me growing up as a kid. I enjoy it today as much as I loved it then.

1½ lb. spinach leaves, thick tough stems removed

1 tbsp olive oil

1 tbsp ghee

4 garlic cloves, each clove cut twice

½ tsp Celtic sea salt, to taste

¼ tsp freshly ground black pepper, to taste

DIRECTIONS:

1. Rinse spinach in a colander and shake colander to remove excess water.

2. In a medium Dutch oven, heat the oil and ghee over medium heat. Add garlic and cook for 1 minute, not letting the garlic get brown (browning garlic makes it bitter). Remove garlic from the oil and set aside in small bowl.

3. Quickly add damp spinach, salt, and pepper to pot with oil, giving it a quick stir and covering it with a lid for about 2 minutes. Remove lid and stir again. Spinach should be slightly wilted but not soggy. Remove from heat, season with salt and pepper to taste.

4. Place spinach in serving bowls and top with reserved sautéed garlic.

Meat and Seafood

Thomas's Bison Meat Loaf

SERVES 6–8 PEOPLE

Recipe (adapted) courtesy of Chef Bobo's Good Food Cookbook by Chef Bobo (a.k.a. Robert Surles) ©2004, Meredith Corporation

This is one of my son's favorite dinners. It's flavorful, juicy, gluten-free, and is made without all the added sugars that often come with traditional meatloaf recipes that are slathered with ketchup or barbecue sauce.

coconut oil cooking spray (look for 100% natural spray oil without added chemicals or propellants)

2 tbsp avocado oil, or ghee

2 small onions, diced*

3–4 medium carrots, grated*

4 garlic cloves, minced*

1½ tbsp dry mustard

1½ tsp salt

1½ tsp black pepper

2 tsp dried thyme

½ c uncooked rolled oats (I use Trader Joe's gluten-free rolled oats)

2 eggs, beaten

2 lb. bison (recipe also works great with hormone-free ground turkey, dark and white meat combined)

** To save time, I throw carrots, onion, and garlic in a mini food processor to chop vegetables before I throw them in the pan.*
Serve with your favorite burger sauce.

DIRECTIONS:

1. Preheat oven to 350°F. Spray an 8 x 4 x 2 in. loaf pan with cooking spray.

2. Heat avocado oil in medium skillet until hot. Add onions, garlic, carrots, mustard, thyme, salt, and pepper. Sauté until onions are translucent. Set aside on cool burner.

3. In a separate bowl, combine oats and egg. Stir to combine. Next add the meat and onion mixture. Mix with hands to thoroughly combine.

4. Place mixture into prepared loaf pan and spread evenly. Bake loaf 40–45 minutes, depending on what type of meat selected. Meatloaf will pull away from sides of pan when it's done. USDA recommends ground meat of any kind be cooked to 160°F.

5. Serve meatloaf with your favorite sauce, or simply gobble it up covered with cauliflower mashed potatoes like we do.

One-Pan Baked Fish and Asparagus

SERVES 4

This is a meal that can be made in under 30 minutes, all in one pan. It's perfect for working families. The fish is simply dressed, but has loads of flavor. As it cooks, it gives off tasty fish juices that lightly season the asparagus, giving it a bright crisp finish.

4 wild-caught white-fish fillets, 5–6 oz. each (tilapia, sole, flounder, mullet, or snapper)

1/2 lemon

4 tbsp grass-fed butter, melted

2–3 garlic cloves, minced

4–5 scallions, white and light green parts only, finely diced

1/2 tsp dried parsley

sea salt

freshly ground pepper

1 bunch asparagus, washed and cut into 2-in. rods

1 tbsp avocado oil

1/4 tsp garlic salt

DIRECTIONS:

1. Preheat oven to 375°F.

2. Place fish fillets on a 12 x 17 in. rimmed sheet pan. Sprinkle each fillet with salt and fresh cracked pepper. Squeeze a little fresh lemon over each fillet.

3. In a small bowl, combine melted butter, scallions, and garlic. Let sit for 1–2 minutes. Evenly divide and spread butter mixture over each fillet.

4. Evenly sprinkle dried parsley over each fillet.

5. Place asparagus in a small bowl and mix with avocado oil. Spread asparagus on sheet pan around fish fillets. Sprinkle asparagus with garlic salt and a pinch of freshly ground pepper.

6. Bake for 10 minutes or until fish is cooked through (it should flake with a fork).

Curry Fish Salad

Let's face it, tuna fish is out. It's just not worth eating a fish with toxic levels of mercury when there are so many other options that are just as tasty and even more nourishing. Canned (or packet) salmon is an obvious alternative and can be used in this dish, but I find that canned smoked trout brings even more flavor to this dish. Freshwater rainbow trout is one of the acceptable farmed fish exceptions because it's raised in an ecologically responsible way and does not come with the PCB risk that the wild-caught trout varieties pose. It's also one of the best sources of omega-3 fatty acids and B12.

7–8 oz. canned (or cooked fresh) smoked trout packed in olive oil, or canned/packet wild-caught salmon, drained and oil discarded

2 tbsp avocado mayo (homemade preferred, recipe page 188) (Primal Kitchen or Sir Kensington's brands)

1 tsp medium yellow curry powder

1 tsp garlic powder

1/8 tsp garam masala

1/8 tsp dill

1/4 tsp chili powder

Salt to taste*

DIRECTIONS:

1. Place all ingredients in a small bowl and stir to combine. I like to eat this salad with 1/2 sliced raw red pepper instead of bread. I simply cut a pepper in half and stuff it with curry fish salad. My kids don't like that method. They prefer to eat the curry fish salad plain with a fork or with crackers and have the raw red pepper slices on the side.

**Taste this salad before you add salt. Canned trout is usually salty enough out of the can. You can reduce some of the sodium by running the fish under water before preparing.*

Chicken Curry with Green Peas

If you don't usually eat Indian food, you are missing out on an explosion of flavor that comes with eating this delicious cuisine. Curry powder is actually made up of several ingredients, which vary depending on which region of the world it comes from. It often will include spices like turmeric, coriander, cardamom, cumin, and cloves, which are responsible for some of curry's most dramatic health benefits.

- 2 tbsp ghee
- 1 tsp avocado oil, or ghee
- 1 onion, diced
- 2 cloves garlic, minced
- 3 tbsp medium yellow curry powder (I get mine from the Savory Spice Shop)
- 1 tsp ground cinnamon
- 1 tsp paprika
- ½ tsp fresh gingerroot, grated
- 1¼ tsp salt
- ¼ tsp black pepper
- 3 skinless, boneless, pastured chicken breasts, cut into ½-in. bite-size pieces (about 1.5 lb.)

- 1 tbsp tomato paste
- 1 can full-fat organic unsweetened coconut milk
- ½ c bone broth, or chicken broth
- ½ tsp local honey
- 2 bay leaves
- 1 c frozen peas
- 1 c broccoli florets, chopped into bite-size pieces (optional)
- 1 c baby spinach, chopped (optional)

DIRECTIONS:

1. In a large saucepan, heat ghee over medium heat. Add onion, ½ tsp salt, and ¼ tsp pepper to pan and sauté until onion is translucent and slightly browned around the edges. Add 1 tsp oil or ghee to pan along with garlic, fresh ginger, curry powder, cinnamon, and paprika. Let spices absorb in oil and roast in pan for 1–2 minutes.

2. Add chicken pieces, tomato paste, coconut milk, bone broth, honey, and bay leaves to pan and stir to combine. Let simmer on medium-low heat for about 15–20 minutes, or until chicken is cooked through. Stir in peas and spinach (if using) until peas are warmed and spinach is wilted. You can add any green vegetable that you like. I sometimes switch it up and use broccoli florets or chopped cauliflower, it just depends on what I have available.

3. Eat as is, or serve over brown basmati rice and enjoy.

Chimichurri Shrimp Skewers

SERVES 4

Even though this dish is frequently enjoyed in the summertime, it really can be a hit all year long. It's a snap to make and is always a crowd pleaser with adults and kids alike.

1.25 lb. wild-caught shrimp	2 tbsp fresh lemon juice
½ c fresh parsley	¼ tsp red pepper flakes
⅓ c fresh basil	2–3 cloves garlic
¼ c fresh chives	½ tsp salt
2 tbsp fresh oregano	¼ tsp pepper
2 tbsp red wine vinegar	¾ c olive oil

DIRECTIONS:

1. First make chimichurri sauce by placing all ingredients except shrimp in the bowl of a food processor. Blend until smooth. Transfer sauce to a bowl and let sit for at least 30 minutes to meld flavors (the longer the better). After flavors have melded, transfer ¾ c of sauce to a separate bowl and combine with shrimp. Marinate together for 30 minutes. Set aside remaining sauce for dipping after shrimp has been cooked.

2. While shrimp is marinating, soak wooden skewers in water for 20–30 minutes.

3. Thread 5–6 shrimp on each skewer, skewering each shrimp twice.

4. Grill shrimp for about 5–6 minutes, flipping halfway through cooking. Shrimp should be firm and opaque. Serve immediately with reserved chimichurri sauce.

Wild Salmon Lollipops with Italian Pesto   SERVES 4

Who doesn't like to eat lollipops? My kids agree, this makes eating salmon way more fun. And since pesto is one of their favorite flavors, it's an all-around win-win. Salmon is one of the best brain-boosting omega-3-rich foods on the planet, so try to get it in your kids' diets at least once a week. Go ahead and give these a try. They are simple to make, and cook in under 10 minutes.

1 lb. wild-caught salmon fillets, skinless

1–2 tbsp extra virgin olive oil

½ lemon (optional)

salt and pepper to taste

¼ c prepared pesto (recipe page 189)

DIRECTIONS:

1. Preheat oven to 375° F.

2. Cut salmon lengthwise and then again into strips so that you have rectangular pieces about 3-in. long and 1-in. wide. Insert wooden skewer into each piece of salmon piercing twice, once at each long end of rectangle.

3. Baste salmon with olive oil and sprinkle salmon skewers with salt and pepper and a squirt of fresh lemon juice.

4. Place tray of salmon in oven and bake for about 8–10 minutes. Watch fish closely to avoid overcooking.

5. Remove fish from oven and baste with fresh pesto.

Beans, Legumes and Grains

Nic's Black Bean Burgers

SERVES 6–7

These burgers are a huge hit with the whole family. For some time now, veggie burgers have gotten a bad rap for their cardboard-like texture and lack of taste. On the contrary! You'll be surprised how packed these are with flavor and how well they stay together. Since we are a family of four, I love that this recipe gives me some extra burgers that I can throw in the fridge for later in the week when I want to prepare a quick meal for myself or the kids.

- ¾ c sunflower seeds (or cashews)
- 2 15-oz. cans black beans, rinsed and drained
- 2 tbsp ghee or coconut oil
- 1 medium-large onion, diced
- 3 large cloves garlic, minced (let sit for 10 minutes before adding to heat)
- 1 large poblano pepper, diced
- 1 tbsp cumin, ground
- ½ tsp chipotle chili pepper, ground powder (optional)
- 1 tbsp Umami Mushroom Powder (see recipe, page 189)
- 1 egg
- ½ c tigernut flour (or teff flour, buckwheat flour, oat flour)
- ½ c shredded raw cheddar cheese (I like imported hormone-free, grass-fed varieties)

DIRECTIONS:

1. Move oven rack to highest position, which is typically about 4 in. from broiler. Turn the broiler on to preheat oven.

2. Place whole sunflower seeds in a small food processor. Pulse 5–8 times until chopped into small pieces. Transfer to large bowl.

3. Place one can of rinsed beans into large bowl with sunflower seeds. Place second can of rinsed beans in a small food processor and pulse until beans are roughly chopped. Transfer to bowl with rest of beans.

4. Heat 1 tbsp of avocado oil in a medium skillet over medium heat. Add onions, poblano pepper, and cumin, and cook for about 5 minutes until softened. Add garlic and mushroom powder and cook for another 1–2 minutes. Transfer to large bowl with beans.

5. Add egg, flour, and cheese to bowl with bean mixture. Mix together gently until all components are combined. Your hands are your best tool here! Form bean mixture into 6 patties and place on tray. At this point, you may cover and refrigerate if making at a later time. Stack with wax paper in between patties and cover completely to prevent patties from drying out. If making immediately, proceed to step 6.

6. Place patties on rimmed sheet pan sprayed with coconut oil cooking spray. Place tray in oven on top rack. Broil for 10 minutes.

7. Transfer to plate and top with condiments as desired. We like lettuce, tomato, guacamole (recipe page 233) and/or chipotle mayonnaise (recipe page 188).

Working Mom's Black Beans   SERVES 6–8

This recipe came to me 20 years ago when I was visiting with a Cuban friend of mine. It has been one of my staple go-to meals on busy weekday nights ever since. This dish can be made in under 45 minutes, which works well in my house when I have ravenous kids who barrel in the door from athletic events. My kids devour these beans and usually prefer pairing them with a little sprouted long-grain brown basmati rice. Sometimes they eat them as a side dish, but most of the time my family prefers them as a nutritious meal by themselves with a side of broccoli or a fresh mixed green salad.

3 tbsp expeller cold-pressed avocado oil	½ tsp pepper
1 large onion, diced	½ tsp oregano
4 cloves garlic, minced	2 bay leaves
1 red bell pepper, diced	2 tbsp maple syrup
2 cans black beans, washed and drained	2 tbsp balsamic vinegar (good quality)
2 tsp sea salt	2 tbsp red wine (good enough to drink)

DIRECTIONS:

1. Heat the oil in a Dutch oven or small soup pot and add onion, garlic, red pepper, salt, pepper, and oregano. Sauté on medium heat until onion is translucent (about 5 minutes).

2. Add beans, bay leaves, maple syrup, balsamic vinegar, and red wine to the pot. Continue to cook covered on medium-low for approximately 15 minutes, until mixture slightly thickens and flavors meld.

Commercial rice products contain 10–20 times more inorganic arsenic than other cereal crops, which can be toxic to humans (especially infants, children, and pregnant moms). Arsenic scientist, Professor Andrew Meharg of Queen's University Belfast, proved that you can reduce 80 percent of the arsenic content in rice by soaking the rice overnight, rinsing, and then cooking it in a covered saucepan with five parts water, one part rice until tender and then draining the excess water off. If you skip the overnight soak, you end up removing about 50 percent of the arsenic with the five to one water to rice cooking method. It's also wise to only buy rice products from California, India, or Pakistan (avoid Arkansas, Louisiana, Texas), as these regions are known to have lower arsenic levels in the soil.

Creamy Herbed White Beans

This warm and cozy dish is quite versatile. It can be eaten as a side dish to fish or meat, paired alongside a crisp green salad, or tossed with steamed broccoli. It also can be served as a snack for your kids when they run in starving after school.

1 tbsp ghee

1 large onion, finely diced

1 tbsp cold-pressed extra virgin olive oil, or avocado oil

5–6 cloves garlic, minced

1 tsp dried rosemary

½ tsp dried thyme

¼ tsp dried red pepper flakes

2 cans organic white northern beans, or cannellini beans

2 c chicken bone broth (see recipe, page 198), or boxed organic chicken broth/stock

salt and pepper to taste

DIRECTIONS:

1. Drain and rinse beans under running water in a strainer.

2. In a medium saucepan on medium, heat the ghee until warm. Then add onions and ½ tsp salt and ¼ tsp pepper and sauté until onions are soft and translucent.

3. Add olive oil, garlic, rosemary, thyme, and red pepper flakes and sauté another minute.

4. Stir in beans and broth and simmer on low for 20–30 minutes, until liquid is reduced by half and begins to thicken. Remember to stir the mixture every 3–5 minutes to prevent the beans from burning or sticking to the bottom of the pan. Add more broth if mixture looks too thick.

5. Season with sea salt and pepper to taste.

Quinoa Pilaf

Quinoa, pronounced "keen-wah," is one of the oldest cultivated grains in the world. It's packed with antioxidant phytonutrients and is a high-quality protein intact with all essential amino acids. It's truly a powerhouse grain containing a great source of heart-healthy magnesium, bone-building manganese, phosphorus, and copper, as well as fiber and iron. You can cook quinoa just like rice, but I find that sometimes it needs a little pick-me-up. This combination of flavors is sure to please your palate and can be paired with just about anything.

2 c cooked quinoa (see cooking method below)

1 tbsp expeller-pressed avocado oil, grass-fed ghee, or virgin coconut oil

4–5 garlic cloves, minced

1 large onion, finely diced

1 large red pepper, diced

1 tbsp dried basil

½ c organic frozen corn

salt and pepper to taste

1–2 tbsp grass-fed butter (I like Kerry Gold)

DIRECTIONS:

1. Heat avocado oil or ghee in a medium-sized skillet on low-medium heat.

2. Add garlic, onion, pepper, basil, ½ tsp salt, and ¼ tsp pepper to pan. Cook approximately 5–10 minutes, or until the onion has softened and becomes more translucent.

3. Add corn and cook for another 2 minutes.

4. Mix in cooked quinoa to the onion mixture and season with additional salt and pepper to taste. Finish by adding 1 tbsp of butter to quinoa mixture. Remove from heat and serve.

Quinoa contains saponins, which are bitter phytocompounds that are part of the plant's natural pest control. Proper cooking methods will reduce some of these anti-nutrients that can interfere with nutrient absorption and potentially damage your gut. To properly prepare quinoa, first soak by adding 1 cup of quinoa to 2 cups of warm filtered water. Add 1–2 tbsp of an acid like apple cider vinegar or lemon juice to a glass bowl and let soak in a warm spot for 12–24 hours overnight. Pour off soaking liquid, rinse with fresh water, and stir to remove foam. Then cook as usual.

Lentil Meatballs

These little meatballs are all about putting a twist on something familiar. They are a delicious plant-based option that provides comfort and a burst of flavor with every bite. They go great with a smooth guacamole dip or paired with your favorite marinara sauce.

- 1 tbsp organic virgin coconut oil or extra virgin avocado oil
- 1 yellow onion, diced
- 4–5 garlic cloves, minced
- 1¼ tsp salt
- ¼ tsp pepper
- 1 jalapeño pepper, diced
- 2 c green lentils, cooked and cooled (cooked in beef, chicken, or vegetable stock until tender but not mushy)
- 1 egg
- 1 tbsp tomato paste
- 1½ tsp cumin
- ½ tsp coriander
- Raw cheddar cheese, grass-fed, antibiotic-free (I like European cheese from Trader Joe's) (optional)

DIRECTIONS:

1. Preheat oven to 400°F, convection if possible.

2. Heat coconut oil in a medium-sized skillet over medium heat. Add onion, jalapeño, ¼ tsp salt, and ¼ tsp pepper, and cook until vegetables are softened and browned around the edges, about 5 minutes. Add garlic and cook 1 minute more. Remove from heat and set aside.

3. In a food processor, add lentils, onion mixture, egg, tomato paste, cumin, coriander, and 1 tsp sea salt. Pulse, mixing until combined but not pureed, leaving some texture to the mix.

4. Line a medium-sized sheet pan with parchment paper. Scoop rounded tablespoon amounts of meatball mixture into palm of hand. Roll gently into balls and place on parchment-lined pan.

5. Bake for 25 minutes, until browned and cooked through. At this point you can remove the meatballs and eat as is, or you can top them with thin squares of cheese and place back in the oven for 3 minutes, or until the cheese melts.

6. Remove from oven and serve with a side of guacamole dip (recipe page 233).

Variations: *You can also serve these with marinara sauce and zucchini noodles.*

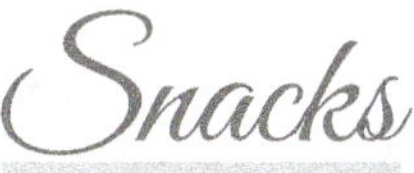

Snacks

Roasted Almonds

MAKES 2 CUPS

Some of the most common commercially available nuts are "roasted." The problem is that most are roasted in highly unstable, polyunsaturated seed oils like cottonseed, soybean, sunflower, canola, or peanut oils and at high temperatures. These fats are easily distorted when exposed to heat and create dangerous free radicals in our bodies. So to get the most nutrition out of your nuts and improve their digestibility, it's beneficial to soak them in salted water and dry roast them at low temperatures. This helps break down some of the nuts' enzyme inhibitors and increases their antioxidant and phytonutrient capacity. Low temperature roasting also helps preserve the nuts' valuable fats and vitamin E content. Try out this simple technique; the end product is delicious!

2 c of raw almonds with skin

Himalayan salt

Warm water

DIRECTIONS:

1. Cover nuts with warm water in a bowl. Add 1 tsp salt and mix to dissolve. Soak for at least 7 hours, or overnight on the kitchen counter.

2. Preheat convection oven to 170°F. Drain water from almonds and dry nuts with paper towel or kitchen towel. Spread nuts on sheet pan and sprinkle with sea salt and/or preferred flavoring, such as garlic and onion powder, curry, cumin, herbs, or seasoned salt. (My favorite is with just sea salt.)

3. Roast for 25–30 minutes (convection oven). Test nuts to make sure they are dried and crisp. Remove from oven and let cool entirely. Store in tightly sealed container in refrigerator.

Avocado Toast

SERVES 1

This healthy and slightly indulgent meal is unbelievably versatile, and best of all, quick! Avocado was my daughter's first food as a baby and has remained one of her favorites for 12 years straight. This yummy meal can be eaten as a simple breakfast or an anytime snack. It provides healthy monounsaturated fat and fiber to help you stay full throughout the day.

½ Haas avocado

½ tsp freshly squeezed lemon juice

sea salt, to taste

freshly ground black pepper, to taste

1 slice of sprouted grain bread, toasted (organic, GMO-free, Ezekiel, Artisan Sourdough, or whole grain gluten-free)

OPTIONAL TOPPINGS:

baby greens

broccoli sprouts

1 egg, pastured, GMO-free

fresh tomato slices

hempseeds

hot sauce

Parmesan cheese

radish

sautéed mushrooms

sliced shallots

DIRECTIONS:

1. Mash avocado in a bowl with a fork. Add lemon juice. Spread avocado on toast, season with salt and pepper (or seasoned salt), and top with desired toppings.

Baked Cinnamon Apple Chips

Bagged fruit chips from the grocery store are expensive, but not when you make them at home! Crunchy, tart, and naturally sweet, these chips combine healthy and tasty into one irresistible snack. Kids love to help make these chips. But beware, there won't be any leftovers.

3 **large organic apples, sliced ⅛ in. thick (I like Fuji or Honeycrisp apples)**

Ceylon cinnamon, to taste

DIRECTIONS:

1. Preheat oven to 225°F. Slice apples with mandolin or sharp knife. With a small round cookie cutter, cut out the hard apple center if needed.

2. Arrange apple slices in single layer (touching but not overlapping) on two parchment-lined sheet pans. Sprinkle each apple slice with cinnamon.

3. Bake for 60 minutes, then flip apple slices and bake 60 minutes more. If apples have not reached desired crispness, simply bake them 10–20 minutes more. Remove from oven and let cool completely. Store in airtight container.

Fresh Berries with Coconut Whipped Cream   SERVES 8–10

Packed with essential vitamins and minerals, fiber, and natural electrolytes, coconut in all its forms is one of the world's healthiest foods. One of the coconut's most important features is its high content of medium-chain fatty acids such as lauric acid, which makes up about 50 percent of the fat in this fruit. It is readily used by the body for energy and is known to enhance immunity. This snack or dessert is quick and easy to prepare. I like to wash a big bowl of berries and leave them in the refrigerator for easy grabbing for smoothies, snacks, or toppings. The coconut cream is a good option for anyone who is sensitive to dairy or lactose intolerant. Although coconut cream has many healthful benefits, it's also quite calorically dense, so only a little bit is needed.

16 oz. fresh strawberries, washed, stems removed, and sliced in half

6 oz. fresh blackberries, washed

1 pint fresh blueberries, washed

1 can full-fat coconut milk or Trader Joe's coconut cream, chilled in refrigerator overnight

1–3 tsp coconut sugar, maple syrup, or 3–5 drops of liquid stevia, to taste (optional)

½ tsp vanilla extract

chopped nuts of choice, optional

DIRECTIONS:

1. Chill a medium metal mixing bowl and whisk attachment in freezer for 10 minutes.

2. Remove chilled can of coconut milk from refrigerator and carefully scoop out solid coconut cream that has solidified at the top of can and place in chilled bowl. Pour out liquid coconut water into separate container and save for later use in smoothies.

3. Add vanilla and coconut sugar (if desired) to bowl. Beat coconut cream mixture with chilled whisk until it becomes whipped and fluffy. If you want a looser, more pourable consistency, add a little reserved coconut milk to mixture 1 tbsp at a time.

4. Spoon some berries into single-sized bowls and top with coconut cream. Sprinkle with chopped nuts or chia seeds.

Miso Tahini Dip** with Veggie Crudités

MAKES ¾ CUP

This is a delicious way to incorporate a fermented food into your family's eating plan. Miso is a fermented soybean product that contains live beneficial lactobacillus bacteria that's great for your gut health. It's been enjoyed in Asia for centuries and is most familiar to Americans as the main ingredient in Japanese miso soup. Always choose a well-sourced, refrigerated organic miso to make sure you are getting a safe, non-GMO product.

2 garlic cloves, minced

½ c raw sesame tahini

1½ tbsp red miso (I like Miso Master, Organic Traditional Red Miso)

¼ c water (approximately)

DIRECTIONS:

1. Mix the tahini and miso in a bowl until well combined. Add the water gradually while stirring. The mixture will first thicken, and then begin to turn smooth and creamy. Add just enough water to get the consistency you want for the dip. Add the mashed garlic and mix well.

2. Serve with vegetable crudités: carrot and celery sticks, cucumber spears, red and orange bell pepper slices, and assorted rice crackers.

   Store leftovers in an airtight container. The dip will keep in the refrigerator for up to a week.

***Reprinted with permission from Fast Food, Good Food. Copyright © 2015 by Andrew Weil, MD. Little Brown & Co., NY.*

Roasted Garlic Hummus

The great thing about hummus is that when made at home, every single ingredient is beneficial for your body. This Mediterranean and Middle Eastern food is a wonderful plant-based protein that also delivers fiber for a healthy digestive system and anti-inflammatory properties that help reduce disease. It's also loaded with essential micronutrients like iron, folate, phosphorus, B vitamins, and immune-boosting vitamin C.

1 15-oz. can chickpeas, rinsed and drained	¾ tsp cumin
2 tbsp lemon juice	¾ tsp salt
¼ c tahini (stirred well)	3 tbsp water
1 head of roasted garlic	paprika, pinch (optional)
2 tbsp extra virgin olive oil	2 tbsp roasted pine nuts (optional)

DIRECTIONS:

1. Roast garlic: Preheat oven to 425°F. Cut the top off of 1 bulb of garlic (about ¼ in.) so that raw garlic cloves are exposed. Lay head of garlic on top of square piece of aluminum foil and pour 1–2 tsp olive oil over the top of the exposed garlic. Wrap garlic head tightly with tin foil and place in hot oven. Roast for 45 minutes, or until garlic cloves are soft and slightly browned. Let cool. (If you don't have time for this step, simply use 1–2 fresh garlic cloves in place of roasted garlic.)

2. If using roasted garlic, combine half head of roasted garlic (about 6 cloves) with remaining ingredients in a food processor. Blend until mixture is smooth and creamy. Add more water if you like a creamier consistency.

3. Transfer hummus to serving bowl and garnish with a sprinkle of paprika and roasted pine nuts, if desired. Serve with vegetable crudités, such as carrots, red peppers, cucumbers, and celery.

Guacamole

"Guac," as we like to call it, is one of the best last-minute healthy snacks you can make. I always keep avocados and lemons in the house. Even if you don't have all the ingredients, or the time, you can make a delicious alternative with avocado, lemon juice, salt, onion powder, and/or garlic powder.

- 2 Haas avocados, ripe
- ¼ c yellow onion, finely diced
- 1 Roma tomato, seeded and finely diced
- 1 jalapeño pepper, stems and seeds removed, finely diced
- 1 small lemon, or lime
- ¾–1 tsp sea salt, or less to taste
- handful of fresh cilantro, about 2–3 tbsp chopped (optional)

DIRECTIONS:

1. Remove skin and seeds from avocados and place green flesh in medium bowl. Mash with a fork. Mix in onion, tomatoes, jalapeño, salt, the juice from one lemon or lime, and cilantro (if using) until combined.

2. Serve with jicama sticks, cucumber slices, bean chips, vegetable crudités, or use it as a spread or accompaniment to meat or seafood.

Homemade Popcorn

SERVE 2–4

If our family has a weakness, it's popcorn! I have a 1950s popper that makes the perfect batch of completely irresistible popcorn. My kids love it too, but they are not allowed to use the electric device by themselves. My kids begged me to buy microwave popcorn, but knowing how harmful it is to our health, I needed to find another solution that they could prepare on their own. Microwave popcorn contains ingredients like partially hydrogenated oils, toxic artificial flavors, artificial coloring, preservatives, and GMO ingredients. And if that isn't bad enough, you also need to worry about the bag. Almost all varieties of microwave popcorn have bags that are lined with perfluorooctanoic acid (PFOA). In fact, the EPA has identified PFOA as a "likely carcinogen," and another study found an acid that can be extracted from the chemical causes cancer in animals and is "likely to cause cancer in humans." Here is a much better alternative. It offers fiber, healthy fat, and a little bit of protein without any toxic ingredients or contaminants.

¼ cup organic popcorn kernels

1 tbsp hempseeds (ground or whole)*

1 tbsp grass-fed butter, ghee, or coconut oil, melted

sea salt, to taste

DIRECTIONS:

1. Place organic popcorn in brown paper bag (lunch box size). Loosely fold the top of the bag two or three times to prevent popcorn from spilling out. Place in microwave on high for 1–2 minutes. (The time varies with microwaves, so it is essential that you listen for when the popping slows, and there are 2–3 seconds between pops. If it pops too long it will burn. You will get the hang of it after making this once or twice. Pour popped kernels into a bowl.

2. Pour butter or ghee over popcorn and then sprinkle with hempseeds and sea salt to taste.

**If you have time, you can grind the hempseeds in a coffee grinder for better coverage on the kernels.*

Optional Toppings:

Everything Bagel seasoning (I like Trader Joe's)

herbs: parsley, chives, rosemary

2 tbsp nutritional yeast, ½ tsp cumin, extra virgin coconut oil

Parmesan cheese

salt and vinegar: spray malt vinegar on popcorn and sprinkle with sea salt

taco seasoning and extra virgin olive oil

toasted sesame seeds

Kale Chips

This is a great recipe to make with your kids. It keeps their attention, allows them to get their hands dirty, and gives them a quick result. The best part is the crispy, crunchy, salty, and, best of all, healthy treat at the end!

1 bunch kale (about 8 oz.), (I like Lacinato or "Dinosaur" Kale but curly kale works great too!)

1 tbsp extra virgin olive oil, avocado oil, or

melted coconut oil

sea salt, to taste (or your favorite flavored salt)

DIRECTIONS:

1. Preheat oven to 300°F.

2. Rinse the kale in fresh water, then carefully cut out the tough stems with a kitchen knife and discard. Cut leaves into large pieces, and place in a salad spinner to remove as much water as possible. Transfer to a kitchen towel to remove any excess water left; drying well will help make the kale chips crispy.

3. Place kale in a clean bowl and toss with olive oil. Your hands are the best tool here to rub each leaf with olive oil to ensure coverage. Arrange leaves flat in a single layer on two large baking sheets lined with parchment paper. Sprinkle each leaf with sea salt to taste. Place in oven and bake for approximately 14–16 minutes, or until thoroughly crisp. These can be a little tricky at first to get them crisp without burning them so watch them closely. Everyone's oven is a little bit different so check on them every 2 minutes to see how fast they are cooking. Enjoy!

Variations:

Sprinkle the kale leaves before roasting with your favorite spice combinations:

- **BBQ kale chips:** ¼ tsp chili powder + ¼ tsp garlic powder + ¼ tsp onion powder + 2 tsp coconut sugar + 1–2 tbsp olive oil + sea salt sprinkle

- **Parmesan kale chips:** 3 tbsp Parmesan cheese + 3 tbsp olive oil + sea salt sprinkle

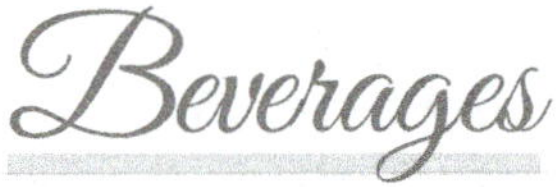

Beverages

Homemade Cashew Milk

MAKES ABOUT 20 OZ.

Most store-bought almond milks are pasteurized, which damages heat-sensitive vitamins and eliminates the almonds' fiber-rich skin. And if you are buying the sweetened varieties, understand that you are consuming mostly sugar water. Making your own nut milk is not only easy but also provides you with more nutrients and less additives, such as genetically modified soy lecithin. Carrageenan is another common emulsifier added to nut milks with questionable safety. If you want a great, easy milk alternative, cashew milk is the way to go. It's creamy, nutritious, and tastes fabulous. Unlike other nut milks, it requires no straining, which means less hassle, more nutrition, and less waste!

1 c raw cashews	1–2 tsp vanilla extract
4 c water*	½ tsp sea salt
3 pitted Medjool dates*	pinch cinnamon (optional)

DIRECTIONS:

1. Soak the cashews in 4 cups of filtered water at least 8 hours, or overnight. Drain the cashews and rinse until the water runs clear. Add the cashews and remaining ingredients to a high-speed blender (a Vitamix works well). Start on a low setting and increase the speed until the cashews are totally pulverized. This could take 2–3 minutes, depending on strength of blender. Milk should be smooth without any lumps or chunks.

2. Pour the milk into Mason jars and store, covered, in the refrigerator. It should keep for 4–5 days.

   **You can adjust the creaminess of the milk by adding more or less water. More water produces a thinner consistency, less water produces a thicker result. The sweetness can also be adjusted with using fewer or more dates.*

Homemade Lemon Ginger Tea

SERVES 1

Ginger is probably one of the top 10 most powerful therapeutic spices. It's used extensively in Ayurveda for its digestive benefits, anti-inflammatory properties, and anti-inflammatory effects. I give this ginger tea to my kids any time they are feeling under the weather or their tummies are "off." This tea is helpful to fight against common kids' viruses like RSV, and some studies show ginger may also help combat bacterial infections. Ginger is also effective for treating nausea from any etiology—seasickness, chemotherapy, morning sickness during pregnancy, or postoperative nausea. Even if you don't have an ailment, this tea is simply delicious and will warm your tummy with "happy."

2 c filtered water

1 tbsp fresh gingerroot, skin removed and roughly chopped

½ lemon, juiced

¼ tsp lemon zest (from an organic lemon)

½ tsp local raw honey, or liquid stevia, to taste

DIRECTIONS:

1. In a small covered saucepan, add water and chopped ginger. Over medium-high heat bring to a boil. Once water boils, turn off heat and let mixture steep, covered, for 10–15 minutes.

2. Pour ginger water into mug through a hand strainer. Squeeze lemon juice and zest into ginger water. Sweeten with ½–1 tsp honey as desired.

3. Grab a blanket, snuggle, and sip this soothing beverage.

Variations:

You can add any herbal tea to the water as it steeps with ginger. I occasionally will add chamomile, dandelion root, or lemon balm tea to the mixture. You can also add healing spices like turmeric or cinnamon for an added health boost.

Fruit Water

This is a fabulous drink for the whole family when plain water gets boring. The flavor combinations are endless. Be aware that herbs generally give off very strong flavors, so a little goes a long way. I keep a batch going in the refrigerator for most of the year. You can also get fancy, and set up a daily fruit water drink station and feel like you are at the spa!

3 qt filtered water

Fresh fruits, vegetables, and herbs of choice

DIRECTIONS:

1. Fill large glass gallon pitcher with water.

2. Add flavor enhancers: ¼-in. sliced fruit, veggies, or herbs. Stir and muddle together.

3. Let chill and infuse in refrigerator for at least 1 hour.

Flavor Combinations

My favorite: 1 Cucumber + 2 Lemons + 1 Orange + 3 Limes + 20 Mint leaves

Blueberries + Peaches

Orange + Grapefruit + Lime + Lemon + Basil

Pineapple + Mint Leaves

Raspberry + Lime

Watermelon + Mint Leaves + Basil

Sensible Soda

In the summertime when it's hot, this is what my kids drink instead of the deleterious bottled drink options that are sold to our kids at every turn. If I could choose one of the worst foods to put in our bodies, soda would be at the top of the list. Aside from the refined sugar, hidden caffeine, and artificial chemicals, soda also contains substantial amounts of phosphorus, which, when excreted, pulls calcium out of the bones, resulting in poor bone mineralization. Not at all what we want for our growing children. This refreshing drink is what I call "sensible soda" because it provides fizz, sweet and sour, but also helps alkalize the body, support bones, keep you hydrated, and gives you a little immune-boosting vitamin C.

8 oz. club soda (or make your own fizzy sparkling water with a SodaStream)

1 lemon or lime (or both)

liquid organic stevia, to taste (I like SweetLeaf or Trader Joe's)

DIRECTIONS:

1. Pour club soda into a tall 12–16 oz. glass.

2. Squeeze lemon or lime (or both) in glass.

3. Place 2–3 drops of liquid stevia in glass and stir. Adjust sweetness to your taste but go slow. A little bit goes a long way. Five drops of liquid stevia is equivalent to 1 tsp of sugar.

4. Add ice and enjoy!

Upgraded Hot Chocolate

SERVES 2

To me, hot chocolate is synonymous with winter, snow skiing, and the holiday season. Unfortunately, if you swing by your local Starbucks or Dunkin' Donuts, a medium hot chocolate will deliver you 10 tsp of sugar and a blood-sugar roller-coaster. This got me thinking, wouldn't it be great if my family could enjoy this old-fashioned drink of the season, but also receive some nourishment at the same time? So instead of stopping at a coffee house or serving them hot cocoa from a packet, I created an upgraded hot chocolate that's dairy-free, contains much less sugar than traditional drinks (only 4.4 g or 1 tsp to be exact), and includes mood-balancing maca powder. (Well-known as a powerful adaptogen and for its ability to regulate hormones, maca has a rich malty flavor that many enjoy with cacao.) This beverage also contains raw cacao powder, which is rich in nutrients and contains nearly 4 times the antioxidant power as cocoa powder and more than 20 times than that of blueberries. Cacao is also one of the highest plant-based sources of iron and magnesium.

- 1 c unsweetened almond milk
- 1 tbsp organic cacao powder (I like Navitas)
- ½ tsp vanilla extract
- 1 tsp maple syrup
- ½ tsp pure monk fruit extract (look for brands without maltodextrin)
- ½ tsp maca powder (optional)

Top with coconut whipped cream if desired.

DIRECTIONS:

1. Add milk, cacao, vanilla, maple syrup, monk fruit extract, and maca powder (if using) to a small sauce pot and whisk while bringing to a boil.

2. Turn off heat, pour into mugs, and enjoy!

**My kids don't care for the unique maca flavor in this, so I leave it out for them. The adults, however, celebrate anything that balances hormones.*

Green Juice*

SERVES 1–2

Although vegetable juice is not a complete meal, it is loaded with vitamins, minerals, and phytonutrients that make it an excellent addition to your family's diet. It's easy to digest and allows your body to absorb nutrients fast. Where people go wrong with juicing, is that they often add too much fruit to the recipe. While no fruit is best, one small apple can add a much more favorable taste and acceptance of the drink without too much sugar. Vegetable juice is highly perishable, so it's best to drink it immediately after juicing, or ideally within 24 hours.

1 bunch kale, organic	1 lemon, organic
1 bunch spinach, organic	1 small green apple, organic
1 -in. piece ginger	2 cucumbers, organic

DIRECTIONS:

1. Wash and trim fruit and veggies.

2. Cut into pieces and run all above ingredients together through juicer.

**Omega and Breville make good juicers.*

Other flavor combinations:

The Disease Fighter: 1 c broccoli +1 cucumber + 2 c Romaine lettuce + ½ c parsley + ½ green apple + 1 lime

Endurance Juice (before an event): 2 beets + 2 carrots + 3 kale leaves + 1-in. piece ginger + 1 lemon

Athlete's Rehydrating Juice: 4 oz. coconut water + 4 celery stalks + 1 cucumber + 1 peeled lemon

**Another great option is to mix the above ingredients in a blender instead of juicing. This way you get all the fiber for your gut health.*

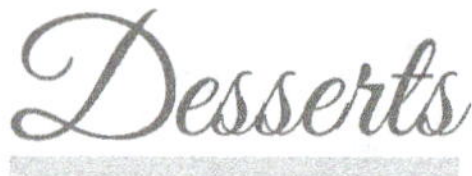

Desserts

Dark Chocolate Bark
with Super Seeds and Sea Salt

SERVES 8–10

Not all chocolate is created equal. When making this recipe, stick to good-quality dark chocolate that has 70% cocoa solids, or higher, to obtain the most potent antioxidants and the least amount of sugar. Milk chocolate has little, if any health benefits, whereas dark chocolate's attributes are quite impressive. Its high antioxidant and anti-inflammatory properties have both neuroprotective and cardioprotective benefits. Making this dark chocolate bark couldn't be easier, and it's so delicious! It combines sweet, salty, and crunchy all in one bite. Mix and match the toppings to whatever your family enjoys.

12 oz. dark chocolate (70% cocoa or higher), melted

2 tbsp sunflower seeds, lightly chopped

2 tsp sesame seeds (white or black)

2 tsp chia seeds

¼ tsp sea salt (finishing salt like Fleur de sel)

coconut cooking spray

DIRECTIONS:

1. Line a 9 x 9 in. pan with waxed paper and lightly spray with cooking spray.

2. Pour melted chocolate in pan and smooth into an even layer.

3. Sprinkle with nuts, seeds, and sea salt.

4. Place pan in freezer for 45 minutes, or until chocolate is hardened.

5. Break into bite-sized pieces and store in refrigerator.

Variations:

Change up the nut and seed toppings as you like. I also enjoy chopped Brazil nuts, pistachios, almonds, unsweetened coconut, and popped amaranth.

Frozen Chocolate Banana Bites

In my house, you won't find many "sweets," to my mother's dismay when she comes to visit. I am, however, a fan of dark chocolate. I admire it not just for its deliciousness, but also its many health benefits. The latest studies show that dark chocolate may be good for the heart and help make blood vessels more flexible. Chocolate contains polyphenols, the same kinds of antioxidants found in red wine and green tea. It also contains stearic acid, a type of saturated fat that doesn't raise cholesterol levels, and flavonoids, which reduce the stickiness of platelets, inhibiting blood clotting and reducing the danger of coronary artery blockages. This recipe serves as a satisfying sweet treat, yet also supplies some valued nutrients, unlike cookies, ice cream, or cake. Your kids will love helping you make these too!

- 4 medium bananas, ripe but firm
- 3 tbsp lightly salted nuts or seeds, finely chopped (macadamias, almonds, pistachios, cashews, sunflower seeds, or hempseeds) (optional)
- 6 oz. good-quality dark chocolate (70% or higher cocoa solids), chopped

DIRECTIONS:

1. Peel, then cut each banana into bite-sized, 1-in. pieces. Place the nuts in a shallow dish or on a small plate.

2. In a small saucepan, melt the chocolate over the lowest possible heat, stirring frequently. Once melted, dip each banana piece into the chocolate, turning to coat, and immediately roll in the nuts or seeds. Place on a tray covered in waxed paper, and freeze for 2–3 hours. Once frozen, serve immediately or store in airtight container in freezer for up to 2 weeks.

Peach Yogurt Ice Pops

You can make these with just about any fruit combination. They make a refreshing summer treat without added sugar.

- 1 c frozen or fresh peaches, organic
- 1 c plain full-fat Greek yogurt, grass-fed, organic (goat yogurt preferred, or non-dairy yogurt)
- 1/4 tsp vanilla extract
- 10–15 drops liquid stevia (start with 5 drops, mix and taste, repeat for desired sweetness)

DIRECTIONS:

1. Combine all ingredients in blender and puree until smooth.

2. Pour the mixture into Popsicle molds and freeze until firm, about 3 hours. When ready to eat, run under hot water for 5 seconds to loosen treat.

Banana Chia Pudding*

SERVES 2

If you want a smooth, delicious, brain-boosting treat that's sweetened naturally with fruit, try this pudding. Unlike traditional pudding, this dessert is dairy-free with healthy medium-chain fats and nutrient-dense chia seeds. The sweetness will depend on the ripeness of the banana you use. If the banana is really green, you may end up with a more bitter tasting pudding. I wouldn't use overly ripe brown bananas either as it creates a bad alcohol-like flavor. Stick to just-ripened yellow bananas for the best result.

½ c full-fat coconut milk

1 egg yolk

½ tsp maple syrup (optional)

½ tsp vanilla

⅛ tsp cinnamon

pinch salt

½ medium banana, mashed with a fork

2 tsp chia seeds**

Fresh blueberries, raspberries, or goji berries, optional topping

DIRECTIONS:

1. Place coconut milk in a small saucepan.

2. Whisk in egg yolk, vanilla, maple syrup (if using), cinnamon, salt, and banana. Heat over medium heat until mixture comes to a boil, stirring constantly with a whisk. Once mixture is slightly boiling, turn heat to low and lightly simmer for 1 minute more, continue to whisk. You will notice the mixture slightly thicken.

3. Remove from heat and stir in chia seeds. Pour mixture evenly into two 4-oz. ramekin cups.

4. Cover with plastic wrap and refrigerate overnight, or for at least 8 hours.

Serve with fresh blueberries, raspberries, or dried goji berries on top. Enjoy!

**You can also make this without the banana, which tastes more like traditional vanilla pudding.*

***To get an extra fiber boost, I sometimes add 2 tbsp of chia seeds instead of 2 tsp. This will make the pudding very thick and a little less sweet tasting but still quite satisfying.*

APPENDIX A: GRAINS AND GLUTEN CONCERNS

Two questions I get asked a lot pertain to whether we should be eating grains at all and if gluten-free is just a fad diet. Here's my take on both subjects.

DO WE REALLY NEED TO EAT GRAINS?

As you've discovered from reading this book, we've been misled by the abysmal nutrition recommendations that have circulated over the last 50 years. Our USDA nutrition guidelines, which have been created at the hands of special interest groups, have been telling us to eat more "healthy whole grains" for years, recommending such foods as bread, bagels, crackers, breakfast cereals, pancakes, rice cakes, and pasta. I couldn't disagree more. First, a whole grain, which is an unprocessed, wholly intact food (think rice, quinoa, or millet), is digested and absorbed far differently than a grain that's been refined into flour. People are always surprised when I tell them that bread raises your blood sugar faster than table sugar. In fact, wheat bread and white bread have close to the same effect on a person's blood sugar.

But when the question comes down to whether we should be eating whole grains at all, I think we need to weigh the pluses and minuses as they pertain to our own personal health. We can exist perfectly fine without grains in our diet. The downside to grains are 1) most people consume *refined* grains instead of consuming them in their *whole* form; 2) many people are sensitive to grains, which disrupt their digestive systems; and 3) grains contain phytates, lectins, and trypsin inhibitors, often referred to as anti-nutrients, which interfere with the absorption of nutrients and challenge our immune system. Certain groups of people, such as infants and vegans, should be careful of anti-nutrient intake. In addition, if you are someone with leaky gut, an autoimmune condition, or have a compromised immune system, then I would consider going without grains, especially those that contain gluten. But for an otherwise healthy adult or child, I think whole grains in reasonable amounts can be part of a healthy eating plan. On the plus side, whole grains offer a great source of fiber, are loaded with B vitamins, and contain key minerals like zinc, iron, and magnesium.

That said, you should always consume grains in their whole forms, in small amounts, and with the right cooking preparation. This means choosing unrefined, non-GMO grains like quinoa, amaranth, millet, steel-cut oats, sorghum, and buckwheat, and eating no more than 1–2 half-cup servings a day combined with quality protein and healthy fat. Soaking and sprouting whole grains is also important to break down some of their nutrient blockers, like lectin and phytate. It's also possible to enhance mineral absorption of grains by consuming them with nutrient-enhancing foods. For example, eating a food with phytic acid along with animal protein or vitamin C has been documented to increase the absorption of iron. Same goes for the allium family of veggies (think garlic and onion). For example, brown rice cooked with 1–2 cloves of garlic or eaten with 1–2 slices of onion has been shown to increase the availability of iron and zinc by up to 50 percent.[229]

IS GLUTEN REALLY A PROBLEM?

The short answer is yes. Let's break this down to what we know.

What Is Gluten?

Gluten is a large family of storage proteins found in wheat, barley, spelt, semolina, kamut, farro, and rye. We often throw oats on that list, simply because commercial brands are often cross-contaminated in facilities that also process gluten-containing grains. People with a serious genetic condition called celiac disease must eliminate gluten entirely from their diet.

What Is Gluten Sensitivity?

It's a syndrome that occurs in people without celiac disease. After they consume foods with gluten, they develop symptoms within the gut or systemically throughout the body. Symptoms vary widely but include painful stomachaches, diarrhea, headaches, joint pain, brain fog, skin conditions, depression, and anemia, just to name a few. These symptoms occur soon after gluten is eaten and usually disappear when gluten is removed from the diet. Non-celiac gluten sensitivity, as it's officially called, is a real issue and has been reported that 30 percent of those with irritable bowel–like symptoms also have gluten sensitivity.[230] There are hundreds of related but distinct gluten proteins, but gliadin—a gluten protein found in wheat, barley, and rye—has been the most extensively studied and for the time being appears to be the most problematic.

What Has Science Taught Us About Gluten?

The first groundbreaking studies came from renowned scientist Dr. Alessio Fasano, who showed that gluten has the potential to impact the intestinal lining in all of us, not just those with celiac disease.[231] His work has taught us that gluten (specifically alpha gliadin) is one of the powerful triggers that releases a protein called zonulin in the small intestine.[232] When zonulin is lurking, it goes to work loosening the tight junctions of our gut. As a consequence, our intestinal lining becomes permeable, meaning the once tightly sealed gut now leaks proteins and toxins into the bloodstream, igniting an immune response.

The consequence of this phenomenon may not show up for a day or two but presents with serious symptoms like joint pain, digestive issues, anxiety, or chronic migraine headaches. This zonulin finding is clearly part of the development of unwanted inflammation in the gut. It adds to the existing paradigm that three key ingredients are needed for the development of autoimmune diseases: 1) a specific genetic makeup, 2) altered gut bacteria, and 3) an environmental trigger such as gluten. Research has shown that zonulin is an integral player in the development of autoimmune diseases such as diabetes, IBD, arthritis, and more.[233] The good news is that for those with non-celiac gluten sensitivity, these conditions can be reversed. This is achieved by removing environmental triggers like gluten to restore intestinal barrier function. Dr. Fasano writes, "Once gluten is removed from the diet, serum zonulin levels decrease, the intestine resumes its baseline barrier function, the autoantibody titers are normalized, the autoimmune process shuts off, and, consequently, the intestinal damage heals completely."[234]

What Has Modern Agriculture Done to Gluten-Containing Grains?

I have a front-row seat to a fictitious healthcare show called "The Human Diet: Pixie Dust or Captain Hook's Greatest Weapon." If I know one thing for sure, something's gone awry, as shown by the 140 pounds of gluten-containing grains that a typical American eats each year.[235] While we know gluten is linked to increased intestinal permeability and a host of chronic diseases, we are not exactly sure why. Taking a look at humankind's manipulations of modern-day grains may provide us with a few more pieces to the puzzle.

We get a lot of our gluten from wheat flour. But the bread of today looks very different from what our ancestors ate centuries ago. In fact, it has only been in the last 50 years that we've seen such an unprecedented change in the growth, structure, nutrient value, and consumption of wheat. As Dr. William Davis points out in his book Wheat Belly, the modern wheat of today is nearly unrecognizable to the emmer wheat of our grandmothers. Agricultural scientists have dramatically transformed our present-day wheat, Triticum aestivum, through hybridization and crossbreeding in order to increase yields, resist drought and pests, and decrease production costs.[236] The problem is hybridization has created new forms of gluten proteins that our bodies do not recognize. Although small, the new biochemical differences in wheat's protein structure may have the potential to turn genes on or off that otherwise would be dormant. This substantial change could very well be the source for the recent and rampant ill reactions to our present-day wheat consumption.

Another huge problem lies with the manner in which modern wheat is grown and harvested by conventional wheat farmers. Wheat harvest protocol since the 1990s has been to drench wheat fields with glyphosate 7-10 days before harvest. This creates an earlier, bigger harvest for the farmer, but leaves the consumer with a toxic food source. We know that glyphosate lethally disrupts the all-important shikimate pathway found in beneficial gut bacteria and contributes to gut permeability. Is it a stretch, then, to connect gluten-containing grains sprayed with herbicides to gluten sensitivity or chronic inflammation? What's equally disturbing is the sheer lack of human safety testing that exists from the US government to determine whether our modern hybrid wheat has the potential to create adverse health effects.

Lastly, gluten is everywhere, and we have the US food and agricultural industries to thank for that. Gluten hides in countless products from cheeses and soy sauce to lunch meats and snack foods. Our consumption is far greater than ever before. Vital gluten, a product extracted from wheat that's 100 percent pure gluten, has also been added to food products to increase baking volume and to add chewiness. Vital gluten consumption has tripled since 1977, and it's interesting that it's the same time period that aligns with the increase in celiac disease.[237] The bottom line is this: modern gluten-containing grains are increasingly challenging our physiology for which we are not genetically prepared. As discussed, food regulates the expression of many of our genes, and we have only scratched the surface in understanding how our modern-day wheat might be signaling our DNA to promote disease.

Is Gluten for You?

As a clinical nutritionist who cares for thousands of patients at risk for diabetes, autoimmune diseases, gastrointestinal disorders, obesity, headaches, brain fog, depression, and a host of other chronic diseases, I have personally witnessed dramatic turnarounds in health in those who have removed gluten and certain grains from their diets. In fact, I would even argue that no other food can be blamed for such an incredible range of disorders. There are clearly some proteins in grains that are immunogenic, which means that although they don't produce an immediate allergic response, they activate other parts of our immune system and cause unwanted inflammation. The overwhelming science behind this shows that modern gluten-containing grains such as wheat, barley, rye, spelt, kamut, and sometimes oats are among the most inflammatory ingredients of our modern era. This teaches us once again that nutrition is much more than just fuel for our bodies. Our gut is the largest interface that we have with our physical environment, and food can either support our bodily functions or trigger a response that harms us.

The point is that many of the most common ailments in today's modern world are the direct result of eating everyday foods such as wheat. Other foods that are most likely to provoke sensitivities are dairy, soy, eggs, peanuts, and corn. Elimination diets still remain the cheapest, quickest, most reliable way to test for food sensitivities or food reactions that are not allergies. If you or your child are struggling with a chronic ailment, are overweight, or if you just want to see if a gluten-free diet can have an effect on your general health, try it for at least 21 days. It's a great place to start to get at the root cause of your issues.

I would also encourage you to speak with an integrative nutritionist or physician who is well-versed in functional medicine so that they can address all the potential inflammatory triggers in your lifestyle and help maximize your nutrient intake. They can also further test for IgG food sensitivities with a simple blood test that measures your degree of sensitivity to a whole panel of foods. Addressing and eliminating food sensitivities can turn around many diseases and can provide for a healthy body and mind.

APPENDIX B: SUPPLEMENTATION BUYING GUIDE

Americans spent roughly $34 billion on supplements in 2015.[238] It's clearly a huge industry, but how can you be sure you are buying the safest, most effective brands? Or a more important question: Do you really need them? Basic nutritional science and experimental data from the world's leading physicians and researchers tell us that nutritional supplementation can be very helpful to achieve optimal health. In fact, nutritional researcher Dr. Bruce Ames believes that due to our poor diets practically every American is deficient at some level of the 40 or so essential nutrients needed to efficiently run our metabolism.[239] Even more alarming, new government research indicates that 9 out of 10 Americans fall short of key nutrients like calcium, vitamin D, and potassium in their diets.[240] Kids might even be more at risk given their high nutrient needs during growth matched with their classically poor eating habits. Kids living on a calorie-rich, nutrient-poor diet simply leaves them overfed and undernourished. It's absolutely possible that your child's bad mood, brain fog, or depression could be caused by a nutrient deficiency.

How can this be? It's pretty straightforward. If your child is growing and doesn't have an overt deficiency disease like scurvy, it simply means they are meeting the *minimum* amounts of nutrients needed for growth. It does *not* mean they are meeting their needs for optimal thriving health. There is a very big difference. Dr. Ames's triage theory explains that if our bodies are nutritionally limited in micronutrients, our bodies will ration them in terms of priority. "The body will always direct nutrients toward short-term health and reproductive capability—and away from regulation and repair of DNA and proteins that increase longevity."[241] What this means is that while your body is keeping your fundamental operations alive, at the cellular level, disease and decay are setting in.

To compound this issue further, even if we ate a really good whole foods diet, there are still real-life obstacles to achieving our optimal nutrient needs, such as:

- An existing chronic disease or ailment will most likely require higher nutrient needs.

- Modern intensive agriculture methods have stripped increasing amounts of nutrients from the earth's soils.[242]

- Our increased exposure to environmental toxins requires higher micronutrient needs to eliminate toxins from the body. An unhealthy diet will lead to key mineral deficiencies needed for detoxification, causing oxidative stress affecting brain function and a whole host of metabolic functions.[243]

- Foods currently fed to modern animals are unnatural and less nutrient-rich than in the past.

- Chronic psychological stress along with chronic excitation from electronic devices changes our metabolism of nutrients as well as increases our adrenal output of mineral corticoids. Nutrient needs will be higher to replace minerals such as calcium, zinc, magnesium, and chromium.[244]

- Our body's nutritional demands are higher in our modern society due to poor sleep habits, low levels of exercise, and chronic inflammation.

- Food that has undergone long-distance transportation along with food refining also have cost nutrient content.

With all that said, it's unlikely that we can obtain all of our needed nutrients from food alone, even with a good diet. Therefore, I recommend that most adults and children take a well-researched whole foods multivitamin and mineral supplement each day, along with a quality omega-3 fat supplement if omega-3 rich foods are not in your weekly eating plan. I also recommend finding a functional medicine practitioner to further test for potential nutrient deficiencies and/or toxicities unique to you, especially if you or your child has an unresolved health issue. The future of medicine is in targeted nutrition therapy. Even though the vast majority of adults and children are deficient in nutrients like vitamin D, magnesium, and iron, it is prudent to obtain a blood test prior to supplementing to avoid toxicity and to obtain proper dosing unique to your own biochemistry.

How to Ensure You're Purchasing a Quality Supplement

Walking down the vitamin aisle shouldn't be a scary thing, but with the hundreds of thousands of choices available to us, how can we be sure we are buying the safest, most effective brands? Today there are very minimal standards in regulating supplements since the federal government categorizes them as food and not drugs. The Dietary Supplement Health and Education Act of 1994 eliminated the need for supplements to go through an FDA approval process, which for the most part allows supplement companies to put anything they want in their products. No pre-market safety or validation program exists. This is of great concern because as consumers, we desire confidence in knowing that when we purchase a supplement, it contains 100 percent authentic ingredients and is free from toxic contaminants. The majority of Americans are purchasing vitamins in one of three places: from a mass-market store like GNC or Walmart, online, or from a health practitioner. After a lot of research, I have assembled a Supplement Buying Guide for Families that explains purchasing guidelines, top brands, safety tips, and key items to look for on labels.

In 2015, the NY State Attorney General's office investigated and DNA-tested herbal products from GNC, Target, Walgreens, and Walmart and found that 79 percent of the products tested did not contain any of the herbs listed on their labels.[245]

Supplement Buying Guide for Families

I highly recommend purchasing supplements through a licensed healthcare professional. Although this doesn't absolutely ensure a perfect product, it greatly increases the chances that it will be pharmaceutical grade, third-party tested, and comply with good manufacturing practices.

SUPPLEMENT BUYING GUIDE

QUESTIONS TO ASK	LOOK FOR	BE AWARE
Where are the ingredients sourced from?	Products sourced from USA, Canada, Australia, or a European nation.	Do not purchase supplements sourced from India, China, Peru, Mexico, or Bolivia. Made in USA and sourced from USA are two different things.
Were the supplements processed in a way that kept nutrients intact?	Opaque bottles that block light from entering	Avoid clear bottle packaging as light denatures nutrients. (Some children's multivitamins are sold in clear containers.)
How are they stored and shipped?	Manufacturers that ship directly from the manufacturing plant and use care with products by using refrigerated packaging when needed.	Heat destroys nutrients. Avoid purchasing from online retailers like Amazon that might have supplements sitting in hot warehouses or in hot packaging left on your front porch.

QUESTIONS TO ASK	LOOK FOR	BE AWARE
Are they pharmaceutical grade supplements, tested for purity and quality?	Third-party certification from companies like USP (US Pharmacopeia), NSF International, COA (Certificate of Analysis), or Consumer Lab.	Do not purchase supplements from mass-market stores such as GNC, Walgreens, Walmart, Target, or grocery stores. Don't get fooled by phrases like "pharmaceutical strength."
What are the inactive ingredients?	Supplements without fillers. Generally safe ingredients are gelatin, fruit extracts, citric acid, ascorbic acid, and glycerin.	Additives, filler and allergens like soybean oil (GMO), carrageenan, artificial sweeteners, HFCS, food dyes, titanium dioxide, potassium sorbate, magnesium stearate
Are they batch tested?	Quality manufacturers include a batch or lot number on their products so that consumers can trace a product back to product origin.	No batch number prevents consumers from tracing a product through the supply chain to determine origin of ingredients.
When is the potency guarantee?	"Best By" or "Use By" dates on labels indicate how long it will last before its potency falls below 100 percent of the listed amount.	"Date of Manufacture" is useless as it only indicates when the supplement was made, not how long ingredients remain potent and stable.
Are they free of toxic metals?	If the country of origin is USA, Canada, Australia, or a European nation, it has a much better chance at being clean. You may ask companies for a heavy metals lab report on the lot number purchased, but you will find many companies do not perform this testing.	USDA allows any level of heavy metals in supplement products, even certified organic products. Avoid product sourced from China, Peru, India, Mexico, or Bolivia.

Once you have ascertained that you have a reputable brand, the next big question is, "Is my vitamin supplement absorbable?" Because really, if it's not absorbable, then what's the point? There are lots of things that get in the way of absorption, so educate yourself prior to spending hundreds of dollars on pills that may serve little benefit to you. A study published in the *Journal of Pharmacy and Pharmaceutical Sciences* proved just how problematic absorption is in everyday multivitamins. Although many factors like gut pH and transport mechanisms play a role in absorption of multivitamins in tablet form, the first critical step is disintegration. The study tested 49 popular multivitamin supplements like Kirkland Signature Formula (Costco's brand) and GNC Mega Men (two of the worst performers) and found 25 did not disintegrate within the optimal 20-minute absorption window.[246] That's 51 percent of well-known multivitamin brands that did not disintegrate within the optimal time frame needed for absorption.

There are three other important factors to evaluate when choosing a multivitamin supplement: beneficial quantities, beneficial forms, and micronutrient competition. When multivitamin manufacturers formulate a multivitamin, the quantities are often determined by cost of a particular vitamin or the amount of space it will take up in the supplement. For example, magnesium and calcium are expensive and bulky and are hard to fit into a compact pill. Next, the vitamin form is equally important to ensure optimal absorption. Vitamin B6 is best absorbed in the bioactive form pyridoxal-5-phosphate, but many inferior products use pyridoxine HCL, which is not the active form of this B vitamin.[247] Lastly, because of many micronutrient competitions, it's wise to choose a multivitamin that does not contain iron or copper. There are other competitions that occur, but these are two big offenders. I recommend consulting with a healthcare practitioner who is up to date on micronutrient synergy and competition before taking multiple supplements.

While there are many great products available, at the moment, here are a few brands that I like:

Fish Oil
Nordic Naturals ProOmega and ProOmega Jr.
Vital Choice Wild Salmon Oil
Barlean's Omega Swirl Fish Oil
Green Pasture Fermented Cod Liver Oil and Butter Oil Blend
Standard Process Cod Liver Oil and Olprima EPA/DHA
Carlson Fish Oil

Vitamin D3 with K2
Life Extension D and K
Ortho Molecular Vitamin D3 with K2
Nordic Naturals Vitamin D3+K2 Gummy
Designs for Health Vitamin D Supreme with Vitamin K1 and K2

Multivitamin
Garden of Life: Vitamin Code and mykind Organics (Prenatal Multi and Kids Multivitamin)
Standard Process Catalyn and Catalyn Chewable
Pure Encapsulations: PreNatal Nutrients (pregnancy) and O.N.E. Multivitamin (for teens)
Pure Encapsulations Nutrient 950 with Vitamin K
Designs For Health DFH Complete Multi

Probiotic

HMF Neuro (babies and kids)

Klaire Labs Ther-Biotic Complete and Children's Chewable

Garden of Life Dr. Formulated

Primal Blueprint Primal Probiotics

Micronutrients (like iron, zinc, and magnesium) and Targeted Nutrient Therapy

Life Extension

Pure Encapsulations

Standard Process

Xymogen

Thorne Research

Nordic Naturals

Metagenics

Designs for Health

RESOURCES AND RECOMMENDED READING

While these are helpful resources, this is by no means a complete list, simply some of my favorites to get you started.

Books

Cure Your Child with Food by Kelly Dorfman, MS, LND

Deep Nutrition by Catherine Shanahan, MD

Digestive Wellness for Children by Elizabeth Lipski, PhD, CCN

Eat Fat Lose Fat by Dr. Mary Enig, PhD, and Sally Fallon

Eating On the Wild Side by Jo Robinson

Food Fight by Kelly Brownell and Katherine Battle Horgen

Food Politics by Marion Nestle

Food: What the Heck Should I Eat? by Mark Hyman, MD

Grain Brain by David Perlmutter, MD

In Defense of Food by Michael Pollan

Making a Good Brain Great by Daniel G. Amen, MD

Nourishing Traditions, by Sally Fallon

Nutrition and Physical Degeneration by Weston A. Price, DDS

Nutritionism by Gyorgy Scrinis

Omnivore's Dilemma: A Natural History of Four Meals by Michael Pollan

Pasture Perfect by Jo Robinson

Salt Sugar Fat by Michael Moss

Super Nutrition for Babies by Katherine Erlich, MD and Kelly Genzlinger, CNC, CMTA

The Autoimmune Solution by Amy Myers, MD

The Big Book of Kombucha by Hannah Crum and Alex LaGory

The Breastfeeding Book by William Sears, MD and Martha Sears, RN

The Disease Delusion by Dr. Jeffrey S. Bland

The Gut Balance Revolution by Gerard E. Mullin, MD

The Inside Tract by Gerard E. Mullin, MD and Kathie Madonna Swift, MS, RD, LDN

The Jungle by Upton Sinclair

The Picky Eating Solution by Deborah Kennedy, PhD

The Toxin Solution by Dr. Joseph Pizzorno

The Virgin Diet by JJ Virgin, CNS, CHFS

What to Eat by Marion Nestle

Wild Fermentation by Sandor Ellix Katz

Cookbooks

Against All Grain by Danielle Walker

Fast Food, Good Food by Andrew Weil, MD

How to Cook Everything Vegetarian by Mark Bittman

Natural Health magazine https://www.naturalhealthmagazine.co.uk/

Nom Nom Paleo by Michelle Tam and Henry Fong

Once Upon a Chef, the Cookbook by Jennifer Segal

100 Days of Real Food by Lisa Leake

Skinnytaste Fast and Slow by Gina Homolka with Heather K. Jones, RD

The Art of Simple Food by Alice Waters

The Food Lab by J. Kenji López-Alt

The Nourishing Traditions Cookbook for Children by Suzanne Gross and Sally Fallon Morell

The Sprouted Kitchen by Sara Forte

True Food: Seasonal, Sustainable, Simple, Pure by Andrew Weil, MD, and Sam Fox

Films

Consuming Kids: The Commercialization of Childhood, directed and written by Adriana Barbara and Jeremy Earp, documentary by The Media Education Foundation, 2008, .

Food, Inc., produced and directed by Robert Kenner and produced by Eric Schlosser, documentary by Participant Media, 2008, .

Sugar, The Bitter Truth, presented by Robert H. Lustig, MD, UCSF Professor of Pediatrics in the Division of Endocrinology, University of California Television, July 30, 2009, https://www.youtube.com/watch?v=dBnniua6-oM.

The Myth of Choice: How Junk-Food Marketers Target Our Kids, presented by Anna Lappé & Food MythBusters, The Real Food Media Project, September 26, 2013, https://www.youtube.com/watch?v=PWOcP-bXuO8.

Food Matters, produced by James Colquhoun and Laurentine Ten Bosch, documentary by FMTV, www.foodmatters.com/films.

Websites

American Grassfed www.americangrassfed.org

Center for Science in the Public Interest www.cspinet.org

Food Marketing Workgroup www.foodmarketing.org

Fooducate www.fooducate.com

Institute for Responsible Technology (GMO awareness) www.responsibletechnology.org

Jamie Oliver, chef and healthy eating advocate www.jamieoliver.com

Local Catch www.localcatch.org

Natural Resources Defense Council www.nrdc.org

Seafood Watch www.seafoodwatch.org

The Cornucopia Institute (organic milk and egg scorecards) www.cornucopia.org

The Environmental Working Group www.ewg.org

The Institute for Functional Medicine www.ifm.org

The Weston A. Price Foundation www.westonaprice.org

Truth in Olive Oil www.extravirginity.com

Products

Bob's Red Mill www.bobsredmill.com

Butcher Box www.butcherbox.com/

Clean Fish www.cleanfish.com

Cultured Food Starters www.thehealthyhomeeconomist.com, www.culturesforhealth.com

Eat Wild www.eatwild.com

Fair Trade Certified www.fairtradecertified.org

Kettle and Fire Bone Broth www.kettleandfire.com

Kombucha Kamp www.kombuchacamp.com

Radiant Life https://www.radiantlifecatalog.com/

Thrive Market www.thrivemarket.com

US Wellness Meats https://discover.grasslandbeef.com/

Vital Choice Seafood www.vitalchoice.com

Resources to find healthy local food near you

Clean Plates www.cleanplates.com

Coop Directory Service www.coopdirectory.org

Eat Well Guide www.eatwellguide.org

Farmers Market Coalition www.farmersmarketcoalition.org

Happy Cow www.happycow.net

Local Harvest www.localharvest.org

ACKNOWLEDGMENTS

I would like to first acknowledge my Creator who has guided me my entire life. It was my faith in Him that gave me the strength to persevere through some tough times in my life. My heart is also filled with gratitude for all the beautiful gifts He has bestowed upon me.

To my sister Michelle Chalfant, my sister-cousin Cara Maddox, my aunt Marilyn O'Connor, and my mom, Nancy Brindisi, who are by far my greatest cheerleaders, ever. I would be nothing without you. Your fierce strength, your loving kindness for humanity, and your quest for personal wholeness are my blueprints for living.

To my father, thank you for showing me what it looks like to love with your whole heart. I will continually strive to make you proud as you look down on me from heaven.

To Georgiana Howe, one of the most brilliant women I know, for giving me a special type of love and support that's been bonded now by four generations. You are the person who reminds me of where I came from, and you inspire me to "keep on keeping on."

To all my family members, I deeply thank you for the constant joy and support that you bring to my life.

I want to thank Laurie Hubbs for her wonderful insights, her excellent business and life coaching, and for keeping me on track all those times I wanted to throw in the towel. Much gratitude, Laurie.

I also want to thank Andrea McKinney for embracing children's health and allowing me to implement school wellness programs that empower parents and students. You taught me one great lesson, which is, "Never stop speaking out, because we all need to be reminded of life-saving truths." You are an amazing example for school administrators across the country.

A special thank you to Dr. John Troup and the staff at Standard Process for believing in this book and helping launch the vital message of whole food nourishment to the world.

I am also grateful to the members and staff at the Arizona Center for Integrative Medicine for leading the way for respectful, practical, evidenced-based integration of natural therapies into the professional care for adults and children.

Thanks are also due to the leaders of the Institute for Functional Medicine and to all the bench researchers like Dr. Randy Jirtle, who have brought cutting-edge science to the world.

I want to send my gratitude and appreciation to nutrition pioneers, namely Weston A. Price, Sir Robert McCarrison, Sir Frederick Gowland Hopkins, and our present-day Dr. Jeffery Bland. The powerful and inspiring conviction of their work has paved the way for optimal human health.

And then there are all those who have taught and inspired me: Dr. Andrew Weil, Dr. Tieraona Low Dog, Dr. Mark Hyman, Dr. Bruce Lipton, Dr. Gerard Mullin, Dr. Liz Lipski, and so many others.

Thank you to John Wear at the Center for the Environment, and others who have invited me to speak on this topic, and whose audiences' questions, comments, and suggestions have helped me make the points here more clearly.

Special thanks to my brilliant editor Paula Sarson for believing in this book and in me from the beginning. Thank you for your laser-like vision, your professionalism, and your guidance to see this project through to the very end.

Thank you to Kimberley Mulder for her professional guidance and expert proofreading skills. And huge thanks to Christina Gaugler for her beautiful interior design and creative counsel. You both were blessings that came to me at just the right time.

To all my mentors, specifically Ana Abad Sinden and Carol Rees Parrish who were two of the best clinical educators during my young training as a clinical dietitian. To Nita Catterton, your gentle yet strong guidance was a gift that will never be forgotten.

Thank you to all those who allowed me to reproduce important charts and pictures to help solidify my information in this book, specifically the EWG for their "Dirty Dozen" and "Clean 15" lists as well as Chef Bobo, The Westin A. Price Foundation, Dr. Randy Jirtle, and Dr. Andrew Weil.

To my brilliant partner in crime Dr. Jennifer Hudson. Your optimism and commitment to making a difference in the lives of children is truly inspiring.

To my dear friends Lisa Druckenbrod, Sarah Joynt, and Beth Pietropaolo for their constant encouragement and support. Heartfelt thanks to each of my dear and trusted friends who have shown nothing but support and faith in me over the past four years.

To Rea Wright, gifted soul healer, empowerment teacher, and friend.

To my patients, for their trust, patience, and mentorship through the many years.

Thanks also to all of the students and attendees of my classes and lectures, and to those friends in my community who over the years persistently inquired, "Where's the book?" I'm finally delivering! Your continued encouragement is deeply appreciated.

To my children, Thomas and Isabella, who bring sunshine to my heart every day and are my life's greatest treasures.

These acknowledgements would not be complete without a most special thank you to my amazing husband, Dr. Christopher Magryta. Chris has been a continued support behind the scenes, encouraging, proofreading, giving needed neck rubs, taking on "kid duties" so I could find time to write, and most of all loving with his huge heart. My journey would not be complete without you. You're the peanut butter to my jelly. Loving you today, yesterday, and always tomorrow.

NOTES

INTRODUCTION

1   Kelly M. Adams et al., "Nutrition in Medicine: Nutrition Education for Medical Students and Residents," *Nutrition in Clinical Practice* 25, no. 5 (2010): 471–80.

CHAPTER 1

2   Dana Dabelea et al., "Prevalence of Type 1 and Type 2 Diabetes among Children and Adolescents from 2001 to 2009," *Journal of the American Medical Association* 311, no. 17 (2014): 1778–1786.

3   Centers for Disease Control and Prevention, "Diabetes Report Card 2014," Atlanta, GA: Centers for Disease Control and Prevention, US Dept. of Health and Human Services, 2015.

4   Rebecca M. Lovell and Alexander C. Ford, "Global Prevalence of and Risk Factors for Irritable Bowel Syndrome: A Meta-Analysis," *Clinical Gastroenterology and Hepatology* 10, no. 7 (2012): 712–721.

5   OECD (Organisation for Economic Co-operation and Development), "Obesity and the Economics of Prevention: Fit Not Fat, Key Facts—United States, Update 2014." http://www.oecd.org/unitedstates/Obesity-Update-2014-USA.pdf.

6   CDC (Centers for Disease Control and Prevention), "About Us," last updated August 7, 2018. https://www.cdc.gov/nccdphp/dnpao/division-information/aboutus/index.htm.

7   CDC, "About Chronic Diseases," last updated August 6, 2018. https://www.cdc.gov/chronicdisease/about/index.htm.

8   Jeanne Van Cleave, Steven L. Gortmaker, and James M. Perrin, "Dynamics of Obesity and Chronic Health Conditions among Children and Youth," *Journal of the American Medical Association* 303, no. 7 (2010): 623–630.

9   Food Allergy Research & Education, "Facts and Statistics," accessed December 7, 2017, https://www.foodallergy.org/life-food-allergies/food-allergy-101/facts-and-statistics.

10 CDC, "Key Findings: Trends in the Parent-Report of Health Care Provider-Diagnosis and Medication Treatment for ADHD: United States, 2003—2011," last updated September 7, 2017. https://www.cdc.gov/ncbddd/adhd/features/key-findings-adhd72013.html.

CHAPTER 2

11 John Ikerd, "Agriculture in the Post-Industrial Era: Challenges and Opportunities for Alaskans,", abstract (presentation at a workshop on Sustainable Livestock Production in Alaska, October 13-14, 2011) accessed January 11, 2017, http://web.missouri.edu/ikerdj/papers/Alaska%20-%20Post-Industrial%20Agriculture.htm.

12 John Ikerd, "Healthy Soils, Healthy People: The Legacy of William Albrecht," abstract (presentation at the William A. Albrecht Lecture, Memorial Union, University of Missouri, Columbia MO, April 25, 2011), last updated July 7, 2016, http://web.missouri.edu/ikerdj/papers/AlbrechtLectureHealthySoilsHealthyPeople.pdf

13 David Wallinga, "Today's Food System: How Healthy Is It?," *Journal of Hunger & Environmental Nutrition* 4, no. 3–4 (2009): 251–281.

14 Grace Communications Foundation, "Antibiotics," accessed August 27, 2018, http://www.sustainabletable.org/257/antibiotics.

15 FAO (Food and Agriculture Organization of the United Nations), OIE (World Organization for Animal Health), and WHO (World Health Organization), "Joint FAO/OIE/WHO Expert Workshop on Non-Human Antimicrobial Usage and Antimicrobial Resistance: Scientific assessment," Geneva, December 1–5, 2003.

16 Grace Communications Foundation, "Animal Feed," accessed on August 27, 2018. http://www.sustainabletable.org/260/animal-feed.

17 Cynthia A. Daley et al., "A Review of Fatty Acid Profiles and Antioxidant Content in Grass-Fed and Grain-Fed Beef." *Nutrition Journal* 9, no. 1 (2010): 10.

18 C. J. Lopez-Bote et al., "Effect of Free-Range Feeding on Omega-3 Fatty Acids and Alpha-Tocopherol Content and Oxidative Stability of Eggs," *Animal Feed Science and Technology* 72 (1998): 33–40.

19 Daley et al., "A Review of Fatty Acid Profiles," 10.

20   APHA (American Public Health Association), "Opposition to the Use of Hormone Growth Promoters in Beef and Dairy Cattle Production," Policy Statements, November 10, 2009, https://www.apha.org/policies-and-advocacy/public-health-policy-statements/policy-database/2014/07/09/13/42/opposition-to-the-use-of-hormone-growth-promoters-in-beef-and-dairy-cattle-production.

21   J. Raloff, "Hormones: Here's the Beef: Environmental Concerns Re-emerge over Steroids Given to Livestock." *Science News* 161, no. 1 (2002).

22   R. W. Stephany, "Hormones in Meat: Different Approaches in the EU and in the USA," *APMIS Supplement* 109 (2001): S357–S363.

23   European Commission, "Opinion of the Scientific Committee on Veterinary Measures Relating to Public Health on[…] Potential Risks to Human Health From Hormone Residues in Bovine Meat and Meat Products," last modified April 10, 2002, https://ec.europa.eu/food/sites/food/files/safety/docs/cs_meat_hormone-out50_en.pdf.

24   F. S. vom Saal et al., "Chapel Hill Bisphenol A Expert Panel Consensus Statement: Integration of Mechanisms, Effects in Animals and Potential Impact to Human Health at Current Exposure Levels," *Reproductive Toxicology* 24, no. 2 (2007): 131–138.

25   Ian R. Dohoo et al., "A Meta-Analysis Review of the Effects of Recombinant Bovine Somatotropin: 2. Effects on Animal Health, Reproductive Performance, and Culling," *Canadian Journal of Veterinary Research* 67, no.4 (2003): 252.

26   American Nutrition Association, "Milk and Health," n.d., accessed September 4, 2018, http://americannutritionassociation.org/toolsandresources/milk-americaâ€™s-health-problem.

27   Hassan Malekinejad, and Aysa Rezabakhsh, "Hormones in Dairy Foods and their Impact on Public Health: A Narrative Review Article," *Iranian Journal of Public Health* 44, no. 6 (2015): 742.

28   A. J. Lanou, "Should Dairy Be Recommended as Part of a Healthy Vegetarian Diet? Counterpoint," *American Journal of Clinical Nutrition* 89, no. 5 (2009): 1638S–1642S.

29   "Current GMO Crops," gmoanswers.com, accessed August 31, 2017, https://gmoanswers.com/current-gmo-crops.

30   John Fagan, Michael Antoniou, and Claire Robinson, "GMO Myths and Truths," Earth Open Source, 2nd edition, last modified 2014, https://earthopensource.org/wordpress/downloads/GMO-Myths-and-Truths-edition2.pdf.

31   Union of Concerned Scientists, "Genetic Engineering in Agriculture," n.d., accessed August 31, 2017, http://www.ucsusa.org/our-work/food-agriculture/our-failing-food-system/genetic-engineering-agriculture#.Wag3662ZM6g.

32   Danny Hakim, "Doubts about the Promised Bounty of Genetically Modified Crops," *New York Times*, October 26, 2016, https://www.nytimes.com/2016/10/30/business/gmo-promise-falls-short.html.

33   S. O. Duke and S. B. Powles, "Glyphosate-Resistant Crops and Weeds: Now and in the Future," *AgBioForum* 12, no. 3 and 4 (2009): 346–357.

34   Philip J. Landrigan and Charles Benbrook, "GMOs, Herbicides, and Public Health," *New England Journal of Medicine* 373, no. 8 (2015): 693–695.

35   Anthony Samsel and Stephanie Seneff, "Glyphosate's Suppression of Cytochrome P450 Enzymes and Amino Acid Biosynthesis by the Gut Microbiome: Pathways to Modern Diseases," *Entropy* 15, no. 4 (2013): 1416–1463.

36   IARC, "Monographs Volume 112: Evaluation of Five Organophosphate Insecticides and Herbicides," March 20, 2015, www.iarc.fr/en/media-centre/iarcnews/pdf/MonographVolume112.pdf.

37   Scitable, "The Darwinian Evolution of Superweeds", last update September 08, 2015, https://www.nature.com/scitable/blog/plantchemcast/the_darwinian_evolution_of_superweeds.

38   Food Democracy Now! and The Detox Project, "Glyphosate: Unsafe On Any Plate", n.p., accessed September 4, 2018, https://s3.amazonaws.com/media.fooddemocracynow.org/images/FDN_Glyphosate_FoodTesting_Report_p2016.pdf.

39   Robin Mesnage et al., "Transcriptome Profile Analysis Reflects Rat Liver and Kidney Damage Following Chronic Ultra-Low Dose Roundup Exposure," *Environmental Health* 14, no. 1, (2015): 70; G. E. Seralini et al., "Republished Study: Long-Term Toxicity of a Roundup Herbicide and a Roundup-Tolerant Genetically Modified Maize," *Environmental Sciences Europe* 26, no. 14 (June 24, 2014), https://doi.org/10.1186/s12302-014-0014-5; T. M. Uren Webster and E. M. Santos, "Global Transcriptomic Profiling Demonstrates Induction of Oxidative Stress and of Compensatory Cellular Stress Responses in Brown Trout Exposed to Glyphosate and Roundup," *BMC Genomics* 16, no. 32 (January 31, 2015), https://doi.org/10.1186/s12864-015-1254-5; K. Larsen, R. Najle, A. Lifschitz, and G. Virkel, "Effects of Sub-lethal Exposure of Rats to the Herbicide Glyphosate in Drinking Water: Glutathione Transferase Enzyme Activities, Levels of Reduced Glutathione and Lipid Peroxidation in Liver, Kidneys and Small Intestine," *Environmental Toxicology and Pharmacology* 34, issue 3 (November 2012): 811–818, https://doi.org/10.1016/j.etap.2012.09.005

40 Global Research, "Monsanto Controls Both the White House and the US Congress", March 6, 2018, https://www.globalresearch.ca/monsanto-controls-both-the-white-house-and-the-us-congress/5336422.

41 Center For Food Safety, "About Genetically Engineered Foods", n.p., accessed September 4, 2018, https://www.centerforfoodsafety.org/issues/311/ge-foods/about-ge-foods.

42 WHO, "Children's Health and the Environment. WHO Training Package for the Health Sector," latest update 2011, http://who.int/ceh/capacity/chemicals.pdf.

43 Monika Krüger et al., "Detection of Glyphosate Residues in Animals and Humans," *Journal of Environmental & Analytical Toxicology* 4, no. 2 (2014): 1.

44 USDA, "Food Prices and Spending", last update July 25, 2018, https://www.ers.usda.gov/data-products/ag-and-food-statistics-charting-the-essentials/food-prices-and-spending/.

45 Lisa A. Sutherland, Lori A. Kaley, and Leslie Fischer, "Guiding Stars: The Effect of a Nutrition Navigation Program on Consumer Purchases at the Supermarket," *The American Journal of Clinical Nutrition* 91, no. 4 (2010): 1090S–1094S.

46 Science Daily, "Highly Processed Foods Dominate U.S. Grocery Purchases", last update March 29, 2015, https://www.sciencedaily.com/releases/2015/03/150329141017.htm.

47 H. Mollie Grow and Marlene B. Schwartz, "Food Marketing to Youth: Serious Business," *JAMA* 312, no. 18 (2014): 1918–1919.

48 UConn Rudd Center for Food Policy & Obesity, "FACTS 2017 Food Industry Self-regulation After 10 Years", November 2017, http://www.uconnruddcenter.org/files/Pdfs/FACTS-2017_Final.pdf.

49 Vivica I. Kraak, Jennifer Appleton Gootman, and J. Michael McGinnis, eds., *Food Marketing to Children and Youth: Threat or Opportunity?* (Washington, DC: National Academies Press, 2006), 8-10.

50 Corinna Hawkes, "Marketing Food to Children: The Global Regulatory Environment," World Health Organization, 2004, http://apps.who.int/iris/bitstream/handle/10665/42937/9241591579.pdf;jsessionid=30212A2F6F9485F78B444D511D42AFB1?sequence=1.

51 Adriana Barbaro, Jeremy Earp, Jason T. Young, and Alex Peterson, *Consuming Kids: The Commercialization of Childhood* (Northampton, MA: Media Education Foundation, 2008), http://www.mediaed.org/transcripts/Consuming-Kids-Transcript.pdf.

52 W. C. Frazier III and J. L. Harris, "Trends in Television Food Advertising to Young People: 2015 Update," UConn Rudd Center for Food Policy & Obesity, last modified July 2016, http://uconnruddcenter.org/files/TVAdTrends2016.pdf.

53 Lisa M. Powell, Jennifer L. Harris, and Tracy Fox, "Food Marketing Expenditures Aimed at Youth: Putting the Numbers in Context," *American Journal of Preventive Medicine* 45, no. 4 (2013): 453–461.

54 Victoria J. Rideout, Ulla G. Foehr, and Donald F. Roberts, "Generation M2: Media in the Lives of 8-to-18-Year-Olds," The Henry J. Kaiser Family Foundation, January 2010, https://kaiserfamilyfoundation.files.wordpress.com/2013/01/8010.pdf.

55 Jennifer L. Harris et al., "A Crisis in the Marketplace: How Food Marketing Contributes to Childhood Obesity and What Can Be Done," *Annual Review of Public Health* vol. 30 (April 21, 2009): 211–225, https://doi.org/10.1146/annurev.publhealth.031308.100304

56 Mary Story and Simone French, "Food Advertising and Marketing Directed at Children and Adolescents in the US," *International Journal of Behavioral Nutrition and Physical Activity* 1, no. 3 (2004), http://doi.org/10.1186/1479-5868-1-3.

57 Jennifer L. Harris and Tracy Fox, "Food and Beverage Marketing in Schools: Putting Student Health at the Head of the Class," *JAMA Pediatrics* 168, no. 3 (March 2014): 206–208.

58 Harris and Fox, "Food and Beverage Marketing," 206–208.

CHAPTER 3

59 I. Hoffmann, "Transcending Reductionism in Nutrition Research," *American Journal of Clinical Nutrition* 78 Supplement (2003): 514S–516S.

60 C. T. McEvoy, N. Temple, and J. V. Woodside, "Vegetarian Diets, Low-Meat Diets and Health: A Review," *Public Health Nutrition* 15, no. 12 (2012): 2287–2294.

61 T. C. Campbell and T. M. Campbell, *The China Study: Startling Implications for Diet, Weight Loss and Long-Term Health* (Dallas, TX: Benbella Books, 2005), 20.

62 Weston A. Price, *Nutrition and Physical Degeneration* (Lemon Grove, CA: The Price-Pottenger Nutrition Foundation 2012), 1-8.

63 The Weston A. Price Foundation, "Weston A. Price, DDS," January 1, 2000, http://www.westonaprice.org/health-topics/

weston-a-price-dds/

64   Price, *Nutrition and Physical Degeneration, 22-252*.

65   The Weston A Price Foundation, "On the Trail of the Elusive X-Factor: A Sixty-Two-Year-Old Mystery Finally Solved", February 14, 2008, https://www.westonaprice.org/health-topics/abcs-of-nutrition/on-the-trail-of-the-elusive-x-factor-a-sixty-two-year-old-mystery-finally-solved/.

66   Poul Erik Peterson, "Challenges to Improvement of Oral Health in the 21st Century: The Approach of the WHO Global Oral Health Programme," *International Dental Journal* 54, no. S6 (2004): 329–343.

67   "Dental Caries (Age 2 to 11)," National Institute of Dental and Craniofacial Research, last modified July 2018, https://www.nidcr.nih.gov/research/data-statistics/dental-caries/children.

68   Steven Lin, *The Dental Diet: The Surprising Link between Your Teeth, Real Food, and Life-changing Natural Health* (Carlsbad, CA: Hay House, 2018).

69   Robert McCarrison, *Studies in Deficiency Disease*, (London: H. Frowde and Hodder & Stoughton, 1921).

70   The Global Dialogue Foundation, "The Hunza Health Secrets," VedicSociety.org, accessed on July 31, 2018, http://www.globaldialoguefoundation.org/files/41.pdf.

71   G. T. Wrench, *The Wheel of Health: The Source of Long Life and Health Among the Hunza* (Mineola, NY: Dover Publications, 2006), 32.

72   Buettner, Dan. *The Blue Zones: 9 Lessons for Living Longer from the People Who've Lived the Longest.* (Washington, D.C.: National Geographic, 2012.)

CHAPTER 4

73   Dr. Jeffrey S. Bland, *Disease Delusion* (Toronto: Harper Wave, 2014), 32.

74   Bland, *Disease Delusion, 32.*

75   Bland, *Disease Delusion, 31.*

76   Robert A. Waterland and Randy L. Jirtle, "Transposable Elements: Targets for Early Nutritional Effects on Epigenetic Gene Regulation," *Molecular and Cell Biology* 23, no. 15 (2003): 5293 - 5300.

77   Dana C. Dolinoy, Dale Huang, and Randy L. Jirtle, "Maternal Nutrient Supplementation Counteracts Bisphenol A-Induced DNA Hypomethylation in Early Development," *Proceedings of the National Academy of Sciences of the United States of America* 104, no. 32 (August 7, 2007): 13056–13061.

78   Bland, *Disease Delusion,*

79   Sang-Woon Choi and Simonetta Friso, "Epigenetics: A New Bridge between Nutrition and Health," *Advances in Nutrition* 1, no. 1 (November 1, 2010): 8–16.

80   Sama F. Sleiman et al., "Exercise Promotes the Expression of Brain Derived Neurotrophic Factor (BDNF) through the Action of the Ketone Body B-Hydroxybutyrate," *eLife* 5 (2016): e15092.

81   A. Baccarelli and V. Bollati, "Epigenetics and Environmental Chemicals," *Current Opinion in Pediatrics* 21, no. 2 (2009): 243–251.

82   M. K. Skinner et al., "Alterations in Sperm DNA methylation, Non-coding RNA and Histone Retention Associate with DDT-induced Epigenetic Transgenerational Inheritance of Disease," *BMC Epigenetics and Chromatin* 11, no. 8 (2018).

83   C. S. Möller-Levet et al., "Effects of Insufficient Sleep on Circadian Rhythmicity and Expression Amplitude of the Human Blood Transcriptome," *Proceedings of the National Academy of Sciences of the United States of America* 110, no. 12 (2013): E1132–E1141.

84   Perla Kaliman et al., "Rapid Changes in Histone Deacetylases and Inflammatory Gene Expression in Expert Meditators," *Psychoneuroendocrinology* 40 (February 2014): 96–107, https://doi.org/10.1016/j.psyneuen.2013.11.004

85   M. K. Bhasin et al., "Relaxation Response Induces Temporal Transcriptome Changes in Energy Metabolism, Insulin Secretion and Inflammatory Pathways," *PLOS ONE* 8, no. 5 (2013): e62817. https://doi.org/10.1371/journal.pone.0062817

CHAPTER 5

86   Max Planck Institute for Chemical Ecology, "The Nutritionists Within: Firebugs Depend on Gut Bacteria for Vitamin Supply," ScienceDaily, accessed January 22, 2018, www.sciencedaily.com/releases/2014/12/141201163239.htm.

87   Rob Stein, "Finally, a Map of All the Microbes on Your Body," Health News from NPR, June 13, 2012, www.npr.org/sections/health-shots/2012/06/13/154913334/finally-a-map-of-all-the-microbes-on-your-body.

88   Judah L. Rosner, "Letters: Ten Times More Microbial Cells than Body Cells in Humans," *Microbe* 9, no. 2 (2014): 47,

accessed January 9, 2017, https://www.asmscience.org/content/journal/microbe/10.1128/microbe.9.47.2; and Ed Yong, "You're Probably Not Mostly Microbes," *The Atlantic,* January 8, 2016, http://www.theatlantic.com/science/archive/2016/01/youre-probably-not-mostly-microbes/423228/.

89   C. Jernberg, S. Lofmark, C. Edlund, et al., "Long-term impacts of antibiotic exposure on the human intestinal microbiota," *Microbiology* (2010), 156, 3216–3223.

90   CDC, "Achievements in Public Health, 1900–1999: Control of Infectious Diseases," *MMWR Weekly* 48, no. 29 (July 30, 1999): 621–629, https://www.cdc.gov/mmwr/preview/mmwrhtml/mm4829a1.htm .

91   G. Vighi et al., "Allergy and the Gastrointestinal System," *Clinical and Experimental Immunology* 153, Supplement 1 (2008): 3–6, https://doi.org/10.1111/j.1365-2249.2008.03713.x.

92   Michaeleen Doucleff, "How Bacteria in the Gut Help Fight Off Viruses," NPR, Noveber 14, 2014, http://www.npr.org/sections/goatsandsoda/2014/11/14/363375355/how-bacteria-in-the-gut-help-fight-off-viruses.

93   F. Karlsson, V. Tremaroli, J. Nielsen, and F. Bäckhed, "Assessing the Human Gut Microbiota in Metabolic Diseases," *Diabetes* 62, no. 10 (2013): 3341–3349, https://doi.org/10.2337/db13-0844

94   M. B. Azad et al., "Gut Microbiota of Healthy Canadian Infants: Profiles by Mode of Delivery and Infant Diet at 4 Months," *Canadian Medical Association Journal* 185, no. 5 (2013): 385–394, https://doi.org/10.1503/cmaj.121189

95   J. Neu and J. Rushing, "Cesarean versus Vaginal Delivery: Long Term Infant Outcomes and the Hygiene Hypothesis," *Clinics in Perinatology* 38, no. 2 (2011): 321–331, https://doi.org/10.1016/j.clp.2011.03.008.

96   Azad et al., "Gut Microbiota of Healthy Canadian Infants," 385-386.

97   Azad et al., "Gut Microbiota of Healthy Canadian Infants," 385-394.

98   Duke Medicine News and Communication, "Breast Milk's Magic Flora," Duke Today, August 28, 2012, https://today.duke.edu/2012/08/breastmilk.

99   Gerard Mullin, *The Gut Balance Revolution* (New York: Rodale, 2015), 20.

100 Genetic Science Learning Center, "Your Changing Microbiome," Learn.Genetics, n.d., accessed February 2, 2017, https://learn.genetics.utah.edu/content/microbiome/changing/.

101 William Parker, "Reconstituting the Depleted Biome to Prevent Immune Disorders," *The Evolution & Medicine Review* (October 13, 2010), https://evmedreview.com/reconstituting-the-depleted-biome-to-prevent-immune-disorders/.

102 Michelle M. Stein et al., "Innate Immunity and Asthma Risk in Amish and Hutterite Farm Children," *New England Journal of Medicine* 375, no. 5 (2016): 411–421.

103 Jeff D. Leach, *Rewild: You're 99% Microbe. It's Time You Started Eating Like It* (CreateSpace Independent Publishing Platform, August 2015), 112.

104 Cheryl S. Rosenfeld, "Gut Dysbiosis in Animals Due to Environmental Chemical Exposures," *Frontiers in Cellular and Infection Microbiology* 7 (September 8, 2017): 396.

105 Jenna Bilbrey, "BPA-Free Plastic Containers May Be Just as Hazardous," *Scientific American,* August 11, 2014. https://www.scientificamerican.com/article/bpa-free-plastic-containers-may-be-just-as-hazardous/.

106 Charles M. Benbrook, "Trends in glyphosate herbicide use in the United States and globally," *Environmental Sciences Europe,* 28.1 (2016): 3. https://www.ncbi.nlm.nih.gov/pmc/articles/PMC5044953/.

107 A. A. Shehata et al., "The Effect of Glyphosate on Potential Pathogens and Beneficial Members of Poultry Microbiota In Vitro," *Current Microbiology* 66, no.4 (April 2013): 350–358.

108 M. Krüger, A. A. Shehata, W. Schrödl, and A. Rodloff, "Glyphosate Suppresses the Antagonistic Effect of *Enterococcus* spp. on *Clostridium botulinum,*" *Anaerobe* 20 (April 2013): 74–78.

109 Centers for Disease Control and Prevention, "Be Antibiotics Aware: Smart Use, Better Care," Healthy Living CDC Feature, last updated December 15, 2017, http://www.cdc.gov/features/getsmart/.

110 F. Imhann et al., "Proton Pump Inhibitors Affect the Gut Microbiome," *Gut* 65 (2015): 740–748; and M. A. Rogers and D. M. Aronoff, "The Influence of Non-steroidal Anti-inflammatory Drugs on the Gut Microbiome," *Clinical Microbiology and Infection* 22, no. 2 (February 2016): 178.e1-178.e9.

111 C. Jernberg, et al., "Long-term Impacts of Antibiotic Exposure on the Human Intestinal Microbiota," *Microbiology* 156, (November 1, 2010): 3216–3223, doi: 10.1099/mic.0.040618-0.

112 M. Blaser, "Stop the Killing of Beneficial Bacteria," *Nature* 476 (August 2011): 393–394.

113 Mullin, *The Gut Balance Revolution,* 23.

114 Mullin, *The Gut Balance Revolution*, 23.

115 M. Blaser, "Stop the Killing of Beneficial Bacteria," 393–394.

116 Moises Velasquez-Manoff, "Among Trillions of Microbes in the Gut, A Few Are Special," *Scientific American*, March 1, 2015, www.scientificamerican.com/article/among-trillions-of-microbes-in-the-gut-a-few-are-special/.

117 M. Conlon and A. Bird, "The Impact of Diet and Lifestyle on Gut Microbiota and Human Health," *Nutrients* 7 (2014): 17–44.

118 Niamh Michail, "Lack of Diversity in Processed Foods May be Causing Obesity and Cancer," FoodNavigator.com, May 20, 2015, https://www.foodnavigator-usa.com/Article/2015/05/20/Lack-of-diversity-in-processed-foods-may-be-causing-obesity-and-cancer?utm_source=RSS_text_news&utm_medium=RSS%2Bfeed&utm_campaign=RSS%2BText%2BNews#

119 Niamh Michail, "Lack of Diversity."

120 MindBodyGreen, "Crave Sugar or Fat? Blame Your Gut Bacteria!," August 18, 2014, www.mindbodygreen.com/0-14975/crave-sugar-or-fat-blame-your-gut-bacteria.html.

121 P. J. Turnbaugh et al., "The Effect of Diet on the Human Gut Microbiome: A Metagenomic Analysis in Humanized Gnotobiotic Mice," *Science Translational Medicine* 1, no. 6 (November 11, 2009): 6ra14.

122 Ellen Ruppel Shell, "Artificial Sweeteners May Change Our Gut Bacteria in Dangerous Ways," *Scientific American*, April 1, 2015, www.scientificamerican.com/article/artificial-sweeteners-may-change-our-gut-bacteria-in-dangerous-ways/.

123 Rob Knight, "Why Microbiome Treatments Could Pay Off Soon," *Nature* 518, no. 7540 (2015): S5.

124 Mark Hyman, "5 Reasons High Fructose Corn Syrup Will Kill You," MarkHyman.com, 2016, http://drhyman.com/blog/2011/05/13/5-reasons-high-fructose-corn-syrup-will-kill-you/.

125 Richard J. Johnson et al., "Potential Role of Sugar (Fructose) in the Epidemic of Hypertension, Obesity and the Metabolic Syndrome, Diabetes, Kidney Disease, and Cardiovascular Disease," *The American Journal of Clinical Nutrition* 86, no. 4 (2007): 899–906.

126 E. Powell, L. Smith, and B. Popkin, "Recent Trends in Added Sugar Intake among US Children and Adults from 1977 to 2010," Abstract presented at The Obesity Society (TOS) annual meeting, 2014.

127 Robert Lustig, "Sugar: The Bitter Truth," University of California TV, July 30, 2009, https://www.youtube.com/watch?v=dBnniua6-oM

128 R.K. Johnson, L.J. Appel, M. Brands, et al., "Dietary sugars intake and cardiovascular health: a scientific statement from the American Heart Association," 120 (2009): 1011-20.

129 Nicole Avena, "This is Your Brain On Sugar," TedEd video, January 7, 2014, https://ed.ted.com/lessons/how-sugar-affects-the-brain-nicole-avena.

130 Rahul Agrawal and Fernando Gomez-Pinilla, "Metabolic Syndrome' in the Brain: Deficiency in Omega-3 Fatty Acid Exacerbates Dysfunctions in Insulin Receptor Signalling and Cognition," *The Journal of Physiology* 590, no.10 (2012): 2485–2499.

131 Agrawal and Gomez-Pinilla, "Metabolic Syndrome' in the Brain," 2485.

132 Jayanthi Maniam et al., "Sugar Consumption Produces Effects Similar to Early Life Stress Exposure on Hippocampal Markers of Neurogenesis and Stress Response," *Frontiers in Molecular Neuroscience* 8 (2015): 86.

133 Alessio Fasano and Terez Shea-Donohue, "Mechanisms of Disease: The Role of Intestinal Barrier Function in the Pathogenesis of Gastrointestinal Autoimmune Diseases," *Nature Clinical Practice Gastroenterology & Hepatology* 2, no. 9 (2005): 416–422.

CHAPTER 6

134 Joanne Slavin, "Fiber and Prebiotics: Mechanisms and Health Benefits," *Nutrients* 5, no. 4 (2013): 1417–1435.

135 Patrice D. Cani, Audrey M. Neyrinck, Nicole Maton, and Nathalie M. Delzenne, "Oligofructose Promotes Satiety in Rats Fed a High-Fat Diet: Involvement of Glucagon-Like Peptide-1," *Obesity* 13, no. 6 (June 2005): 1000-1007.

136 Gary B. Huffnagle and Sarah Wernick, *The Probiotics Revolution* (New York: Bantam Dell, 2008), 275.

137 J. Pérez-Jiménez, V. Neveu, F. Vos, and A. Scalbert, "Identification of the 100 Richest Dietary Sources of Polyphenols: An Application of the Phenol-Explorer Database," *European Journal of Clinical Nutrition* 64, (2010): s112–s120.

138 Gretel H. Schueller, "How Good Gut Bacteria Could Transform Your Health," *Eating Well*, July/August 2014, www.eatingwell.com/nutrition_health/nutrition_news_information/how_good_gut_bacteria_could_transform_your_health.

139 Sarah Reece, "Pass the Potato Salad This Summer," PR Newswire, July 12, 2016, http://www.prnewswire.com/news-releases/

pass-the-potato-salad-this-summer-300297327.html; Diane F. Birt et al., "Resistant Starch: Promise for Improving Human Health," *Advances in Nutrition: An International Review Journal* 4, no. 6 (2013): 587–601; "Resistant Starch in Foods," http://freetheanimal.com/wp-content/uploads/2013/08/Resistant-Starch-in-Foods.pdf; Murphy, Douglass, and Birkett, "Resistant Starch Intakes in the United States," 67–78; Alejandra García-Alonso, Isabel Goñi, and Fulgencio Saura-Calixto, "Resistant Starch and Potential Glycaemic Index of Raw and Cooked Legumes (Lentils, Chickpeas and Beans)," *Zeitschrift für Lebensmitteluntersuchung und-Forschung A* 206, no.4 (1998): 284–287; Geoff E. Bednar et al., "Starch and Fiber Fractions in Selected Food and Feed Ingredients Affect their Small Intestinal Digestibility and Fermentability and their Large Bowel Fermentability In Vitro in a Canine Model," *The Journal of Nutrition* 131, no. 2 (2001): 276–286; and Li-Yong Chen et al., "Sources and Intake of Resistant Starch in the Chinese Diet," *Asia Pacific Journal of Clinical Nutrition* 19, no. 2 (2010): 274–282.

140 Fred Brouns, Bernd Kettlitz, and Eva Arrigoni, "Resistant Starch and 'the Butyrate Revolution,'" *Trends in Food Science & Technology* 13, no.8 (2002): 251–261.

141 Mary M. Murphy, Judith Spungen Douglass, and Anne Birkett, "Resistant Starch Intakes in the United States," *Journal of the American Dietetic Association* 108, no. 1 (2008): 67–78.

142 Mullin, *The Gut Balance Revolution*, 90.

143 Jyoti P. Tamang et al., "Functional Properties of Microorganisms in Fermented Foods," *Frontiers in Microbiology* 7, no. 578 (April 26, 2016): 1-13.

144 Chris Kresser, "Treating SIBO, Cold Thermogenesis, and When to Take Probiotics," ChrisKresser.com, March 12, 2013, https://chriskresser.com/treating-sibo-cold-thermogenisis-and-when-to-take-probiotics/

145 Mershen Govender et al., "A Review of the Advancements in Probiotic Delivery: Conventional vs. Non-conventional Formulations for Intestinal Flora Supplementation," *Journal of the American Association of Pharmaceutical Scientists* 15, no. 1 (2013): 29–43.

146 Dr. Mercola, "Nourishing Your Gut Bacteria is Critical for Health and Mental Well-Being," March 13, 2016, http://articles.mercola.com/sites/articles/archive/2016/03/13/nourishing-gut-bacteria.aspx.

147 Johan D. Söderholm and Mary H. Perdue, II, "Stress and intestinal barrier function," *American Journal of Physiology-Gastrointestinal and Liver Physiology* 280, no. 1 (2001): G7–G13.

CHAPTER 7

148 D. L. Katz and S. Meller, "Can We Say What Diet Is Best for Health?," *Annual Review of Public Health* 35 (2014): 83–103.

149 David Zeevi et al., "Personalized Nutrition by Prediction of Glycemic Responses," *Cell* 163 no. 5 (2015): 1079–1094.

150 Sharon Palmer, "Nutrients of Concern for Individuals Following a Plant-Based Diet," *Today's Dietitian*, June 2014, http://www.todaysdietitian.com/pdf/courses/PBDNutritentsofConcern.pdf.

151 Keeve E. Nachman et al., "Roxarsone, Inorganic Arsenic, and Other Arsenic Species in Chicken: A U.S.-Based Market Basket Sample," *Environmental Health Perspectives* 121, no. 7 (2013): 818–824.

152 A. J. Lanou, S. E. Berkow, and N. D. Barnard, "Calcium, Dairy Products, and Bone Health in Children and Young Adults: A Reevaluation of the Evidence," *Pediatrics* v115, no. 3 (March 2005):736–743.

153 Amy Joy Lanou, "Should Dairy Be Recommended as Part of a Healthy Vegetarian Diet? Counterpoint," *The American Journal of Clinical Nutrition* 89, no. 5 (May 1, 2009): 1638S–1642S.

154 Lanou, "Should Dairy Be Recommended," 1640S.

155 "Welcome to the Chicken and Egg Page," Mother Earth News, n.d., www.motherearthnews.com/homesteading-and-live-stock/eggs-zl0z0703zswa.

156 Zachary S.Clayton et al., "Egg consumption and heart health: A review," *Nutrition* 37 (May 2017): 79-85. https://doi.org/10.1016/j.nut.2016.12.014

157 Donghao Zhou et al., "Nut consumption in relation to cardiovascular disease risk and type 2 diabetes: a systematic review and meta-analysis of prospective studies," *The American Journal of Clinical Nutrition* 100, no. 1 (July 1, 2014): Pages 270–277. https://doi.org/10.3945/ajcn.113.079152

158 L. U. Thompson, R. L. Rea, and D. J. A. Jenkins, "Effect of Heat Processing on Hemagglutinin Activity in Red Kidney Beans," *Journal of Food Science* 48 (1983): 235–236, https://doi.org/10.1111/j.1365-2621.1983.tb14831.x

159 Yakov I. Yashin et al., "Creation of a Databank for Content of Antioxidants in Food Products by an Amperometric Method," *Molecules* 15, no. 10 (2010): 7450–7466.

160 Thomas Bøhn et al., "Compositional Differences in Soybeans on the Market: Glyphosate Accumulates in Roundup Ready GM Soybeans," *Food Chemistry* 153 (2014): 207–215.

161 Sophie Richard et al., "Differential Effects of Glyphosate and Roundup on Human Placental Cells and Aromatase," *Environmental Health Perspectives* (2005): 716–720; Siriporn Thongprakaisang et al., "Glyphosate Induces Human Breast Cancer Cells Growth via Estrogen Receptors," *Food and Chemical Toxicology* 59 (2013): 129–136.

162 Fumio Watanabe et al., "Vitamin B12-containing Plant Food Sources for Vegetarians," *Nutrients* 6, no. 5 (2014): 1861–1873.

163 Rajiv Chowdhury et al., "Association of Dietary, Circulating, and Supplement Fatty Acids with Coronary Risk: A Systematic Review and Meta-analysis," *Annals of Internal Medicine* 160, no. 6 (2014): 398–406.

164 Patty W. Siri-Tarino et al., "Meta-analysis of Prospective Cohort Studies Evaluating the Association of Saturated Fat with Cardiovascular Disease," *The American Journal of Clinical Nutrition* 91, no. 3 (2010): 535–546, https://doi.org/10.3945/ajcn.2009.27725.

165 V. L. Veum et al., "Visceral Adiposity and Metabolic Syndrome after very High-Fat and Low-Fat Isocaloric Diets: A Randomized Controlled Trial," *American Journal of Clinical Nutrition* 105, no. 1 (2017): 85–99.

166 . Uffe Ravnskov, "The Questionable Role of Saturated and Polyunsaturated Fatty Acids in Cardiovascular Disease," *Journal of Clinical Epidemiology* vol. 51, no. 6 (1998): 443–460; and Andrew Mente, Lawrence de Koning, and Harry S. Shannon, "Supporting a Causal Link between Dietary Factors and Coronary Heart Disease," *Archives of Internal Medicine* 169, no. 7 (2009):659–669, doi:10.1001/archinternmed.2009.38.

167 D. Mozaffarian et al., on behalf of the American Heart Association Statistics Committee and Stroke Statistics Subcommittee, "Heart Disease and Stroke Statistics—2016 Update: A report from the American Heart Association [published online ahead of print December 16, 2015], Circulation 133, no.4, https:doi.org/10.1161/CIR.0000000000000350.

168 Ian A. Prior et al., "Cholesterol, Coconuts, and Diet on Polynesian Atolls: A Natural Experiment: The Pukapuka and Tokelau Island Studies," *The American Journal of Clinical Nutrition* 34, no. 8 (1981): 1552–1561.

169 British Heart Foundation, "European Cardiovascular Disease Statistics 2008," https://www.bhf.org.uk/publications/statistics/european-cardiovascular-disease-statistics-2008.

170 S. L. Malhotra, "Epidemiology of Ischemic heart disease in India." *Indian Journal of Industrial Medicine* 14, no. 4 (1968): 219-241.

171 Gupta R, Joshi P, Mohan V, et al., "Trends in Coronary Heart Disease Epidemiology in India." *Annals of Global Health* 82, no. 2 (March-April 2016): 307-15.

172 Kang-Jey Ho et al., "The Masai of East Africa: some unique biological characteristics." *Archeological Pathology* 91 (1971): 387-410; G. V. Mann et al., "Atherosclerosis in the Maasai," *American Journal of Epidemiology* 95 (1972): 26–37; W. C. Willett et al., "Mediterranean diet pyramid: a cultural model for healthy eating." *American Journal of Clinical Nutrition* 61, no. 6S (June 1995): 1402S–1406S; F. Perez-Llamas et al., "Estimates of food intake and dietary habits in a random sample of adolescents in southeast Spain," *Journal of Human Nutrition Diet* 9, no. 6 (December 1996): 463–471; A. Alberti-Fidanza et al., *European Journal of Clinical Nutrition* 48 no. 2 (February 1994): 85–91; Weston Price, *Nutrition and Physical Degeneration*, (San Diego, CA: Price-Pottenger Nutrition Foundation, 1945), 59–72; G. Z. Pitskhelauri, *The Long Living of Soviet Georgia*, (New York, NY: Human Sciences Press, 1982); D. Franklyn, "Take a Lesson from the People of Okinawa," *Health*, September 1996, 57–63.

173 Mary Enig and Sally Fallon, "The Skinny on Fats," The Weston A Price Foundation, January 1, 2000, https://www.westonaprice.org/health-topics/know-your-fats/the-skinny-on-fats/

174 Mary Enig and Sally Fallon, *Eat Fat, Lose Fat* (New York: Hudson Street Press, 2005); and Weston A. Price Foundation, "Know Your Fats Introduction," December 6, 2017, www.westonaprice.org/health-topics/know-your-fats/know-your-fats-introduction/.

175 E. Hämäläinen, H. Adlercreutz, P. Puska, and P. Pietinen, "Diet and Serum Sex Hormones in Healthy Men," *Journal of Steroid Biochemistry.* 20, no. 1 (January 1984): 459–464.

176 R. R. Wolfe et al., "Dietary Fat Composition Alters Pulmonary Function in Pigs," *Nutrition* 18 (2002): 647–653.

177 A. Wijga et al., "Association of Consumption of Products Containing Milk Fat with Reduced Asthma Risk in Pre-School Children: The PIAMA Birth Cohort Study," *Thorax* 58, no. 7 (2003): 567–572.

178 Ramón Estruch et al., "Primary Prevention of Cardiovascular Disease with a Mediterranean Diet," *New England Journal of Medicine* 368, no.14 (2013): 1279–1290.

179 Leah G. Gillingham, Sydney Harris-Janz, and Peter J. H. Jones, "Dietary Monounsaturated Fatty Acids Are Protective against Metabolic Syndrome and Cardiovascular Disease Risk Factors," *Lipids* 46, no. 3 (2011): 209–228.

180 Bengt Vessby et al., "Substituting Dietary Saturated for Monounsaturated Fat Impairs Insulin Sensitivity in Healthy Men and Women: The KANWU Study," *Diabetologia* 44, no. 3 (2001): 312–319.

181 Ji-Hua Yang et al., "Effects of Different Amounts and Types of Dietary Fatty Acids on the Body Weight, Fat Accumulation, and Lipid Metabolism in Hamsters," *Nutrition* 32, no. 5 (2016): 601–608.

182 Meera Penumetcha, Nadya Khan, and Sampath Parthasarathy, "Dietary Oxidized Fatty Acids: An Atherogenic Risk?," *Journal of Lipid Research* 41, no. 9 (2000): 1473–1480.

183 Artemis P. Simopoulos, "The Importance of the Ratio of Omega-6/Omega-3 Essential Fatty Acids," *Biomedicine & Pharmacotherapy* 56, no. 8 (2002): 365–379.

184 . Rachel V. Gow and Joseph R. Hibbeln, "Omega-3 Fatty Acid and Nutrient Deficits in Adverse Neurodevelopment and Childhood Behaviors," *Child and Adolescent Psychiatric Clinics of North America* 23, no. 3 (2014): 555–590.

185 Ines Banjari, Ivana Vukoje, and Milena L. Mandić, "Brain Food: How Nutrition Alters our Mood and Behaviour," *Hrana u zdravlju i bolesti* 3, no. 1 (2014): 13–21.

186 Chris Kresser, "How too much omega-6 and not enough omega-3 is making us sick," *Chris Kresser - Let's Take Back Your Health,* May 8, 2010, https://chriskresser.com/how-too-much-omega-6-and-not-enough-omega-3-is-making-us-sick/.

187 Emilio Ros, "Health Benefits of Nut Consumption," *Nutrients* 2, no. 7 (2010): 652–682.

188 Chun-Yi Ng et al., "Heated Vegetable Oils and Cardiovascular Disease Risk Factors," *Vascular Pharmacology* 61, no. 1 (2014): 1–9.

189 George Mateljan Foundation, "What is the Special Nutritional Power found in Fruits and Vegetables?," The World's Healthiest Foods, n.d., accessed July 31, 2018, http://www.whfoods.com/genpage.php?tname=faq&dbid=4

190 Vijaya Lobo et al., "Free Radicals, Antioxidants and Functional Foods: Impact on Human Health," *Pharmacognosy Reviews* 4, no. 8 (2010): 118.

191 Jo Robinson, *Eating on the Wild Side* (New York: Little, Brown and Company, 2013), 5.

192 Emanuele-Salvatore Scarpa and Paolino Ninfali, "Phytochemicals as Innovative Therapeutic Tools against Cancer Stem Cells," *International Journal of Molecular Sciences* 16, no. 7 (2015): 15727–15742.

193 Robinson, *Eating on the Wild Side,*13.

194 Robinson, *Eating on the Wild Side*, 13.

CHAPTER 8

195 L. I. Hou, X. Zhang, D. Wang, and A. Baccarelli, "Environmental Chemical Exposures and Human Epigenetics," *International Journal of Epidemiology* 41, no. 1 (February 2012): 79–105.

196 Roundtable on Environmental Health Sciences, Research, and Medicine; Board on Population Health and Public Health Practice; Institute of Medicine, *Identifying and Reducing Environmental Health Risks of Chemicals in Our Society: Workshop Summary* (Washington (DC): National Academies Press, October 2, 2014).

197 "Why this matters - Cosmetics and your health," *EWG's Skin Deep Cosmetic Database*, n.d., accessed August 11, 2018, http://www.ewg.org/skindeep/2011/04/12/why-this-matters/

198 Douglas Main, "Glyphosate Now the Most-Used Agricultural Chemical Ever," *Newsweek*, February 2, 2016, http://www.newsweek.com/glyphosate-now-most-used-agricultural-chemical-ever-422419

199 "Body Burden: The Pollution in Newborns," The Environmental Working Group, July 14, 2005, http://www.ewg.org/research/body-burden-pollution-newborns.

200 "Body Burden," The Environmental Working Group

201 "Toxic Chemicals Found in British Celebrities' Bodies," The Environmental Working Group, May 20, 2005, https://www.ewg.org/enviroblog/2005/05/toxic-chemicals-found-british-celebritiesâ€™-bodies#.W5cWjC2ZOu4.

202 "Third National Report on Human Exposure to Environmental Chemicals," Department of Health and Human ServicesCenter for Disease Control and Prevention, July 2005, https://biomonitoring.ca.gov/sites/default/files/downloads/NHANES%20Exposure%203rd%20report.pdf.

203 Open Access Council on Environmental Health, "Iodine Deficiency, Pollutant Chemicals, and the Thyroid: New Information on an Old Problem," *Pediatrics* 133, no. 6 (June 2014): 1163–1166.

204 "Consumer Reports Issues New Consumption Guidelines Based On Analysis of Arsenic Levels in Rice Products & Other Grains" Consumer Reports, November 18, 2014, https://www.consumerreports.org/media-room/press-releases/2014/11/my-entry-3/.

205 "Interior Landscape Plants for Indoor Air Pollution Abatement," National Aeronautics and Space Administration, September 15, 1989, https://ntrs.nasa.gov/archive/nasa/casi.ntrs.nasa.gov/19930073077.pdf.

206 Joseph E. Pizzorno, *The Toxin Solution: How Hidden Poisons in the Air, Water, Food, and Products We Use Are Destroying Our Health--and What We Can Do to Fix It* (New York: HarperOne, 2017); Jenny L. Carwile et al., "Canned Soup Consumption and Urinary Bisphenol A: A Randomized Crossover Trial," *JAMA* 306, no. 20 (2011): 2218–2220.

207 "National Study: Toxic Nonstick Chemicals Still Found in Many Fast Food Wrappers," The Environmental Working Group, February 1, 2017, https://www.ewg.org/release/national-study-toxic-nonstick-chemicals-still-found-many-fast-food-wrappers#.

208 A. J. Cross, and R. Sinha, "Meat-Related Mutagens/Carcinogens in the Etiology of Colorectal Cancer," *Environmental and Molecular Mutagenesis* 44, no. 1 (2004): 44–55.

209 Kanithaporn Puangsombat and J. Scott Smith, "Inhibition of Heterocyclic Amine Formation in Beef Patties by Ethanolic Extracts of Rosemary," *Journal of Food Science* 75, no. 2 (March 2010): T40-T47.

210 Kenji Oishi et al., "Effect of Probiotics, *Bifidobacterium breve* and *Lactobacillus casei*, on Bisphenol A Exposure in Rats," *Bioscience, Biotechnology, and Biochemistry* 72, no.6 (May 2014): 1409-1415, https://doi.org/10.1271/bbb.70672.

211 Laura J. Stevens et al., "Amounts of Artificial Food Colors in Commonly Consumed Beverages and Potential Behavioral Implications for Consumption in Children," *Clinical Pediatrics* 53, no. 2 (Feb 2014): 133-40, https://doi.org/10.1177%2F0009922813502849.

212 Nicholas A. Bokulich and Marin J. Blaser, "A Bitter Aftertaste: Unintended Effects of Artificial Sweeteners on the Gut Microbiome," *Cell Metabolism* 20, no.5 (November 4, 2014): 701-703, https://doi.org/10.1016/j.cmet.2014.10.012.

213 Dana Flavin, "Metabolic Danger of High-Fructose Corn Syrup," *Life Extension Magazine* (2008), https://www.lifeextension.com/magazine/2008/12/Metabolic-Dangers-of-High-Fructose-Corn-Syrup/Page-01.

214 R.B. Ervin, C. L. Ogden, and U.S. Department of Health and Human Services, Centers for Disease Control and Prevention. "NCHS Data Brief, No. 122: Consumption of Added Sugars Among U.S. Adults, 2005–2010," May 2013, www.cdc.gov/nchs/data/databriefs/db122.pdf.

215 Leon Ferder, Marcelo Damián Ferder, and Felipe Inserra, "The Role of High-Fructose Corn Syrup in Metabolic Syndrome and Hypertension," *Current Hypertension Reports* 12, no. 2 (2010): 105–112.

216 Hwan Goo Kang et al., "Evaluation of Estrogenic and Androgenic Activity of Butylated Hydroxyanisole in Immature Female and Castrated Rats," *Toxicology* 213, no.1 (2005): 147–156; Sang-Hee Jeong et al., "Effects of Butylated Hydroxyanisole on the Development and Functions of Reproductive System in Rats," *Toxicology* 208, no. 1 (2005): 49–62.

217 M. J. Dennis et al., "The Determination of the Flour Improver Potassium Bromate in Bread by Gas Chromatographic and ICP-MS Methods," *Food Additives & Contaminants* 11, no. 6 (1994): 633–639.

218 Joanne K. Tobacman, "Review of harmful gastrointestinal effects of carrageenan in animal experiments." *Environmental Health Perspectives* 109, no.10 (Oct 2001): 983-994.

219 "Carrageenan: How a "Natural" Food Additive is Making Us Sick," The Cornucopia Institute, March 2013, https://www.cornucopia.org/wp-content/uploads/2013/02/Carrageenan-Report1.pdf.

CHAPTER 9

220 "Super-Tasting Science: Find Out If You're a "Supertaster"!," Scientific American, December 27, 2012, https://www.scientificamerican.com/article/super-tasting-science-find-out-if-youre-a-supertaster/.

221 Valentina De Cosmi et al., "Early Taste Experiences and Later Food Choices," *Nutrients* 9, no.2 (February 2017): 107, http://doi.org/10.3390/nu9020107.

222 Mark Hyman, "How Eating At Home Can Save Your Life," HuffPost, last modified May 25, 2011, https://www.huffingtonpost.com/dr-mark-hyman/family-dinner-how_b_806114.html.

223 Annemarie Olsen et al., "Serving Styles of Raw Snack Vegetables: What Do Children Want?" *Appetite* 59, no. 2 (2012): 556–562.

224 Brian Wansink et al., "Attractive Names Sustain Increased Vegetable Intake in Schools," *Preventive Medicine* 55, no. 4 (2012): 330–332.

225 Carine Vereecken, Alisha Rovner, and Lea Maes, "Associations of Parenting Styles, Parental Feeding Practices and Child Characteristics with Young Children's Fruit and Vegetable Consumption," *Appetite* 55, no. 3 (2010): 589–596.

226 "Parent Toolkit", NEDA (National Eating Disorders Association), 2015, www.nationaleatingdisorders.org/parent-toolkit

227 Daniel G. Amen, *Making a Good Brain Great: The Amen Clinic Program for Achieving and Sustaining Optimal Mental Performance* (New York: Three Rivers, 2006), 90.

228 "2017 State of The Industry," National Restaurant Association, accessed September 11, 2018, https://www.restaurant.org/News-Research/Research/soi.

APPENDIX A

229 S. Gautam, K. Platel, and K. Srinivasan, "Higher Bioaccessibility of Iron and Zinc from Good Grains in the Presence of Garlic and Onion," *Journal of Agricultural and Food Chemistry* 58, no. 14 (July 28, 2010): 8426–8429.

230 D. V. Digiacomo et al., "Prevalence of Gluten-Free Diet Adherence among Individuals without Celiac Disease in the USA: Results from the Continuous National Health and Nutrition Examination Survey 2009–2010," *Scandinavian Journal of Gastroenterology* 48 (2013): 921–925.

231 Sandro Drago et al., "Gliadin, Zonulin and Gut Permeability: Effects on Celiac and Non-Celiac Intestinal Mucosa and Intestinal Cell Lines," *Scandinavian Journal of Gastroenterology* 41, no. 4 (2006): 408–419.

232 Alessio Fasano, "Zonulin, Regulation of Tight Junctions, and Autoimmune Diseases," *Annals of the New York Academy of Sciences* 1258, no. 1 (2012): 25–33.

233 Alessio Fasano, "Zonulin and its Regulation of Intestinal Barrier Function: The Biological Door to Inflammation, Autoimmunity, and Cancer," *Physiological Reviews* 91, no. 1 (2011): 151–175.

234 Alessio Fasano, "Leaky Gut and Autoimmune Diseases," *Clinical Reviews in Allergy & Immunology* 42, no. 1 (2012): 71–78.

235 Donald D. Kasarda, "Can an Increase in Celiac Disease Be Attributed to an Increase in the Gluten Content of Wheat as a Consequence of Wheat Breeding?," *Journal of Agricultural and Food Chemistry* 61, no.6 (February 2013): 1155-1159, http://doi.org/10.1021/jf305122s.

236 William Davis, *Wheat Belly* (New York: Rodale, 2011), 22-24.

237 D. D. Kasarda, "Can an Increase in Celiac Disease be Attributed to an Increase in the Gluten Content of Wheat as a Consequence of Wheat Breeding?" *Journal of Agricultural and Food Chemistry* 61, no. 6 (2013): 1155–1159, https://doi.org/10.1021/jf305122s

APPENDIX B

238 "Retail Sales of Vitamins & Nutritional Supplements in the United States from 2007 to 2017 (in billion U.S. dollars)," *The Statistics Portal*, accessed January 2, 2018, www.statista.com/statistics/235801/retail-sales-of-vitamins-and-nutritional-supplements-in-the-us/.

239 Philip Smith, "Life Extension® Interview with Dr. Bruce Ames," *Life Extension Magazine*, August 2011, www.lifeextension.com/magazine/2011/8/Interview-with-Dr-Bruce-Ames/Page-01.

240 "Nine Out of 10 Americans Fall Short of Key Nutrients They Need, New Study Concludes," Cision PR Newswire, January 11, 2011, www.prnewswire.com/news-releases/nine-out-of-10-americans-fall-short-of-key-nutrients-they-need-new-study-concludes-113273399.html.

241 Philip Smith, "Life Extension® Interview with Dr. Bruce Ames."

242 Roddy Scheer and Doug Moss, "Dirt Poor: Have Fruits and Vegetables Become Less Nutritious?" *Scientific American,* n.d., accessed June 5, 2018, https://www.scientificamerican.com/article/soil-depletion-and-nutrition-loss/

243 Renee Dufault et al., "Mercury Exposure, Nutritional Deficiencies and Metabolic Disruptions May Affect Learning in Children," *Behavioral and Brain Functions* 5, no.1 (2009): 1.

244 Jess Armine, "Finally Get a Perfect Night's Sleep," DC Medicinal Supplements Summit, September 17, 2016, http://medicinalsupplementsummit.com.

245 "AG Schneiderman Asks Major Retailers to Halt Sales of Certain Herbal Supplements as DNA Tests Fail to Detect Plant Materials Listed on Majority of Products Tested," Attorney General Barbara D. Underwood, February 3, 2015, https://ag.ny.gov/press-release/ag-schneiderman-asks-major-retailers-halt-sales-certain-herbal-supplements-dna-tests.

246 Raimar Löbenberg and Wayne Steinke, "Investigation of Vitamin and Mineral Tablets and Capsules on the Canadian Market," *J Pharm Pharm Sci.* 9, no. 1 (2006): 40–49.

247 Jayson Calton and Mira Calton, *The Micronutrient Miracle: The 28-Day Plan to Lose Weight, Increase Your Energy, and Reverse Disease* (New York: Rodale, 2015), 168.

INDEX

Locators in **bold** refer to tables and those in *italics* to figures.

ABOUT THE AUTHOR

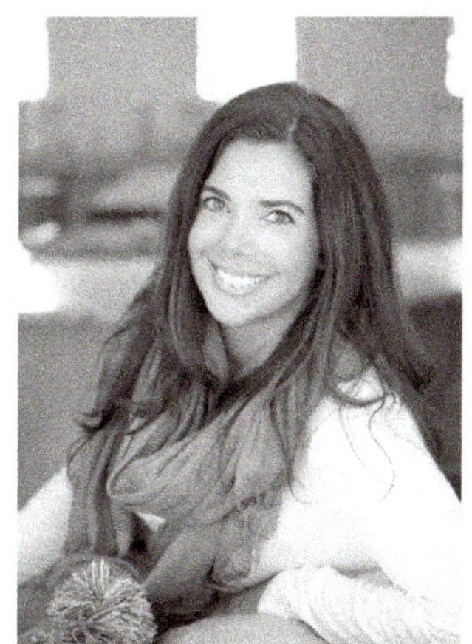

Nicole Magryta, MBA, RDN, LDN, is a nutrition consultant, educator, certified integrative health coach, and author specializing in integrative and functional medicine therapies for children. In her private practice today, Nicole has changed the lives of children and adults by tackling chronic disease from the root and not the leaves. She can be found throughout her community transforming school wellness programs, guiding large corporate wellness plans for companies such as GE and Conagra, as well as sitting on the board of directors of Live Healthy Carolinas. With additional culinary training, she spends her spare time transforming food in her test kitchen, teaching, inspiring, and developing quality, nutrient-dense foods for corporate and community clients. Nicole lectures extensively to academic, business, and community audiences on integrative nutrition, family and children's health, disease prevention, and healthy cooking techniques. She lives in Davidson, NC, with her husband and two children. Find out more about Nicole at www.nicolemagryta.com.

 CPSIA information can be obtained
at www.ICGtesting.com
Printed in the USA
LVHW101339120820
662995LV00009B/1261